WHEN RESEARCH GOES OFF THE RAILS

When Research Goes Off the Rails

Why It Happens
and What You Can Do About It

EDITED BY
DAVID L. STREINER
SOURAYA SIDANI

THE GUILFORD PRESS
New York   London

© 2010 The Guilford Press
A Division of Guilford Publications, Inc.
72 Spring Street, New York, NY 10012
www.guilford.com

Printed in the United States of America

This book is printed on acid-free paper.

Last digit is print number: 9   8   7   6   5   4   3   2   1

Library of Congress Cataloging-in-Publication Data
When research goes off the rails : why it happens and what you can do about it /
edited by David L. Streiner and Souraya Sidani.
     p. cm.
   ISBN 978-1-60623-410-5 (pbk.: alk. paper)
   ISBN 978-1-60623-411-2 (hbk.: alk. paper)
     1. Psychology—Research—Methodology.   2. Medical sciences—Research—
Methodology.   I. Streiner, David L.   II. Sidani, Souraya.

   BF76.5.W475 2010
   150.72—dc22

                                                          2009033166

Preface

Welcome to the wonderful world of research. Actually, as a reader of this book, you probably don't need a welcome; you're already in it, as a researcher or a student learning the ins and outs of design, methodology, sampling, statistics, focus groups, and all of the other arcane arts that are necessary to be successful. As researchers and teachers of research ourselves, for more years than either of us would like to admit, we know about these things and how they're presented, both in the classroom and in published papers. But we also know what's *not* told—that research is not a smooth, paved superhighway leading from the idea, to the proposal, through the funding agency, the execution of the plan, and ending in eventual publication. It's more like a rutted back road, full of dead ends, potholes, detours, and branching side roads. We also know that highways may be fast and efficient, but they're boring; the back roads are far more unpredictable and scenic. You never know what you'll find; sometimes it will be little more than a nondescript backwater town, but more often than not it will be a vista that takes your breath away.

There are many textbooks that act as tour books for the superhighway, but none that are guides to the back roads; this book is such a guide. It tells what *really* happens on the bumpy road of research; things you find out about only over a beer in the campus pub with a seasoned researcher who's in a melancholy mood. Each of the 42 vignettes describes how a carefully crafted, well-thought-out study has been derailed by Murphy's law—"If anything can go wrong, it will." In a few cases, the chapters are as cathartic as they are educational, with the authors sadly relating how the derailment was disastrous. What comes through in all of the chapters, though, is ingenuity, flexibility, resourcefulness, and—most of all—the love of research. Projects may have been derailed, at least for a while, but the researchers weren't. These vignettes describe how issues were resolved, problems overcome, and, in some cases, projects modified to meet the exigencies of reality.

Most research goes through a number of stages: Approval must be granted by an ethics board—in some cases, a number of boards; participants have to be accessed, recruited, and retained; the study itself must be implemented; the data collected and then analyzed. Through it all, it's often necessary to maintain working relationships with collaborating agencies and institutions. The parts of this book are arranged in this order, so that the reader (or the instructor) can match the chapters to the phases in which research is done, although, as you'll see, most of the vignettes cover two or more topics. Each of the parts has its own introduction, placing the particular aspect of research in context and highlighting where things can go off the rails. Within each part, most of the chapters follow a common format: a description of the project (at least as it was initially intended); the problems that were encountered; how they were (or, in a few cases, were not) overcome; and the lessons that were learned from the experience. Key annotated references are included at the end of the chapters so that the reader can delve deeper into the topics. In order to make it easier to find specific readings, there's a matrix following the table of contents, tying key methodological issues to specific chapters in which they're discussed.

These 43 stories were written by 63 contributors. The authors come from a variety of backgrounds (e.g., psychology, nursing, evaluation, medicine, sociology, epidemiology, anthropology), from six countries (Brazil, Cameroon, Canada, the United States, the United Kingdom, and Venezuela), and range in experience from graduate students to seasoned (and well-traveled) researchers. The examples, though, transcend the specifics of the studies, and even of the disciplines—ethics boards constitute a troubling hurdle that must be overcome by most people studying humans and animals, and breakdowns in collaboration are universal.

So, we hope you enjoy reading the book as much as we enjoyed putting it together. Learn from others' mistakes and be forewarned, but mainly be heartened—despite the setbacks described here, all of the authors are still enthusiastic about research and look forward to doing more of it.

In conclusion, we'd like to thank those who made the book possible and better. There were three reviewers—Paul R. Swank, University of Texas Health Science Center; Amanda L. Garrett, University of Nebraska–Lincoln; and Jessica G. Irons, James Madison University—each of whom made excellent suggestions regarding the format, such as the matrix and annotated reading lists. Mainly, though, our thanks to C. Deborah Laughton at The Guilford Press, whose support from the very beginning gave us hope that we could carry this off.

DAVID L. STREINER
SOURAYA SIDANI

Contents

WHEN RESEARCH GOES OFF THE RAILS

A GUIDE TO THE CONTENTS OF EACH CHAPTER

Part	Chapter	University	School	Hospital/Clinic	Community	Industry/Other	Qualitative	Quantitative	2° Data/Meta-Analysis	Delays	Modification	Risk	Payment
		Setting					Method			Ethics Issues			
I. Ethics	1		✓				✓	✓		✓	✓		
	2	✓						✓		✓		✓	
	3				✓		✓	✓				✓	
	4				✓			✓				✓	✓
II. Accessing the Participants	5				✓		✓						
	6			✓			✓	✓		✓	✓		
	7				✓		✓						
	8					✓			✓				
	9	✓						✓	✓	✓			
III. Recruitment and Retention	10	✓											
	11			✓				✓					
	12				✓		✓						
	13				✓			✓				✓	
	14			✓				✓				✓	
	15				✓			✓			✓		
	16			✓				✓					
	17				✓			✓					
	18				✓			✓					
IV. Study Implementation	19			✓				✓					
	20			✓				✓					
	21	✓						✓					
	22			✓				✓					
	23			✓		✓		✓					
V. Data Collection	24				✓			✓					
	25		✓					✓					
	26				✓			✓					
	27		✓					✓		✓		✓	
	28				✓		✓	✓				✓	
	29			✓				✓					
	30				✓		✓						
	31					✓		✓	✓				
	32							✓					
VI. Data Analysis	33				✓		✓						
	34				✓				✓	✓		✓	
	35			✓				✓					
	36				✓			✓					
	37						✓						
	38							✓					
	39							✓					
VII. Collaboration	40		✓					✓					
	41		✓					✓					
	42				✓			✓					

| Treatment | | | Other Issues | | | | | | | | | | | |
Implementation	Adherence	Safety	Access	Recruitment	Retention	Security	Data Collection	Missing Data	Modification	Technology	Analysis	Collaboration	Funding	Vulnerable Groups
												✓		
														✓
				✓								✓		✓
				✓								✓		✓
			✓			✓						✓		✓
			✓	✓								✓	✓	
			✓	✓										✓
			✓			✓		✓	✓			✓		
			✓			✓								
				✓					✓					
				✓										
				✓								✓		
			✓	✓					✓			✓		✓
			✓	✓					✓			✓		
				✓										
		✓		✓										
				✓	✓									✓
	✓			✓										✓
✓				✓								✓		
✓				✓	✓							✓		
✓					✓			✓		✓				
✓					✓		✓					✓		
✓												✓		
				✓										✓
							✓			✓		✓		
							✓			✓				
			✓				✓					✓		
			✓				✓	✓		✓				
							✓						✓	
			✓				✓					✓		✓
							✓	✓						
							✓	✓		✓	✓			
											✓			
			✓								✓			
											✓			
							✓							✓
										✓	✓			
								✓		✓				
							✓	✓			✓			
			✓	✓			✓					✓		
												✓	✓	
												✓		

Going Off the Rails
An Introduction

SOURAYA SIDANI
DAVID L. STREINER

THE IMPORTANCE OF CAREFULLY DESIGNING
RESEARCH STUDIES

It is hard to overemphasize the importance of research (especially to researchers). Both quantitative and qualitative research help us to discover new phenomena, to develop and validate theories that explain the relationships between variables, and to better understand behavior in general. In the clinical realm, it can uncover the nature, prevalence, determinants, and consequences of problems encountered by people—both healthy and ill—in daily life; by professionals in their day-to-day practice; and determine the effectiveness of interventions that address these issues. The goal is to improve individuals' well-being, whether those people are students, homeless persons, new immigrants requiring social assistance, healthy people who want to change their behaviors, or patients looking to improve their physical and psychological functioning.

However, in order to come to accurate conclusions and be useful, research studies must be carefully crafted and implemented. We cannot correctly understand phenomena, the problems professionals encounter, or how to deliver high-quality and safe interventions unless our studies are well designed and competently executed. There is much at stake: the well-being of people presenting with a problem, the credibility of professionals, and the respect of our colleagues. No professional wants to be known for developing a theory of limited applicability, generating a measure that

1

does not tap what it purports to, misdiagnosing a problem, or prescribing the wrong treatment. In carefully designing and implementing quantitative studies, the aim is to eliminate or minimize bias, which threatens the validity of findings; with qualitative studies, the findings should provide in-depth information about the phenomena of interest, as perceived by participants.

Many books and articles have been written describing how to carefully design and carry out research. Often, they describe in great detail the research process, starting with how to frame the research question; moving on to how to search, review, critically appraise, and synthesize the literature; then discussing selection of a research design and a sample, collecting and analyzing the data; interpreting the findings; and ending with the reporting of the results. In addition to books and texts (e.g., Lincoln & Guba, 1985; Shadish, Cook, & Campbell, 2002), some publications present an in-depth analysis of specific issues associated with designing and conducting research, with a particular focus on the types and sources of bias. Researchers are forewarned of possible threats to validity and are offered strategies to prevent them, and to manage them if they do occur. But despite all our best efforts to carefully plan and execute a study, and to minimize bias, things can (and will) go wrong; at some point, our study will go off the rails.

THE CHALLENGE: MURPHY'S LAW

As we suggested in the Preface, in all of the books about research and articles reporting study findings, research is described as a straightforward, smooth process, starting with an idea; going through a clear, explicit, sound, and easy-to-follow plan that incorporates useful strategies for minimizing bias; an uneventful execution of the plan; and culminating a short while later with glasses of champagne celebrating the end of a successful endeavor and the publication of relevant findings. How realistic is this scenario?

Murphy's law offers a clear and certain answer to this question, as it states, "If anything can go wrong, it will." Novice researchers are perhaps dimly aware of Murphy's law. They may remember reading about it somewhere, probably in a paragraph or a footnote in some research text. Experienced investigators, though, those actually involved in research, acknowledge its universal applicability and immutability. Any study, no matter how well designed, will face challenges in its execution. Reality is not always (or even usually) as neat as implied in any book's description of the research process or any publication's report of the study protocol and its findings.

Traditional research textbooks may mention Murphy's law, but if they do so, it is only *en passant*. Almost none show how the law may cause problems in implementation or execution, or provide examples illustrating these stumbling blocks, or discuss the ingenious preventative or post hoc solutions researchers must take to get around it. Further, research reports published in journals tell stories of successful studies, giving the impression that carrying out the research plan was easy and in conformity with the original design at each stage. Researchers are left to discover these stumbling blocks through experience and to improvise, on the spot, strategies to address them effectively. However, sit down with almost any researcher over a glass of beer, and stories will quickly emerge of the multitude of unanticipated problems that have occurred during a study. Very few, though, venture to share their experiences on paper. A limited number of journals have published articles presenting challenges encountered during the conduct of a study. These are usually published as part of the methodology section of a research-oriented journal or of a methods-focused issue of the journal. This book is a collection of stories about unanticipated problems encountered by researchers from a number of disciplines conducting studies using various designs within the quantitative and qualitative research approaches. The stories provide ample evidence of the existence of Murphy's law. We should note that although some of the authors are graduate students, the majority are seasoned and published researchers. These are not the follies of novices venturing into a new area; they are the quotidian experiences of those who toil in the field for their livelihood.

WHERE DOES MURPHY'S LAW STRIKE?

The short answer is: It can (and does) strike anywhere!

The unanticipated problems encountered during a study appear at every stage of the research process: obtaining approval from a research or institutional ethics board; designing the study; recruiting and selecting research staff; enrolling, selecting, and retaining participants; carrying out the study protocol; collecting the data; storing and analyzing the data; and even when the results are finally presented.

Ethics Approval

With the increasing concern about the ethical conduct of studies and the generation of new guidelines (e.g., HIPPA in the United States, Tri-Council Policy in Canada), Research Ethics Boards (REBs) review study protocols for their scientific merit as well as their conformity with ethical principles. They can make seemingly impossible demands regarding the design or execution of a study or impose modifications of the original study design. For instance, one of our students was informed by the ethics board that she could not have a research assistant observe participants in a focus group session and take notes of the group dynamics, owing to concerns about privacy and confidentiality. The student had no choice except to eliminate this useful source of information, which prevented data triangulation that is essential for validity of findings in some qualitative research designs. The situation may get complicated in multisite projects. REBs at different institutions may have different perspectives on how the research should be carried out and therefore demand changes that may not be acceptable to other participating sites, resulting in variability of the protocol. In one of our multisite studies, the ethics board at one site rejected, whereas the ethics board at another site allowed, screening of participants for eligibility (i.e., cognitive and psychological impairment) during the initial interview conducted over the phone. Thus, at the first site, screening took place after obtaining written consent; at the second, it was done once participants provided verbal agreement over the phone. However, the ethics board at the second site did not approve of using any data collected from participants who may have been eligible but did not sign a consent form. Yet these data would have been useful in comparing enrollees to nonenrollees to determine the extent of selection bias at the second site. In a different study, one hospital required a consent form to discuss financial compensation in case anything untoward happened, but another hospital absolutely forbade mention of this. We ended up with different consent forms at the various institutions.

Overall Research Design

Logistical problems at the site where a study is being conducted, as well as a host of other issues, can interfere with implementing the original design and lead to modifications in some of its aspects. We ran into this problem when we were doing a study in long-term care settings evaluating the effectiveness of an educational intervention. Its purpose was to enhance nursing staff members' knowledge and skills in providing personal care to persons with dementia, in order to reduce patients' agitation and promote their involvement in this aspect of care. We decided to use a wait-list control group design. The plan was to give the intervention to a randomly selected group of nurses immediately after obtaining pretest data, and to the other group once posttest data collection was completed; the latter group would serve as control in the pretest to posttest comparisons. Several factors prevented us from collecting the data as we had planned: (1) *characteristics of people with dementia*: because of their cognitive status, we had to get consent for their participation from their significant others, many of whom were not available (e.g., out of town, too busy, or not visiting the institutionalized person) to meet with the research assistant and provide consent within the allotted time period; (2) *the unit's culture*: most staff members did not value research and viewed it as an "add-on" that only increased their workload—consequently, they were unwilling to change their work schedule to accommodate gathering the pretest data; and (3) *unforeseen events*: the sudden death of the unit manager required us to allow staff members a grief period, which delayed data collection. These difficulties required us to change to a one-group pretest–posttest design if the study were to be completed within the funding period. In a different study, the pharmaceutical company refused to make placebo pills that looked like their drugs, so that this arm of the randomized controlled trial had to be dropped.

Recruiting and Selecting Research Staff

Careful selection and training of research staff members is critical for a study, inasmuch as they're the ones actually doing the work. Possible personnel include research assistants (RAs) responsible for recruiting the participants and for data collection and entry, and therapists who deliver the interventions. Despite carefully interviewing these people, selecting them on the basis of personal characteristics and professional qualifications, and a period of intensive training, some degree of "slippage" in performance will likely occur. In our experience, RAs differ in their level of success in recruiting participants or in their accuracy in entering data, and therapists in implementing the intervention as designed, despite having similar professional preparation and being given the same training. In one of our studies, for example, we saw a difference between two RAs working at the same site in the number of hospitalized patients who consented to take part. In another study, one of us (S. S.) listened to phone interactions of two therapists with participants. The interactions focused on delivering a self-management intervention designed to assist women with breast cancer in adjusting to their illness and its treatment. As originally planned, the therapists were to assess the women's concerns, explore their understanding of these concerns, and offer strategies to help the women address them. We noted differences between the therapists in their tone of voice, how they handled participants' concerns, and how they provided the intervention; for example, one therapist was very brief, did not explore the women's concerns in any depth, and suggested few strategies without discussing how to carry them out. These differences translated into variability in the participants' exposure to the intervention and reaching the desired outcome. At the end, we found no significant differences between the women assigned to one therapist (i.e., the one who was brief) and the control group, and significant differences between the women assigned to the other therapist and the control group.

Recruiting, Selecting, and Keeping Participants

Enrolling and retaining participants are essential for achieving the required sample size and minimizing potential biases. However, stories of challenges in recruitment are abundant. The problems are further exacerbated in studies addressing certain topics or targeting specific populations, or being carried out in clinical settings, where the pool of eligible persons is restricted. There are endless examples illustrating recruitment challenges; here are just a few. An outbreak of an infectious disease resulted in one hospital involved in a study banning participants coming in for data collection or to attend therapy sessions, which happened to us a few years ago when SARS hit several cities. One of the other hospitals allowed participants to come in, but insisted that both they and the therapist wear hospital gowns and masks—not an ideal way to build rapport with borderline patients. In another study, we had to recruit people admitted to complex continuing care units (these provide treatment for acute conditions in persons with chronic, debilitating illness). The aim of the study was to examine the reliability and validity of different methods for assessing health-related subjective outcomes. Accordingly, participants had to be cognitively intact, able to read English, and present with specific disease conditions. Within few months of beginning recruitment, administrative changes took place in the units, resulting in changes in the characteristics of the patients who were admitted. As a consequence, the majority of patients were no longer eligible, requiring us to revise the selection criteria and to include additional sites. In another study, where recruitment was to take place in the emergency room (ER) of a hospital that handled all psychiatric cases in the city, a new ER opened up just as the study began. The flow of patients was cut in half, and the characteristics of those who were enrolled changed, because the two ERs handled different catchment areas. Note that very few of these mishaps were under the control of the researchers; they simply reflect the real world.

Even having a large pool of subjects to draw on may not help if there are many inclusion and exclusion criteria, because these will reduce the size of the participant pool (Haidich & Ioannidis, 2001). For instance, Spiro, Gower, Evans, Facchini, and Rudd (2003) reported that of 680 potential participants (patients with lung cancer) who were identified, 161 were deemed ineligible for logistical reasons and 274 for clinical reasons (total = 435). About 64% were considered to have not met the study selection criteria. Further, only 25% (n = 63) of those eligible actually enrolled in the clinical trial. Thus, the yield of participants was less than 10%.

In clinical studies, an additional impediment is identifying the potential participants. Gurwitz et al. (2001) described healthcare professionals as "active gatekeepers" in recruiting research participants. Because of ethical concerns researchers are in a Catch-22 situation: They cannot review patients' medical records to determine eligibility on the basis of the type of illness or demographic factors without consent, and they can't get consent if they don't know which patients meet the criteria. It is up to the clinicians looking after the patients to introduce the study briefly and refer them to researchers. Unfortunately, clinicians often interfere with recruitment: They do not have time to carry out these research activities, which are viewed as burdensome and extra work; they may not be willing to refer "their" patients to clinical trials evaluating treatments because of concerns about the ethics of randomization, or fears of interference with their relationships with patients (Barrett, 2002), or their perception of the treatments being studied. One researcher told us that clinicians refused to refer patients attending their clinic to the clinical trial because they did not hold a positive or favorable view of the study and the intervention under evaluation; only a handful of patients were referred over a period of 6 months, even though a larger number of patients were considered potentially eligible (based on the registry maintained by the clinic).

Much has been written about attrition or loss of participants over the course of longitudinal studies, both experimental and nonexperimental, and about strategies to improve retention. That participants will drop out of a study is as certain as the sun will rise, thus supporting Murphy's law. Attrition rates vary across studies, with rates as low as 0.2% in one 2-year study of more than 19,000 patients (CAPRIE Steering Committee, 1996) and as high as 60%. Part of the reason has to do with characteristics of the participants (over which we have little control); other factors include the study protocol and, in clinical studies, the treatment itself. Characteristics of participants that affect a tendency to drop out of a study include (1) sociocultural characteristics, such as ethnicity (non-white), age (older), and education or socioeconomic status (low level); (2) health status (severely ill people with limited functional capacity and many health problems tend to withdraw); and (3) psychological distress (participants experiencing increased life stress, indicated by depression and anxiety, opt out more often). The complexity of the study protocol also affects attrition. The number and timing of contacts, how much the person has to do (e.g., completing many or long questionnaires or keeping a daily diary), and the invasiveness of some data collection measures, such as blood tests or brain scans, may deter some participants from completing the study. In clinical studies, participants tend to drop out if they view the treatment as complex, demanding (i.e., its implementation requires changes in behaviors, habits, or lifestyle), or not meeting their expectations in terms of personal benefits (Harris, 1998; Lindsay, Davis, Broome, & Cox, 2002; Moser, Dracup, & Doering, 2000). In addition to their direct main effects, these three categories of factors may interact in determining who drops out. In particular, interactions between participants and treatment characteristics have been reported to affect attrition, in that certain types of people may not like and become dissatisfied with their assigned treatment. For instance, Wingerson et al. (1993) found that those who dropped out within the first 2 weeks of a randomized trial that evaluated the effectiveness of anxiolytic medications had high scores on impulsiveness and disorderliness. This showed that they were overenthusiastic at the beginning of the study, did not give attention to logistical issues (such as time away from work that would prevent them from attending), and did not like the structure the study required, such as regimented, predictable, and time-consuming visits, interviews, filling out of forms, and complex drug regimens.

Carrying Out the Protocol

Once all the background work has been done—getting through the ethics board, hiring staff members, training them, modifying the protocol, enrolling participants—Murphy's law really has a chance to kick in. In one of our studies, participants were to fill out health diaries for 3 consecutive days, every 2 weeks. To increase compliance, we mailed them a reminder that should have arrived just prior to when the people would fill out the forms. Just as the study started, postal workers went on strike, requiring a change in strategy for sending the reminder. In another of our studies, which has just started, the protocol involved giving a $10 gift certificate to participants, who included patients admitted to long-term care facilities. Some of them have limited mobility and spend part of the week in bed. So, it was only considerate on our part to buy the certificates from the gift shop located at the facility, making it easier for the participants to redeem them. As soon as recruitment began, the gift shop manager decided that it was no longer profitable to sell the certificates. To change the incentive to a cash payment means going back to the ethics board, potentially delaying recruitment until (and if) approval is granted. Modifying the protocol is sometimes necessary, probably more often than not, once the beautiful design meets ugly reality.

In some cases, Murphy's law strikes after a study has been carried out, but its consequences are recognized only at the time of data analysis and interpretation. Shapiro et al.'s (2002) study is an interesting example. It consisted of an experimental condition involving mindfulness-based stress reduction that instructed participants in the use of meditation in six structured group sessions. Participants in the comparison group were told to engage in stress management activities of their choice. The researchers had to inform the participants to which treatment they were assigned so that they could make necessary arrangements to attend the sessions. The researchers disclosed group assignments before obtaining baseline data. This premature disclosure, which was necessary for logistical reasons, resulted in a selection bias. Participants in the experimental group had higher levels of psychological distress and need for control than those in the comparison group.

Uncontrolled events can take place at the site where the study is carried out, as Morse, Durkin, Buist, and Milgrom (2004) discovered. The study was set to evaluate brief training for nurses in the early detection and management of depression in new mothers. During the study period there were changes in staffing, which resulted in upheaval and unrest among nurses owing to increased workload, and computerized health records were introduced, which required additional training in how to use them. These events interfered with the nurses' attendance at the training session and their ability to use their new skills, thus mitigating the effects of the intervention.

Data Collection

Examples of unanticipated problems encountered during the data collection phase of a study are abundant, yet rarely, if at all, published. In quantitative studies, such problems can relate to:

1. *Acceptability and relevance of a measure's content to the target population.* Participants may feel uncomfortable with, and be reluctant to respond to, items with sensitive content such as sexual orientation or practices, particularly in the presence of interviewers. For others, the items' content may not be relevant (e.g., a religious coping scale for atheists), leading to nonresponse or missing data.

2. *Format of presentation.* A cluttered questionnaire may make it difficult to read, potentially resulting in frustration and nonresponse. Not having the response options line up could lead to selecting the wrong response, as might have happened in the 2000 presidential election in the United States. (A somewhat different problem highlighted by a number of elections is the absence of the option many people want—"None of the above.") Linear analogue scales with no gradations on the lines may be misinterpreted by some participants, particularly elderly people, resulting in inappropriate responses. Questions with yes/no responses may cause some people to get frustrated when they want to be able to say, "It all depends."

3. *Typographical errors.* For example, after reviewing a prototype questionnaire several times to ensure that the content was correct, having it printed (by a printing company that was paid for its services!), and administering it to a substantial proportion of participants, investigators found typographical errors in the questionnaire. In one study, the word "bushed," which is a rather old term for "fatigued," was printed as "blushed," a typo that was not picked up by the researcher or the RA, for whom English was not their first language. When completing this item (which was part of an established scale), some respondents identified the typing mistake, recognized that the correct term was "bushed," and responded accordingly. Others were puzzled and responded haphazardly. In another study, a particular item on a scale was reproduced twice, on two separate pages. At least

this gave an unplanned opportunity to test consistency in the participants' responses. Probably the most egregious example we know of was a questionnaire that asked about sexual practices. In one question, the phrase "such as" came out as "suck as," which provided for a lot of amusement, if not usable answers.

4. *Duplication mistakes.* Duplicating questionnaires is often done in bulk to save on costs. Photocopying machines can fail us. In some instances, a whole page or part of a page can go missing, increasing the amount of missing data. This is a particular problem with pages printed on both sides; forgetting to press the "back printed" button on the machine will result in half the pages disappearing into the void.

5. *Inaccurate contact information.* Participants' contact information (e.g., regular or electronic mail address, phone number) are needed in studies of all kinds. The inaccuracy of contact information is likely when it is taken from an organization database (e.g., the information may not be up-to-date) or even from the participants themselves (e.g., some may provide incomplete information, or information may have been incorrectly recorded because of problems with pronunciation or a poor phone connection).

6. *Rescheduling appointments.* In some instances, participants may not be able to make it to a session for various reasons, such as illness, family problems, difficulties with transportation, inclement weather, sudden emergencies at work, or a host of other problems. This can throw off the timing of the assessment, which can be a concern when data collection is time sensitive, such as in following up with patients who have received a treatment or evaluating people after exposure to a traumatic event.

7. *Distractions during data collection.* Distracters during data collection can range from a fire alarm going off to an electrical blackout. This happened a few years ago when one of us (S. S.) was in a session. The loss of power shut off the lights, which made it difficult to read the questionnaire, and the lack of air-conditioning made it uncomfortable to continue in a closed room in the middle of a hot summer. Even when participants complete a mail-out or phone survey at home, conditions may be far from ideal. Some people may fill out a questionnaire or respond when they're also watching TV, the baby is screaming in the background, or while they are having a meal—hardly conducive situations for concentrating on the questions.

8. *Equipment failures.* Murphy's law tells us that not only will equipment fail, it will fail at the worst possible time. In qualitative studies, where it is necessary to tape-record interviews, batteries will die, resulting in a loss of data; in a focus group session, the microphone will be placed so that the voices of participants won't be heard, but chuckles and coughs will come through clearly. If you're using a computer to present stimuli, it is guaranteed that, right in the middle of a session, the dreaded message "This program has performed an illegal operation and will abort" will

appear, requiring a techie to reset the machine (and he just left for a 2-week holiday). If you're storing vials of blood for later analysis, the refrigerator will break down during the hottest day of the summer (and on a long week-end when there's no one there to notice).

Data Storage and Analysis

We are all familiar with cases of irreparable computer crashes and/or damage to diskettes or USB memory keys, leading to the loss of data. We heard another story in which data were lost. A researcher decided to save the hard copies of completed questionnaires in preparation for data entry into a computerized database. When getting ready for data entry, the researcher found out that rodents had gotten to the questionnaires before she did. (Sounds like a variant of "The dog ate my homework.") Another issue is that various standards require us to save our data for some time after a study ends (often 7–10 years). During that time, programs and storage media change. How many people have data stored on 3½" disks, or—for those of us who've been in this business for many years—5" floppies, computer tapes, or even punch cards? Problems with data analysis include using different computer programs to analyze the same dataset and coming up with different results, owing to a combination of inaccuracies in one of the programs and an inability to determine what algorithm was being used. This isn't much of a problem for the widely used programs like SAS or SPSS, but spreadsheets, for example, are notorious for giving the wrong answers.

THE IMPACT OF MURPHY'S LAW ON VALIDITY

The unanticipated problems in the execution of studies influence the validity of the conclusions to various degrees. Some problems merely delay the start or completion of a project; others may cause the study to take far more time and resources than initially anticipated and budgeted for; others require modifications of the design study and methods, which can potentially introduce bias; and still others make it impossible for the project to be carried out as originally planned. What are possible biases or threats to validity that unanticipated problems may introduce?

Modifications in Research Design

Whether imposed by demands of an ethics board or by constraints within the settings, modifications in the design of a study may affect the quality of the results, and hence the conclusions. We've discussed one example in which the comparison group had to be dropped, resulting in a much weaker before–after study rather than a true experiment. In other studies presented in this book, researchers were kept from examining records that were necessary to get vital information and others were prevented from contacting groups of potential participants because of ethical concerns. In some cases, the researchers were able to work around the problem, but often they could not, so that the project either had to change focus or be abandoned completely.

Recruiting and Selecting Research Staff

RAs and therapists who carry out the interventions are neither automatons nor clones of one another. They are individuals and, as such, their personal and professional characteristics may influence an outcome. For example, Crits-Christoph and Mintz (1991) examined the effects of therapists on outcomes of psychotherapy. The results of this systematic review showed a significant main effect of therapist and a therapist-by-treatment interaction, meaning that therapists directly affect and moderate the effectiveness of interventions. Moreover, in Project MATCH (Matching Alcoholism Treatments to Client Heterogeneity; Project MATCH Research Group, 1998), significant differences were observed between therapists in implementing the treatment, which could potentially lead to differences in outcomes. Even more important, in light of a significant interaction, it is impossible to say which intervention is better; the answer is, "It all depends on who's delivering it."

Recruiting, Selecting, and Retaining Participants

Unanticipated problems in recruiting, selecting, and retaining participants may result in sample selection bias and/or low statistical power. Sample selection bias threatens the representativeness of the sample, so that it no longer reflects the target population (e.g., underrepresentation of non-whites in research, or of people with low levels of severity of some condition), thereby limiting the generalizability of the findings—what Cook and Campbell (1979) refer to as the *external validity* of a study. Low statistical power is most often due to inadequate sample size, which can be a result of low enrollment and/or high attrition rates. In turn, low power increases the probability of a Type II error: not seeing a difference between groups when in fact it's there. Attrition, especially differential attrition (in which people withdraw from the various groups at different rates) results in differences between the groups on baseline characteristics, whether the groups occur naturally or are formed experimentally. If these baseline differences are associated with the outcome, they are confounders, meaning that any differences at the end of the study could be due to them, rather than to the intervention.

Running the Study

Problems in carrying out the protocol as designed may lead to erroneous conclusions, particularly when it involves some intervention. In some situations, some aspects of the treatment or program may have to be modified to make it more applicable within the constraints of the setting or to fit the particular characteristics of the participants. If the treatment is not carried out as originally planned, then you can be committing a Type III error (concluding that an intervention is not effective when it has not been implemented as designed; Basch & Gold, 1986).

Data Collection

Data collection problems may produce inaccurate responses (for example, when an item on a questionnaire is not clear or relevant) or loss of data. As with data entry errors, inaccurate responses mean that the numbers cannot be trusted. Missing data may result in a smaller sample size than was planned or, even worse, a biased sample if those who omitted items differ in some way from those with complete responses.

OVERCOMING THE CHALLENGES

The research literature does present some strategies and recommendations to enhance the design and validity of a study. For instance, critical multiplism (Cook, 1985) suggests using a number of designs (both quantitative and qualitative), ways of obtaining the data, methods for collecting them, and approaches to data analysis. Using this general strategy in research is efficient in that if something goes off the rail in one part of the study, it can be saved with another. Further, strategies for recruiting and retaining participants have been recommended, some of which have empirical evidence supporting them. Examples of these strategies include:

1. Contacting potential participants ahead of time, such as with a prenotification letter to tell them about the study, clarify why it's being done, and let them know what it will entail (Barribal & While, 1999; Moser et al., 2000).
2. Assuring potential participants about confidentially (Singer, von Thurn, & Miller, 1995).
3. Using monetary or nonmonetary incentives (Church, 1993).
4. Maintaining contact at regular times between visits in longitudinal studies (Moser et al., 2000).
5. Making participants' involvement convenient and rewarding.
6. Training research staff in research and interpersonal skills so they

can develop and maintain a trusting relationship with participants.

7. Selecting staff who are similar to the target population, particularly in terms of gender and culture.
8. Using more than one site to recruit people.

Monitoring the fidelity of treatment implementation is becoming a standard requirement in evaluation research (Bellg et al., 2004). It can identify deviations from the protocol and factors that could contribute to these deviations. Such knowledge provides feedback for refining the design, modifying the delivery of the intervention as needed, and accounting for these deviations in the data analysis in order to enhance the validity of the conclusions.

Using validated short versions of measures reduces the response burden and improves the quality and completeness of answers. Within the past decade or so, sophisticated techniques for handling missing data have become available to address this prevalent problem in research, and they should be used. It is also extremely prudent to save your data in a few different locations, such as on different computer hard drives and at least two diskettes or USB keys kept in different places. This is much easier now than in the old days of punched cards, when we kept one copy of our data in the refrigerator, wrapped in foil, just in case the house burned down.

The best way to avoid the consequences of Murphy's law is to anticipate it ahead of time. However, the literature in this regard is limited. This book presents a range of problems that researchers have encountered and has a number of strategies that investigators can use to overcome the unexpected but inevitable challenges. These are derived from researchers' actual experiences. They are feasible, simple, easy to implement, and helpful—they are "tried, tested, and true"!

REFERENCES

Barrett, R. (2002). A nurse's primer on recruiting participants for clinical trials. *Oncology Nursing Forum, 29,* 1091–1096.

Barriball, K. L., & While, A. E. (1999). Non-response in survey research: A methodological discussion and development of an explanatory model. *Journal of Advanced Nursing, 30,* 677–686.

Basch, C. E., & Gold, R. S. (1986). The dubious effects of Type V errors in hypothesis testing on health education practice and theory. *Health Education Research, 1,* 299–305.

Bellg, A., Borelli, B., Resnick, B., Hecht, J., Minicucci, D. S., Ory, M., et al. (2004). Enhancing treatment fidelity in health behavior change studies: Best practices and recommendations from the Behavior Change Consortium. *Health Psychology, 23,* 443–451.

CAPRIE Steering Committee. (1996). A randomised, blinded trial of clopidigrel versus aspirin in patients at risk of ischaemic events. *Lancet, 348*, 1329–1339.

Church, A. H. (1993). Estimating the effect of incentives on mail survey response rates: A meta-analysis. *Public Opinion Quarterly, 57*, 62–79.

Cook, T. D. (1985). Postpositivist critical multiplism. In L. Shotland & M. M. Marks (Eds.), *Social science and social policy* (pp. 21–62). Beverly Hills, CA: Sage.

Cook, T. D., & Campbell, D. T. (1979). *Quasi-experimentation: Design and analysis for field settings*. Chicago: Rand McNally.

Crits-Christoph, P., & Mintz, J. (1991). Implications of therapist effects for the design and analysis of comparative studies of psychotherapies. *Journal of Consulting and Clinical Psychology, 59*, 20–26.

Gurwitz, J. H., Guadagnoli, E., Landrum, M. B., Silliman, R. A., Wolf, R., & Weeks, J. C. (2001). The treating physician as active gatekeeper in the recruitment of research subjects. *Medical Care, 39*, 1339–1344.

Haidich, A-B., & Ioannidis, J. P. A. (2001). Patterns of patient enrollment in randomized controlled trials. *Journal of Clinical Epidemiology, 54*, 877–883.

Harris, P. M. (1998). Attrition revisited. *American Journal of Evaluation, 19*, 293–305.

Lincoln, Y. S., & Guba, E. G. (1985). *Naturalistic inquiry*. Beverly Hills, CA: Sage.

Lindsay Davis, L., Broome, M. E., & Cox, R. P. (2002). Maximizing retention in community-based clinical trials. *Journal of Nursing Scholarship, 34*, 47–53.

Morse, C., Durkin, S., Buist, A., & Milgrom, J. (2004). Improving the post-natal outcomes of new mothers. *Journal of Advanced Nursing, 45*, 465–474.

Moser, D. K., Dracup, K., & Doering, L. V. (2000). Factors differentiating dropouts from completers in a longitudinal, multicenter clinical trial. *Nursing Research, 49*, 109–116.

Project MATCH Research Group. (1998). Therapist effects in three treatments for alcohol problems. *Psychotherapy Research, 8*, 455–474.

Shadish, W. R., Cook, T. D., & Campbell, D. T. (2002). *Experimental and quasi-experimental design for generalized causal inference*. Boston: Houghton-Mifflin.

Shapiro, S. L., Figueredo, A. J., Caspi, O., Schwartz, G. E., Bootzin, R. R., Lopez, A. M., et al. (2002). Going quasi: The premature disclosure effect in a randomized clinical trial. *Journal of Behavioral Medicine, 25*, 605–621.

Singer, E., von Thurn, D. R., & Miller, E. R. (1995). Confidentiality assurances and response. A quantitative review of the experimental literature. *Public Opinion Quarterly, 59*, 66–77.

Spiro, S. G., Power, N. H., Evans, M. T., Facchini, F. M., Rudd, R. M., on behalf of the Big Lung Trial Steering Committee. (2005). Recruitment of patients with lung cancer in a randomised clinical trial: Experience at two centers. *Thorax, 55*, 463–465.

Wingerson, D., Sullivan, M., Dagner, S., Flick, S., Dunner, D., & Roy-Byrne, P. (1993). Personality traits and early discontinuation from clinical trials in anxious patients. *Journal of Clinical Psychopharmacology, 13*, 194–197.

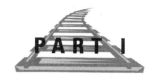

PART I

ETHICS APPROVAL

Perhaps no aspect of research with humans (and animals) is as universal—and as dreaded—as getting approval from the ethics board (usually called the Institutional Review Board, or IRB, in the United States, and Research Ethics Board, or REB, in Canada). You can do a study without having to enroll participants (e.g., secondary data analysis) or use statistics (just ask any qualitative researcher), but with rare exceptions, it's almost impossible to get started without that piece of paper from the board giving its approval. No one can argue that such boards are necessary. The need for ethical standards was first highlighted by the revelations of the inhuman "experiments" performed on inmates of the concentration camps in Nazi Germany, the later revelations of the infamous Tuskegee Study, in which African Americans who had syphilis were left untreated in order to study the natural history of the disease, and the Willowbrook Study in 1963, in which healthy retarded children in an institution were deliberately inoculated with hepatitis to determine if gamma globulin was an effective treatment. Indeed, difficult as it is to imagine today, the few ethical standards that existed until the middle of the 20th century dealt mainly with physician–patient relationships within a clinical context.

The first explicit guidelines were promulgated in 1947 with the *Nuremberg Code* (Weindling, 2001). This was then expanded in 1964, with the *Declaration of Helsinki* (World Medical Organization, 1996), which has subsequently been amended three times, and the *Belmont Report*, which was sponsored by the Department of Health, Education, and Welfare (now the Department of Health and Human Services) in the United States (National Commission for the Protection of Human Subjects of Biomedical and Behavioral Research, 1979). The core ethical principles of the Belmont Report are (1) respect for persons, (2) beneficence, and (3) justice. In practical terms, this translates into the requirement for each study participant to give free and informed consent. "Free" means that there is no coercion, such as having to participate as a course requirement, or being enrolled by the clinician who is also treating the person, as this places undue pressure on the person ("If I don't agree, will the doctor still give me the best care?"), or offering excessive monetary inducements to take part in dangerous or uncomfortable experiments. "Informed" means that the person is told about all serious risks, even if they are rare, as well as less serious but more common ones.

Simple as these guidelines appear, they are open to broad interpretation. How much monetary inducement is "excessive"? Is the same amount reasonable for some groups (e.g., business executives) but excessive for others (e.g., homeless people)? If the treating clinician is the researcher, then he or she is in the best position to explain the study to the potential participant, so how can we balance that function of fully informing the participant with its countervailing coercive effect? Is deception allowable if it is necessary for a study? The problems are magnified when dealing with particular cultural groups. In some, it would be unthinkable for a member to participate without the permission of the elder (and, among some religious groups, for a woman to take part without her husband's permission); and, conversely, they could not refuse to participate if the authority figure says they must. How can we balance these cultural norms against the Western ideal of individual freedom of choice?

It is not surprising, then, that different IRBs come to opposite conclusions about the same study—not surprising, but extremely frustrating for the investigator who must work with two or more institutions. Further, as "risk managers" play an increasingly important role in a risk-averse and litigious environment, it is not surprising either that IRBs can seem picky to the point of punctiliousness, seeming to argue about every clause, if not every comma, in the consent form. (As you read this, bear in mind that one of us (D. L. S.) chaired an REB in one institution for about 15 years and was the deputy chair at another for 10 years; he knows whereof he speaks.)

In Part I, Hwalek and Straub (Chapter 1) address the problems caused when an IRB takes what appears to be an inordinate amount of time to grant approval. Although they were not dealing with a university-based board, the difficulties they faced are (unfortunately) universal. In Chapter 2, Sherry and Amidon deal with a number of problems: differences between two IRBs within the same institution (departmental and university), protection of vulnerable groups (in this case, minors), and varying interpretations of risk. Meyer and her coauthors (Chapter 3) deal with the issue of recruitment of marginalized groups: how ethical concerns about confidentiality conflict with practical problems about contacting people, and the conflicting needs of different minority groups. Finally, in Chapter 4, Rush and Morisano face the problem of incentives: Would payment in cash to substance abusers result in their spending the money for drugs or alcohol?

REFERENCES

National Commission for the Protection of Human Subjects of Biomedical and Behavioral Research. (1979). *The Belmont report: Ethical principles and guidelines for the protection of human subjects of research.* Washington, DC: U.S. Department of Health, Education and Welfare.

Weindling, P. (2001). The origins of informed consent: The International Scientific Commission on Medical War Crimes, and the Nuremberg Code. *Bulletin of the History of Medicine, 75,* 37–71.

World Medical Organization. (1996). Declaration of Helsinki. *British Medical Journal, 313,* 1448–1449.

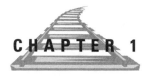

CHAPTER 1

When Mountains Move Too Slowly

MELANIE A. HWALEK
VICTORIA L. STRAUB

BACKGROUND OF THE STUDY

In 1974, the National Research Act of 1974 was passed by the U.S. Congress. The Act was a response to unethical research practices involving human subjects and followed similar international legislation such as the Nuremberg Code and the Declaration of Helsinki (National Commission for the Protection of Human Subjects of Biomedical and Behavioral Research, 1979). The National Research Act aimed to protect human subjects of research. It established the National Commission for the Protection of Human Subjects of Biomedical and Behavioral Research and charged it with summarizing the ethical principles and guidelines for conducting research with human subjects (Public Law 348, 93rd Congress, 2nd Session, July 1974). The Act also created regulations that established Institutional Review Boards (IRBs) as one mechanism by which human subjects would be protected (Penslar, 1993).

In 1979, the Commission released its findings as the Belmont Report. The Belmont Report summarizes the ethical principles and guidelines that should be followed in conducting research with human subjects. By 1991, almost all U.S. federal departments and agencies were governed under common rules for the protection of human subjects (Federal Register, 1991).

Taken together, the Belmont Report and IRB regulations provide the major guidance for researchers and program evaluators wanting to collect data from or about human subjects. Although IRBs are the most well established bodies that monitor the protection of human subjects in research, other similar bodies have also been created to serve essentially the same protective function. Some school districts, for example, have created administrative offices whose purpose is to ensure that any research or evaluation conducted within its schools meets the Belmont Report guidelines for protection of human subjects.

All of these rules and regulations are a good thing. They ensure that subjects know the risks and benefits of participating in the research. They require that subjects give full and informed consent to participate. Informed consent means that the subjects know what the research is about and what data they are being asked to provide. However, when the process of putting these protections into practice is inefficient, it can result in poorer-quality evaluation data and less usefulness of evaluation findings. This is what happened in our project.

Our company is a social research and evaluation organization headquartered in the United States. We were contracted by a college to evaluate the outcomes of a 3-year arts integration program being implemented in six elementary public schools and one charter school. The program pairs artists with elementary school teachers to jointly plan and teach the mandated core elementary reading curriculum using arts as the teaching method. Program implementation is monitored by a project director located at the college, along with four art organization partners who identify, train, and support the artists who are paired with the teachers.

Some empirical evidence suggests that using the arts as a method to teach core academic subjects could motivate students to pay more attention to their lessons (Catterall, 2002). A logical extension of this evidence is that if students pay more attention to their lessons, they will do better on standardized tests of reading, writing, and math. Our evaluation set out to determine whether these outcomes occur for elementary students participating in this collaborative arts integration program.

In addition to providing defensible evidence that arts-integrated teaching helps students achieve academic outcomes, the college wanted to use the evaluation as a learning opportunity for graduate students in education. Therefore, the evaluation design called for graduate students to be responsible for the collection of most of the evaluation data.

The evaluation design used mixed methods. It included observations of teacher–student interactions in a sample of classroom sessions receiving arts-integrated teaching, and of a sample of comparison classroom sessions in the same school that did not use the program. The design involved focus group interviews with a random sample of students in each of the program and comparison classes. It also called for the collection of report card grades, student academic behavior, and standardized test scores for a random sample of 15 students in each of the program and comparison classrooms. The evaluation was to occur over a 3-year time period, with year 1 used for planning and instrument design and then years 2 and 3 for data collection, analysis, and reporting.

THE CHALLENGES

As in many regions in the United States, any evaluation conducted within public schools in this community must first obtain approval from the school district. There is a research approval application process that we had to complete and submit to the appropriate office at least 6 weeks prior to the desired start date of data collection. The application required a full description of the research methods, questions, instruments, and consent forms. In other words, we were required to list every question we wanted to ask from every data source in order to get the district office to approve the conduct of this evaluation.

Applications for the following school year are due in July. There is a notice on the application form stating that the review process takes 4 to 6 weeks to complete. After district office approval, the research plan must then be approved by the participating school principals and teachers. Principal and teacher approvals cannot be solicited until the district office officially approves the research. However, from the onset of the project, all of the school staff involved with the program knew about and supported the research.

We submitted the required application by the required due date. After 6 weeks, we had not received a response from the district office. A call to the office revealed that our application was still somewhere in a pile with many other applications. We were told that we would be notified when the application was reviewed. Every month or so, we called the office, inquiring about the status of our application. We would receive the same "don't call us, we'll call you" response. We finally got to meet with relevant staff members from the office after some behind-the-scenes calls were made to influential persons. This resulted in the review of our application and several back-and-forth modifications and re-reviews. In May—10 months later and almost at the end of year 2 of the evaluation—our modified application was approved, after we had removed any reference to obtaining data on student academic behaviors (i.e., suspensions, attendance, etc.), assuring the district office that the graduate students' observations would not be videotaped, and guaranteeing that the only classrooms that would be observed were those in which 100% of the parents gave consent.

By the time we received approval, programming in the schools was over for the school year. Graduate courses were about to end. The evaluation report for year 2 was due in 3 months.

OVERCOMING THE DIFFICULTIES

Luckily, the district office differentiates between data collected in the normal course of program delivery and data collected for the purpose of evaluation and research. Permission is not needed to collect data if the assessment is part of program delivery. Therefore, given the uncertainty of gaining district office approval, we worked with the program staff and looked to other ways to obtain evaluation data that would be collected primarily for the purpose of monitoring program delivery. Instead of having graduate students conduct focus groups with the elementary students, group interviews were conducted with samples of students by the four artist partner organizations responsible for coordinating the program within each school. The group interviews were audiotaped. The artist partner organizations used the student focus group information for making program improvements and then provided it to the evaluators as secondary data for the evaluation.

Instead of having graduate students go into the schools to observe classrooms, we used existing videos. We learned that the program director routinely videotaped artists while they were delivering the program. The videotapes were used for professional development purposes—showing what good program delivery looks like and teaching new artists about the program. Although each videotape lasts only about 15 minutes, they provided at least some observational data that the program could use to teach graduate students about observational assessment. Students were able to rate the tapes. Then we were given the ratings of students who met proficiency standards in using the rating tool to use for evaluative analyses.

LESSONS LEARNED

Anticipate challenges, know the rules, and be creative! When dealing with a large and complex organization, add an additional 10 months to the time frame of the research project!

We made the assumption before the school year ended that approval from the district office would not be obtained in time for primary data collection by the graduate students. Because of this, we were able to switch gears and work with the program staff to identify other ways to obtain some data for year 2. Had we waited until we heard from the office to make alternate plans, the school year would have ended and we would have had no data to analyze or report for year 2.

Although the office does not state this on the research approval application, because we have been doing evaluations in public schools for many years, we were aware of the rules differentiating data collected for research from data collected in the normal course of program implementation. It is important to read the fine lines and between the fine lines when working with research review bodies.

We were creative in our ability to identify existing sources of data. We were able to reframe the collection of new data to align with the rules and regulations of the district office. We were able to use data collected by the college and its art partner organizations for purposes of program monitoring as secondary data in the second year of the evaluation. Although the data were possibly biased because they were not collected by third-party evaluators, there was at least some evidence obtained about program outcomes. The data were presented in the second year's report acknowledging the potential biases.

A FINAL WORD

We thought it worth noting that our evaluation's ability to produce relevant and useful information has been somewhat constrained because of the rules and regulations promulgated by the Belmont Report. In order to obtain approval, the evaluation had to state all of the research questions up front. This means that the evaluation is bound by the research questions and methodologies that were eventually approved by the district office. This prescribed preidentification of program goals and evaluation questions precludes the ability of the evaluation to have any goal-free attributes. "Goal-free evaluation" is a term coined by Scriven (1991). It refers to the value of having evaluators observe and assess a program without knowledge of the intervention's goals. Having a goal-free evaluator collecting information about a program allows for the emergence of effects that may otherwise not be identified when the evaluator collects data through the lens of preidentified research questions. It is unlikely that our evaluation would have been approved by the district office had we proposed a more goal-free approach.

TO READ FURTHER

Howe, J., & Moses, M. (1999). Ethics in educational research. *Review of Research in Education*, 24, 21–60.

This article is a comprehensive review of the relationship of traditional and contemporary research approaches to the protection of human subjects and the misconduct of research. The article also discusses various rules and regulations of oversight bodies, particularly in relation to educational research. This article convinced me of the need for boards of ethics to maintain oversight over research.

Simons, H. (2006). Ethics in evaluation. In I. A. Shaw, J. C. Greene, & M. M. Mark (Eds.), *The Sage handbook of evaluation* (pp. 213–232). London: Sage.

The Belmont Report and its underlying principles related to protection of human subjects in research are different from the principles of the ethical practice of evaluation. This article differentiates the IRB-type of standards reviews from the ethical conduct of evaluation. It challenges the reader to go beyond concepts of ethical research to the concept of thinking ethically about the work that evaluators do.

REFERENCES

Catterall, J. S. (2002). The arts and the transfer of learning. In R. J. Deasy (Ed.), *Critical links: Learning in the arts and student social and academic development* (pp. 151–157). Washington, DC: Arts Education Partnership.

Federal Register. (1991). *Rules and Regulations,* Vol. 56 #117 Tuesday, June 18.

National Commission for the Protection of Human Subjects of Biomedical and Behavioral Research. (1979). *The Belmont report: Ethical principles and guidelines for the protections of human subjects of research.* Washington, DC: U.S. Department of Health, Education and Welfare.

Penslar, R. L. (1993). *Institutional Review Board Guidebook.* Retrieved January 16, 2008, from *www.hhs.gov/ohrp/irb/irb_introduction.htm.*

Public Law 348, 93rd Congress, 2nd Session. (July 12, 1974). *National Research Act of 1974.*

Scriven, M. (1991). Prose and cons about goal-free evaluation. *American Journal of Evaluation, 12,* 55–62.

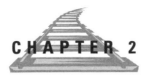

CHAPTER 2

The Ethics of Sex Research on the Internet

ALISSA SHERRY
AMY AMIDON

BACKGROUND OF THE STUDY

Infidelity in relationships is fairly common. Conservative estimates indicate that between 15 and 45% of Americans have engaged in extramarital sex (Glass & Wright, 1985; Kinsey, Pomeroy, Martin, & Gebhard, 1953; Treas & Giesen, 2000). In addition, studies have found that sex differences are gradually diminishing, with men and women under the age of 40 showing similarly high levels of infidelity (Wiederman, 1997). Studying infidelity in psychology research is important because it has been linked to spousal battery and homicide and mental health problems (Amato & Previti 2003; Daly & Wilson, 1988) and is the most commonly reported reason for divorce in America and cross-culturally (Amato & Previti 2003; Amato & Rogers, 1997; Betzig, 1989).

However, infidelity is difficult to research. Prior research has often failed to examine actual experiences of infidelity, looking at predicted experiences of infidelity (Buss & Shackelford, 1997) or vignettes presented to college students (Parker, 1997; Sprecher, Regan, & McKinney, 1998). Furthermore, studies that have assessed actual experiences of infidelity have traditionally done so in a dichotomous manner, asking whether or not individuals had engaged in infidelity and ignoring the type and level of involvement (Atkins, Baucom, & Jacobson, 2001; Treas & Giesen, 2000). Researchers appear to be coming to a better understanding of the complex nature of infidelity and have recently begun to look at both the type and degree of involvement (Banfield & McCabe, 2001; Drake & McCabe, 2000). However, probing these issues with participants can be tricky. As research issues become more personal and charged with socially judgmental overtones, the likelihood of socially desirable responses increases and study validity decreases.

Our study attempted to look at the nuances of relationship infidelity in 250 men and women, over the age of 18, who had been in at least one committed relationship at some point in the last 5 years. The goal was not only to contribute to the minimal amount of prevalence data, but also to explore infidelity from an attachment theory (Bowlby, 1969/1982, 1973, 1980) perspective in order to understand the behavior from a theoretical context. Therefore, the content of the items in the questionnaire covered sexual behavior as well as the general relationship and emotion characteristics of participants. Of issue here is the context and the specifics of the sexual behavior items. The general categories included emotional, physical, and anonymous involvement with others. However, in order to provide the participant with behavioral anchors, specific examples of these categories were suggested. These included having romantic feelings for another person; watching porn; and kissing, oral sex, or intercourse with someone other than your current romantic partner.

In addition, it was decided the best place to collect these data was on the Internet, for several reasons. First, the anonymity provided through Internet data collection solved one of the primary threats to this kind of research: socially desirable responding. Research has indicated that the reporting of socially undesirable behaviors increases with greater anonymity (Levine, Ancill, & Roberts, 1989; Locke & Gilbert, 1995; Turner et al., 1998). Second, we wanted a population old enough to have had a serious, committed relationship with some level of maturity. Internet samples are older and more diverse than typical college subject pools (Gosling, Vazire, Srivastava, & John, 2004). Finally, because this study was in the context of a dissertation project, time and financial resources were limited. Internet studies have been shown to be lower in cost (Schleyer & Forrest, 2000) and faster in-response time (Lazar & Preece, 1999; Franceschini, 2000) than mail, phone, or in person data collection techniques. This is not to say that Internet-based studies do not have their own methodological problems. Although the researcher essentially "casts a wider net" in order to capture participants, it is unclear as to the extent to which participants self-select on the basis of the topic of the study or other variables. There is also no way of knowing at this time how technical difficulties interfere with data collection or how the format influences measurement errors (Granello & Wheaton, 2004). However, when compared with the highly selective average undergraduate psychology subject pool, the Internet provided an excellent alternative for collecting our infidelity data.

THE CHALLENGES

The singular challenge for this study: lack of Institutional Review Board (IRB) approval. However, it was a bit more complicated than that. Our institution has gatekeepers at the departmental level who decide whether a study is ready to be reviewed at the university level. In this particular instance, the departmental gatekeeper was concerned that the study would be viewable by minors if posted on the Internet even though the method and electronic consent specifically invited those 18 and older to participate. Looking more deeply into this issue, we noted a discrepancy between the departmental and university governing bodies on both the general knowledge of Internet research and the ethics surrounding data collection through this avenue. The IRB officials at the university level were fine with the study design and proposal. In fact, other studies from different departments on campus had been approved with much more graphic sexual content than ours, and various gatekeepers within the department had allowed this as well in the past. What's more, the timing of the study was on the heels of the national public debate about MySpace allowing anyone to join without attempts to protect minors.

Our departmental gatekeeper was clear: She would not sign off on the study unless we could *guarantee* that no children would be exposed to the data collection, citing university liability as one of several reasons. What was less clear was how this should be done. She was okay with placing a weblink ad in a local alternative newspaper, placing the link on Facebook, and providing the link to the student subject pool. However, this seemed inconsistent in that placing an ad in the newspaper was no more protective than placing one on a Listserv for nonprovocative adult topics (like one we found for women aged 40 and over who are pursuing their PhDs). What's more, when the study finally did get to the IRB committee meeting, one member was concerned that participants would potentially be asked to respond about relationships they had when they were younger than 18 years old. For example, the study requested information about a relationship that occurred over the last 5 years. If some participants were 20 years old, they could be discussing a relationship that had happened when they were 15 years old. At this point, it seemed as if this issue was getting out of hand, in that many studies rely on retrospective data from adults about childhood experiences. We were unclear why this issue should be treated differently.

As the faculty member who teaches a course on American Psychological Association (APA) ethics in our training program, one of us (A. S.) was intrigued by the overall ethical dilemma. Protection of minors in research is an important issue. However, does this extend to all minors everywhere (e.g., the public at large), or just the minors we invite to participate in our studies? Particularly with regard to the Internet, where does the researchers' responsibility end and parental responsibility begin? And finally, did our questions and research format really constitute a risk, or was this a by-product of the current media frenzy surrounding MySpace? The Belmont Report (1978) outlines the minimum standards for research with human subjects. It has been interpreted by most to regard the protection and care of subjects *invited* to participate in research (whether or not they are then chosen to participate depends on their ability to consent). However, The Belmont Report could be interpreted more generally. In Part B, it states, "Persons with diminished autonomy are entitled to protection." The use of the word "persons" instead of "potential research subjects" or another similar term seems to place a broader responsibility on the research in terms of public protection. We suspect this was the position of our gate keeper.

OVERCOMING THE DIFFICULTIES

Regardless of the reasons, we had to convince our gatekeeper that such a study should be allowed or it would never reach the university IRB officials. The original IRB proposal was submitted in July but not approved until October, and because this was a dissertation, time was of the essence. We agreed to the gatekeeper's terms that the weblink be placed in the alternative newspaper, on Facebook, and provided to the subject pool. Our results were in the expected direction of the hypotheses, but the generalizability of the results was seriously compromised. Although we were able to overcome the social desirability concerns by conducting the study on the Internet, we had to compromise on our population. The majority of subjects ended up coming from the subject pool because of our limitations in advertising the study to a broader base.

LESSONS LEARNED

Given these experiences, we have learned a lot about Internet research, and if we had to do it all again, would proceed differently to address our gatekeeper's concerns. We still have the same looming questions about parental versus researcher responsibility on the Internet as well as whether including written questions about intercourse and oral sex constitute placing someone at risk. Please don't make us use the Clinton–Lewinski example, with its 24-hour news coverage to make this latter point! However, the broader ethical concern remains: It behooves us as researchers to do everything we can to protect the public, regardless of whether or not it directly involves our research participants. Our conduct has implications for how the public perceives, values, and trusts us, as well as our work. A perfect example of this is the controversy the American Psychological Association endured after publishing an article that appeared to minimize (and some would say support) the effect of adult men having sex with supposedly willing boys. The public outcry and subsequent congressional hearings on the matter prompted an APA apology and recognition that the APA should have done more to prevent the publication of such articles that clearly undermined the public trust in psychology. While in the context of working hard to get the research done, it is easy sometimes to become wrapped up in that goal and lose perspective of some of these broader ethical issues. The general concerns of our gatekeeper were valid ones, and we encourage all researchers to always practice some perspective taking when differing opinions like this one come to light. The concerns of such monitoring bodies are frequently for the betterment of the public and the profession.

Since the onslaught of Internet use for research purposes, there have been several suggestions for protecting both the public and our research subjects. Nosek, Banaji, and Greenwald (2002) outline a number of ethical issues that can arise in working through the Internet. Specifically, in regard to protecting the public, they suggest (1) designing the website to maximize its appeal to adults and minimize its appeal to children; (2) targeting adult-dominated venues in advertising for recruiting; (3) requiring a password for participants that is available only through adult-targeted advertisements; and/or (4) implementing an adult-check system, requiring individuals to register with a centralized database by providing evidence of their adult status. The authors also suggest that Internet researchers review the Children's Online Privacy Protection Act of 1998 (*www.ftc.gov/ogc/coppa1.htm*). Reviewing this material and implementing these suggestions may assist you in ensuring the ethical treatment of participants, although it won't necessarily ensure IRB approval!

TO READ FURTHER

Locke, S. D., & Gilbert, B. O. (1995). Method of psychological assessment, self-disclosure, and experiential differences: A study of computer, questionnaire, and interview assessment formats. *Journal of Social Behavior and Personality, 10,* 255–263.

Electronic data-gathering techniques may increase the likelihood that socially undesirable behavior will be more accurately reported owing to the increased anonymity associated with this data-gathering technique. Respondents also noted they enjoyed the electronic data-gathering process more than questionnaire or interview formats.

Granello, D. H., & Wheaton, J. E. (2004). Online data collection: Strategies for research. *Journal of Counseling and Development, 82,* 387–393.

Great review article that discusses the benefits and limitations of online data collection.

REFERENCES

Amato, P. R., & Previti, D. (2003). People's reasons for divorcing: Gender, social class, the life course, and adjustment. *Journal of Family Issues, 24,* 602–626.

Amato, P. R., & Rogers, S. J. (1997). A longitudinal study of marital problems and subsequent divorce. *Journal of Marriage and the Family, 59,* 612–624.

Atkins, D. C., Baucom, D. H., & Jacobson, N. S. (2001). Understanding infidelity: Correlates in a national random sample. *Journal of Family Psychology, 15,* 735–749.

Banfield, S., & McCabe, M. P. (2001). Extra relationship involvement among women: Are they different from men? *Archives of Sexual Behavior, 30,* 119–142.

Betzig, L. (1989). Causes of conjugal dissolution: A cross-cultural study. *Current Anthropology, 30,* 654–676.

Bowlby, J. (1969/1982). *Attachment and loss: Vol. 1. Attachment.* New York: Basic Books.

Bowlby, J. (1973). *Attachment and loss: Vol. 2. Separation.* New York: Basic Books.

Bowlby, J. (1980). *Attachment and loss: Vol. 3. Loss.* New York: Basic Books.

Buss, D. M., & Shackelford, T. K. (1997). Susceptibility to infidelity in the first year of marriage. *Journal of Research in Personality, 31,* 193–221.

Daly, M., & Wilson, M. (1988). *Homicide.* Hawthorne, NJ: Aldine de Gruyter.

Drake, C. R., & McCabe, M. P. (2000). Extrarelationship involvement among heterosexual males: An explanation based on the theory of planned behavior, relationship quality, and past behavior. *Journal of Applied Social Psychology, 30,* 1421–1439.

Franceschini, L. A. (2000). *Navigating electronic survey methods: Three pilot studies.* (ERIC Document Reproduction Service No. 448183)

Glass, S., & Wright, T. (1985). Sex differences in the types of extramarital involvement and marital satisfaction. *Sex Roles, 12,* 1101–1119.

Gosling, S. D., Vazire, S., Srivastava, S., & John, O. P. (2004). Should we trust web-based studies: A comparative analysis of sex preconceptions about Internet questionnaires. *American Psychologist, 59,* 93–104.

Granello, D. H., & Wheaton, J. E. (2004). Online data collection: Strategies for research. *Journal of Counseling and Development, 82,* 387–393.

Kinsey, A., Pomeroy, W., Martin, C., & Gebhard, P. H. (1953). *Sexual behavior in the human female.* Philadelphia: Saunders.

Lazar, J., & Preece, J. (1999). Designing and implementing web-based surveys. *Journal of Computer Information Systems, 39,* 63–67.

Levine, S., Ancill, R. J., & Roberts, A. P. (1989). Assessment of suicide risk by computer-delivered self-rating questionnaire: Preliminary findings. *Acta Psychiatrica Scandinavica, 80,* 216–220.

Locke, S. D., & Gilbert, B. O. (1995). Method of psychological assessment, self-disclosure, and experiential differences: A study of computer, questionnaire, and interview assessment formats. *Journal of Social Behavior and Personality, 10,* 255–263.

Nosek, B. A., Banaji, M. R., & Greenwald, A. G. (2002). E-research: Ethics, security, design, and control in psychological research on the Internet. *Journal of Social Issues, 58,* 161–176.

Parker, R. G. (1997). The influence of sexual infidelity, verbal intimacy, and gender upon primary appraisal processes in romantic jealousy. *Women's Studies in Communication, 20,* 1–24.

Schleyer, T. K. L., & Forrest, J. L. (2000). Methods for the design and administration of web-based surveys. *Journal of the American Medical Informatics Association, 7,* 416–425.

Sprecher, S., Regan, P. C., & McKinney, K. (1998). Beliefs about the outcomes of extramarital sexual relationships as a function of the gender of the "cheating spouse." *Sex Roles, 38,* 301–311.

The Belmont Report. (1978). *Ethical principles and guidelines for the protection of human subjects research.* DHEW Publication No. (OS) 78-0012.

Treas, J., & Giesen, D. (2000). Sexual infidelity among married and cohabiting Americans. *Journal of Marriage and the Family, 62,* 48–60.

Turner, C. F., Ku, L., Rogers, S. M., Lindberg, L. D., Pleck, J. H., & Stonenstein, F. L. (1998). Adolescent sexual behavior, drug use, and violence: Increased reporting with computer survey technology. *Science, 280,* 867–873.

Wiederman, M. (1997). Extramarital sex: Prevalence and correlates in a national survey. *Journal of Sex Research, 34,* 167–174.

CHAPTER 3

When Safeguards Become Straitjackets

How Ethics Research Board Requirements Might Contribute to Ethical Dilemmas in Studies with Marginalized Populations

MECHTHILD MEYER
ALMA ESTABLE
LYNNE MACLEAN
NANCY EDWARDS

BACKGROUND OF THE STUDY

Health and social research involving people generally requires review and approval by a Research Ethics Board (REB) at a university and may call for additional review by boards in other institutions. This process is essential to protect the confidentiality of research participants and to prevent harm. When the focus of the research is the experience of marginalized populations, however, the ethical review procedures and standard requirements may not be sufficient, may be targeting the wrong type of risks, or may be embedded in a power structure that a marginalized population seeks to address or overcome (Berg, Evans, Fuller, & the Okanagan Aboriginal Health Research Collective, 2007).

What ethical challenges can be expected in straightforward program evaluation studies focusing on hard-to-reach communities? We provide two examples from community health research studies with marginalized groups, one in which the challenges were successfully resolved and another for which no satisfying solution was found.

THE CHALLENGES

Example 1

As part of a larger research team, we undertook the qualitative component of an evaluation study to identify barriers to primary healthcare services as experienced by a number of specific marginalized and isolated population groups in one Canadian province. The qualitative component consisted of face-to-face interviews with mothers of young children who had used the program and with leaders closely connected with their communities who knew about service barriers experienced by women in their communities.

The original ethics protocol submitted for this project specified that a health professional involved in service delivery at each site would provide the researchers with a contact list of clients who had agreed to consider participating in the study and were willing to allow the research team to contact them about taking part. In a second step, a research team member would randomly select names of clients from the list and contact them to arrange for a place and time for the interview. It was anticipated that interpreters would be present at interviews with clients who did not speak English and would also verbally translate information letters and confidentiality forms at that point. However, we did not anticipate that we would need to involve interpreters during the recruitment phase.

The REB reviewed this protocol and raised the concern that clients might feel coerced into participating if a health professional was asking them to share their names as potential participants. The REB suggested an alternative protocol: The health professional was to hand each client who came for an appointment during the recruitment time period an information and recruitment letter, written in English. Clients who were interested in participating were to contact the university-based research team directly by telephone or e-mail to express an interest in being interviewed.

From the start, we were doubtful about whether the REB-suggested procedure would work in recruiting the intended target population for this study. Although we all had extensive experience involving marginalized populations in research, we were somewhat unprepared for the compounded ways in which marginalization actually played out with one of the target groups: The women did not speak English, were illiterate in their own language, lived on isolated farms, had no access to telephones, did not use motor vehicles or electricity, and spoke with noncommunity members only if they were permitted to do so by their religious leaders. Adding to these challenges was an unexpected technical glitch: The university's telephone system did not permit collect calls, nor could we offer a 1-800 (free long distance) number. Most of the women in the target population would not have the financial resources to make a long-distance call, and many did not have access to a telephone. We realized that the planned recruitment letters were clearly inadequate and handing them out would waste both time and resources.

We went back to the drawing board and reconsidered our recruitment strategy and informed consent procedures. These were our questions: How were women without access to a telephone, who did not speak English and/or were illiterate—some in their own language—supposed to read a recruitment letter detailing the procedure? And how likely would it be that these women would call us long-distance, or call their local health agency, especially when many in their communities refuse government services? Even in urban areas, would newcomer mothers who spoke no English and had little knowledge of the system be willing or able to attend an interview at the health agency? How could we maintain the confidentiality of individuals when religious leaders in some communities mediated access to women informants? Would women from the isolated farms ever learn that there was a study and they could be interviewed? Even if they still wished to participate, how realistic was it to expect they would commandeer the family horse and buggy to drive themselves and their children into town for individual, confidential interviews? Even if women had expressed an interest in participating and permitted their names to be entered into the contact list, how could we, sitting at the university in a distant city, confirm their interest in participating and set up an interview time and place, as part of the recruitment procedure, if we did not speak their language or if they did not have a telephone?

In practice, the health service providers in the program that we were evaluating were already working with interpreters to deliver their services. In some of the regions, the interpreters also were playing the role of lay health workers and had been hired by local health agencies to provide interpretation and other support services to new mothers. They had also built trusting relationships with the women, especially because they were often members of the same community and thus acted as gatekeepers. With their help, the women might feel comfortable talking with us, who were strangers and outsiders. Logically, and from a practical perspective, including advice we sought from the local health agencies, involving the lay health workers in the outreach to potential participants seemed a good solution. However, the research protocol approved by the REB did not include these intermediaries as recruiters.

Overcoming the Difficulties

We had to rethink the recruitment procedures in a way that was consistent with ethical principles. We had three options:

1. Abandon the qualitative interview component of the project, because the recruitment dilemmas could not be resolved. Without

a different recruitment strategy, we would not be able to reach the most marginalized section of the population of interest.

2. Recruit only those women who could be reached by phone and who were able to communicate in English to set up an in-person interview at the time we were going to be present at their site.

3. Adjust the ethics protocol for recruitment to involve interpreters in recruiting women, explaining the project and confidentiality proce dures, and setting up times and places for the interviews.

We chose the last option, because it seemed unethical, in a study that was supposed to explore service access barriers, to exclude yet again the most marginalized and silenced segment of the population: those who did not speak English or did not have access to a telephone or transportation.

We discussed at great length whether the women might feel coerced into participating if a lay health worker who spoke their language, was already known to them, and was also providing support services to the family, contacted them. We approached a member of our REB and explained the dilemma. We were fortunate that the REB understood the issue: The originally approved protocol did not actually create the conditions for noncoercive informed consent with the target population. A large portion of our target group would be unable to read an information letter and would not be able to contact us because of three factors: inability to communicate in English, lack of access to telephones, and lack of money to make long-distance calls. Our alternative protocol used third-party recruiters who were members of the community, could approach potential participants in person, but were not the providers of the health services that were being evaluated. The REB granted verbal approval for the changed recruitment and consent procedures. We worked with interpreters and/or lay health workers, who contacted potential participants face-to-face, explained the project and confidentiality procedures, and, if the participants agreed, set up a time for us to interview them in person. A first level of consent, to participate in the study and to meet with us, was obtained verbally by the interpreter and/or lay health worker. A second level of consent was obtained by the interviewer at the time of the interview, verbally with those who did not read and through interpreters for those who did not speak English. If this had not happened, our study would have recruited only the least marginalized women in the population.

In the end, the qualitative study included interviews with both "better connected" women and those who were more isolated. For example, in two communities the lay health workers accompanied the interviewer to the women's homes, located in remote rural areas. Without the lay health workers, we would not have been able to find their homes, let alone speak with 6 of the 18 women. At both sites, as part of the recruitment process, the lay health worker had taken time to meet with the women beforehand to explain the lengthy and complicated recruitment letter and consent form in their own language and to answer questions to the best of her knowledge. The interviews with these informants were particularly rich in their descriptions of how the program had been able to provide access to health services for these extremely isolated women.

This study also included interviews with community leaders who had knowledge about service access barriers experienced by members of their community. Our original protocol stated that the health agency at each site would provide a list of community leaders, and we would select from this list the particular leaders to approach. Upon review, we found that some of the community leaders identified were not as close to the communities as we had thought.

Although the lay workers had not been originally identified by the health agencies as community leaders, as we got to know them and their role in the community, it became apparent that they did fit the intention of our definition of community leaders. In fact, these workers had been hired because of their location and active participation within their communities: The characteristics of the leaders were consistent with the defining characteristics of "community leaders," even though they were not explicitly on the list of potential informants. Thus, they were invited to be interviewed. The lay health workers enthusiastically agreed, and we followed the standard procedures to receive informed consent. These interviews provided a particularly deep understanding about community needs and issues as compared with other informant interviews, which we likely would not have been able to access.

Example 2

Ethical dilemmas can occur when limited resources force researchers and REBs to weigh the relative benefits of accommodating the needs of one minority group over those of another. In another study initiated by a health organization in a bilingual community and targeting a very different minority population, we were not successful in obtaining REB approval for a portion of the research. The study focused on assessing a lifestyle change program that was being piloted with a specific minority population. The program was innovative and targeted a high-risk minority population. Our study was intended to shed light on the types of health promotion interventions that might improve outreach and programming for this population. We had approval from the organization to collect the pre–post intervention data as part of the program evaluation. Because the program served both English- and French-speaking clients, our survey instruments, confidentiality forms, and information letters were written in both languages. To strengthen the evaluation design we suggested adding a control group to the study, drawn from patients at a clinic that had agreed to refer clients to the pilot program. The program to be evaluated did not take place at the clinic, nor was it part of the work of the clinic or funded by it. We wanted to survey patients at the clinic prior to their attending the program or getting onto a waiting list for the program, and again after a certain time period had elapsed. This survey required additional approval, this time from the REB where the clinic was situated.

The REB had no problems with the design of the whole study, or so we were told informally; the only issue was that the submission itself would have to be officially translated into French. The project timelines and translation resources could not be stretched that far. Even the advocacy efforts of one of the investigators, a medical doctor involved in the clinic, who was very committed to the control group research design, failed to produce an exemption. As a result, the control group portion of the study was canceled.

The REB requirement that all formal documentation be submitted in both official languages is clearly, and justifiably, intended to safeguard and acknowledge the rights of the French minority population in the community. Nevertheless, we felt caught on the horns of an ethical dilemma. On one hand, the results of the research might help develop effective programming for a marginalized at-risk population; on the other hand, the REB also had concerns about meeting the policies of the bilingual institution, intended to safeguard the rights of the Francophone population. As a result, the needs of one minority group appeared to be in conflict with those of another.

(Not) Overcoming the Difficulties

We had already stretched resources to ensure that survey instruments, recruitment letters, and confidentiality protocols were available in both official languages. However, the requirement to translate the proposal itself for the REB was an insurmountable barrier—we lacked the resources, and the time, to successfully negotiate this last hurdle. As a consequence, the effects of a program intended to assist another minority population (which, ironically, also included French speakers), were not studied, or communicated to the health service sector, as well as they might have been with a control group design.

LESSONS LEARNED

In the future, when designing studies on marginalized populations, we will try even more actively to include people from these communities at the research design stage. Recruitment and consent issues can therefore be addressed proactively. Suggestions by Khanlou and Peter (2005) for conducting participatory research with minority populations include consultation processes with community members about potential risk. They conclude that involving members of minority communities on REBs is a necessary step to improve the approval process.

Another set of recently developed ethical guidelines addresses the specific issues of conducting research with Aboriginal communities (Canadian Institute for Health Research, 2007). Patterson, Jackson, and Edwards (2006) suggest checking assumptions about literacy levels and preferred methods of communication with participating communities prior to developing recruitment and consent protocols. We encourage REBs to include members of the communities that will be "studied" in their assessment of the ethical risks and benefits of various research approaches, especially when the research involves or is intended to benefit marginalized sectors of the population.

Ensuring that the recruitment and informed participation processes truly protect the rights of participants is a laudable goal. In community-based research with minority populations, recruitment often requires creativity and trust-building activities within a community development framework. It may be difficult for members of REBs who are more accustomed to drug trials, clinical research, or randomized controlled trials, to assess which community-based processes are appropriate and which are likely to endanger the participants. While respecting the importance of clear and rigorous mechanisms to ensure that participants in research are kept from harm, it would be interesting for REBs to examine ways that the protocols might include some flexibility and evolve as the study progresses, especially in community-based social research (Khanlou & Peter, 2005). For example, several authors have pointed out that many information letters and consent forms are written in a way that is hard to understand by the average person (Green, Duncan, Barnes, & Oberklaid, 2003; Ham et al., 2004), let alone someone who is struggling with the English language or has minimal literacy skills. Despite researchers' best efforts, it may be that once they are in the field they may find that there is a need to adjust consent forms when it becomes evident that participants are unable to understand them.

Our second example illustrates how a lack of flexibility in applying a language policy, originally designed to protect the rights of one minority population, resulted in stalling research on another underresearched minority population. We suggest that there are important benefits to community-based studies conducted in both official languages. Such studies, however, may not have the financial resources to permit translation of a lengthy and formal document, such as an ethics proposal. If it was impossible for the board to understand the language in which the proposal was written, perhaps the REB could have provided assistance with the translation of the document that they needed to read, given that the project team had already developed the client-contact information in both languages.

Another solution would have been to grant an exemption in this situation. REBs might want to consider including a clause in their policies that would make it possible to approve studies under certain circumstances—for example, when a research study on an understudied and underserved segment of the population will stall otherwise.

In summary, we all appreciate the work REBs do. We are aware that the work is demanding, with constant requests to respond to time constraints set out in different research projects. Those of us who are community-based researchers and have never participated in an REB would like to be able to informally ask questions about possible changes as the project progresses. Owing to the nature and consequences of social marginalization, it is unlikely that most REB members will have an intimate and personal understanding of the realities lived by marginalized communities. Nor would most REB members know the implications that specific medical conditions or psychiatric illnesses might have for recruitment procedures and confidentiality agreements. Their challenge is to seek ways of expanding their understanding through involving other members of society in their deliberations and decision making and to maintain the interest and well-being of those populations, as they define it themselves, as the key ethical concern.

TO READ FURTHER

Government of Canada. Tri-Council Policy Statement: Ethical Conduct for Research Involving Humans. Retrieved December 8, 2008, from *www.pre. ethics.gc.ca/english/aboutus/aboutus.cfm.*

Overview of ethical guidelines for conducting research involving humans, including conducting research on and with aboriginal people. The website provides a five-module online tutorial about key issues: Section 1, Ethics Review; Section 2, Free and Informed Consent; Section 3, Privacy and Confidentiality; Section 4, Conflict of Interest; and Section 5, Inclusion in Research. Completion is estimated to take 2 hours.

Alberta Research Ethics Community Consensus Initiative. Retrieved December 8, 2008, from *www.ahfmr.ab.ca/ programs.php.*

The website provides sample consent forms written in plain language and other useful information regarding preparing ethics proposals. An online tool is provided that is easy to use and helps researchers to assess whether their research projects should undergo an ethics procedure.

Smith, L. J. (2008). How ethical is ethical research?: Recruiting marginalized, vulnerable groups into health services research. *Journal of Advanced Nursing* 62, 248–257.

Good overview from another country of the ethical issues that are involved in conducting research with and on vulnerable populations.

REFERENCES

Berg, L. D., Evans, M., Fuller, D., & the Okanagan Aboriginal Health Research Collective (2007). Ethics, hegemonic whiteness, the contested imagination of "Aboriginal community" in social science research in Canada. *ACME: An International E-Journal for Critical Geographies, 6*(3), 395–409.

Canadian Institute for Health Research. (2007). CIHR Guidelines for Health Research Involving Aboriginal People. Retrieved January 25, 2008, from *www.cihr-irsc.gc.ca/cgi-bin/print-imprimer.pl.*

Green, J. B., Duncan, R. E., Barnes, G. L., & Oberklaid, F. (2003). Putting the "informed" into "consent": A matter of plain language. *Journal of Paediatrics and Child Health, 39*, 700–703.

Ham, M., Jones, N., Mansell, I., Northway, R., Price, L., & Walker, G. (2004). "I'm a researcher!" Working together to gain ethical approval for a participatory research study. *Journal of Learning Disability, 8*, 397–407.

Khanlou, N., & Peter, E. (2005). Participatory action research: Considerations for ethical review. *Social Science and Medicine, 60*, 2333–2340.

Patterson, M., Jackson, R., & Edwards, N. (2006). Ethics in aboriginal research: Comments on paradigms, process and two worlds. *Canadian Journal of Aboriginal Community-Based Research, 1*, 47–57.

CHAPTER 4

Going Off the Rails for "Love or Money"

Implementation Issues Related to Payment of Research Participants in an Addiction-Research Project

BRIAN R. RUSH
DOMINIQUE MORISANO

BACKGROUND OF THE STUDY

Since the 1970s, researchers, service providers, and healthcare administrators and funders have become increasingly aware of the high degree of overlap of mental and substance use disorders among adults and youth in the community at large, as well as among people seeking help from mental health, substance abuse, and other health and social services. Individuals with concurrent disorders generally have worse treatment outcomes than individuals with "one or the other" (i.e., a substance use or mental disorder alone), and risk factors that are associated with the comorbidity (e.g., homelessness, victimization, HIV/AIDS, incarceration) tend to be more prevalent and serious. Economic studies clearly show that the "double trouble" of concurrent disorders has a significant financial impact on health, social, and justice systems.

As a result of the limitations of our screening tools, huge variations in assessment and treatment techniques, and attitudinal factors among service providers related to stigma and discrimination, there is considerable underdetection of the co-occurrence of mental and substance use disorders. In turn, this has resulted in widespread failure to develop integrated treatment and support plans, an issue that has spurred international interest in identifying, and widely disseminating, empirically supported treatments and best practice guidelines for assisting people with concurrent disorders. With further research, we aim to increase identification rates, improve outcomes, and reduce the consequences and costs associated with improperly assessed and treated concurrent disorders.

Best practice reviews, including those undertaken in Canada (Health Canada, 2001), have provided exhaustive overviews of the relevant literature and consistently recommended universal screening of mental disorders among clients entering treatment for substance use problems. At the same time, making strong evidence-based recommendations for routine practice in this area presents significant challenges. First and foremost, there is a dearth of screening measures validated within the substance abuse treatment population and against a recognized gold standard. Furthermore, because the measures that are available to service providers also vary extensively in regard to content, comprehensiveness, administration time, and contribution to subsequent diagnostic assessment and treatment planning, the relative benefits of the various options need to be systematically compared in this population.

The main objectives of our study were twofold. We aimed to both validate and compare four mental health-screening tools in a heterogeneous substance abuse treatment population at the point of treatment entry. Recruitment was planned across three large substance abuse treatment centers in Ontario. After informed consent was obtained, the protocol called for completing the screening tools and other study measures in the context of a research interview. In order to meaningfully assess and compare tool performance, all participants were administered the research version of the Structured Clinical Interview for DSM-IV Disorders (SCID), a tool that is widely regarded as the gold standard for establishing a diagnosis of a mental disorder for research purposes and validating mental health-related screening tools (First, Spitzer, Gibbon, & Williams, 2002).

In this chapter we discuss the main challenge that arose in the early stage of implementing this multisite research study. In effect, our project nearly went "off the rails" as soon as it was launched, and in retrospect, we have some insights about what we might have done differently.

THE CHALLENGES

Surprisingly, the main obstacle arose before data collection even began. Issues related to ethics and research design were unexpectedly broached by staff at the various project sites around our decision to provide cash honoraria to the research participants. In order to highlight how the issue unfolded, we created the following retrospective timeline of project events. We vetted our retrospective account through the three site directors of our study locations, and each individually approved the general summary of the following events.

In July 2005 our grant was approved by the Canadian Institutes for Health Research (CIHR), albeit with a "routine" 18% across-the-board budget cut. The investigators were a multidisciplinary team of four researchers who were well versed in clinical, pharmacological, and health services research. The accepted research protocol stated that participants would each be given $50 in cash for completing the study, and the reviewers raised no issues with the form or amount of the remuneration. In March 2006 we submitted the application to our institutional Research Ethics Board (REB), which, by agreement, uses procedures common to all of the 10 teaching hospitals of the University of Toronto.

In terms of potential risks, harms, and benefits to participants that were addressed in the REB application, we identified risks as including "interview fatigue" and the possible evoking of difficult memories prompted by interview questions. Potential benefits included results from the SCID interview, which were to be made available to participants via their treatment providers. We also included a section in the ethics proposal describing several possibilities for remuneration: (1) reimbursement for expenses incurred, (2) gifts for participation, (3) payment for time, and (4) other. Our choice was "payment for time," which we considered to be most closely aligned ethically with the "wage model" of compensation as compared with a "risk model." Given an adjustment that had to be made in the final approved budget with CIHR, and because the expected time commitment was estimated at 2 to 3 hours, we reduced the original $50 payment per participant to $35. The REB application had not specifically required us to justify our choice of remuneration, and we did not offer further explanation, as we felt that our choice was straightforward. In our protocol and assorted consent forms, we did not offer potential participants a choice of mode of compensation other than cash, nor did we identify specific risks associated with receiving a cash payment. In our Letter of Information to participants, however, we listed the $35 payment under the heading "Benefits/Risks of Participating." Although we implied that this was a potential study benefit, presumably it could have been interpreted by readers as representing either a risk or a benefit. In August 2006 we received ethics approval, with no comments on our choice of cash reimbursement as the mode of remuneration.

In early January 2007 we had our first visit to Site 1, where one of us, the principal investigators (B. R. R.) and the project's research coordinator met with the site director and staff to introduce the study and the protocol details and to outline the roles of staff members and a project research assistant (RA) who would be located there during the subject recruitment phase. Although few issues were raised, staff members did ask about participant compensation, with most stating a strong preference for the planned form of remuneration (i.e., cash). They unanimously agreed that a cash payment best respected the autonomy and dignity of their clients.

A similar visit was made to Site 2 a few days later. Here, the staff members also raised issues with respect to participant remuneration, but indicated that they strongly preferred *noncash* alternatives (e.g., vouchers) because they felt that cash might be a trigger for substance use. After considerable discussion, staff members ultimately agreed that although they would approve cash payments as a potential option for remuneration in order to keep the study going smoothly, they would prefer vouchers (e.g., gift cards or certificates). They also indicated that they would like to have access to information about which clients chose to be paid in cash, so that they might provide special targeted counseling to those clients about the receipt of the money, triggers, and substance use. A decision on this aspect was deferred for more discussion among the entire research team.

Two weeks later, the principal investigator (PI) and research coordinator met with the staff at Site 3. At this meeting the site director was unable to attend. As at the other two sites, however, staff members raised questions about participant remuneration. They also expressed that they strongly preferred vouchers to be used in lieu of cash payments. They stated that, in their opinion, cash payments were almost certain to act as triggers for substance abuse and consequent harm. As the issue was now salient in all three study sites, the research team elected to defer further discussion of subject remuneration until a thorough literature review had been conducted and we could prepare a solid rationale for the cash payment approach. A follow-up meeting between the PI and the site director of Site 3 was scheduled.

The literature we drew upon was culled from published expert opinion and empirical research on research participant payment within the substance abuse field (see Fry, Hall, Ritter, & Jenkinson, 2006, for a comprehensive review), as well as broader health-related research (e.g., Grant & Sugarman, 2004; also see Grady, 2005, for a review). Relevant literature was also sourced from within the substance abuse treatment domain, where contingency management (including cash, vouchers, lotteries) is often used as a therapeutic approach to reinforce abstinence (e.g., Vandrey, Bigelow, & Stitzer, 2007).

Our conclusion from the literature review and analysis of current guidelines was similar to that drawn by Fry et al. (2006) in their much more exhaustive overview. It is important to note that there is no consensus or specific guidelines on what constitutes an ethical approach to the compensation of people with severe substance use problems for participation in research, and Institutional Review Boards (IRBs) vary widely in their decisions regarding participant recruitment (Dickert, Emanuel, & Grady, 2002; Fry et al., 2005). However, we identified several points in the literature that provide considerable guidance to researchers. Research offers empirical support for subject payments in terms of improved subject participation (Seddon, 2005; Fry et al., 2006), as well as evidence of such payments as "standard practice" among researchers (McCrady & Bux, 1999; College on Problems of Drug Dependence, 1995; Wright, Klee, & Reid, 1998; Fry et al., 2005). There is certainly no basis for denial of reward or fair compensation based on negative assumptions about drug user motivations for participating. Many factors over and above monetary gain appear to underlie these motivations (Fry & Dwyer, 2001; Wright et al., 1998; Slomka, McCurdy, Ratiff, Timpson, & Williams, 2007). Further, cash payment, the preferred option among the individuals concerned, has little bearing on participants' subsequent drug use or perceptions of coercion (Festinger et al., 2005; Kurlander, Simon-Dack, & Gorelick, 2006; Rothfleisch, Ronith, Rhoades, & Schmitz, 1999).

In short, our review identified no major ethical barriers to the provision of cash payments to participants in substance abuse research, provided that the investigators remain vigilant to circumstances in which they might add to the risk of harm or other negative consequences (above and beyond the day-to-day risks to which participants and others are normally exposed). Indeed, researchers may even have a duty to provide such payments to be consistent with the ethical principles of autonomy, distributive justice, and beneficence.

OVERCOMING THE DIFFICULTIES

In February 2007 the resolution process for our study began. Basing it on a review of the literature, we prepared a brief summary of potential ethical issues surrounding participant remuneration, which we distributed among the study investigators for review at a team meeting. The team members were unanimous in their support for the cash payment option. We also reviewed the budget again, and interview time was estimated in more detail based on the likelihood of multiple mental disorders needing to be covered in detail in the SCID. Given our new estimate of approximately 4 to 5 hours, the payment was increased back to the original amount of $50. One of the co-PIs then began a series of consultations with managers and frontline staff/counselors at the three sites. These sessions were used both to inform the staff about concerns related to making changes to the study methods (postethics approval and receipt of the grant) and to probe more deeply into the staff's concerns about cash compensation. Both the initial site meetings with the research team and the follow-up staff consultations highlighted the differences of opinion across and even within sites and made it clear that a consensus decision had to be made. In light of the literature review, the consensus of the research team itself, and several rounds of discussion and consultation surrounding the logistics, ethics, and recruitment potential of different forms of remuneration, the final decision was made to use only cash payments, as originally planned. The other requests to accommodate the staff concerns, namely, informing clinicians of a client's payment choice, were rejected on ethical grounds, in that the approved study protocol did not include informing the clinicians about client payment choices. We thought that including this stipulation could blur the line between research and clinical functions. The co-PI relayed the final decision to each of the site directors, and they agreed to proceed with the cash remuneration on the basis of the underlying rationale and knowledge that a uniform decision needed to be made across the sites. The decision was conveyed to site staff members by their managers, and they complied with the decision.

Shortly thereafter we obtained additional ethics approval for minor changes to the informed consent form; wording changes had been made on the basis of comments from the grant reviewers, site-specific adaptations about poststudy contact, and framing of the SCID results as research results (as opposed to clinical results). Furthermore, the cash honorarium amount was changed from $35 back to $50 as agreed upon in the team meetings. The REB did not make any comments about the changes that had been made.

Between late February and mid-March 2007, the study began at all sites with full agreement on remuneration procedures. From that point on, there were two "blips" that came to our attention with regard to participant payments. One event occurred about halfway through the recruitment phase. At this time, the RA from Site 1 sent an e-mail to the research team members to let them know about an incident that had occurred at her site. She said that she had been approached by a friend of one of the study participants, and that this friend had been extremely angry to learn about the $50 cash payment. The friend told the RA that the research staff members had been irresponsible and that they should not have been "handing out cash to addicts." The friend did not, however, go into detail about whether or not specific harm had been caused to the study participant in question as a result of the cash payment. The friend was given contact information for one of the co-PIs, as well as the head of the REB committee, in case she wanted to pursue the issue. However, she was not heard from again.

The second issue was one that arose at Site 2 near the end of the recruitment phase; it concerned the loss of an envelope containing a substantial amount of cash for participant payment ($750). The envelope had been inadvertently left on the intake counter by the courier. We later determined that it wasn't clear to all staff members as to who was responsible for looking after the money when it arrived, and that this responsibility should have rested solely with the on-site RA.

We decided to ask our site directors for their thoughts on the overall payment issue and the resolution process. The director of Site 1 told us that the consultations held between the PIs and the three sites had been important, but that the selling point had been the fact that the method and amount of client payment was established and approved by the CIHR. The director at Site 1 also noted that the final decision had fallen in line with this site's philosophy on emphasizing client choice, empowerment, and ability and therefore was an easy one to accept. The director of Site 2 pointed to the need for consistency among study sites as being key to the resolution process. This director noted that although the staff members at this site would still have preferred to use vouchers, ensuring consistency in methodology across sites was the "correct choice." When the other sites decided to accept cash payments, Site 2 did as well, in order to avoid being an "outlier." The director of Site 3 told us that although his staff members had had some concerns about cash payment, they had been flexible with their concerns and had simply accepted the final decision of the research team.

When asked if the final decision to go with "cash only" had resulted in any negative impacts on the study, their program, or the clients/participants, the site directors didn't raise any issues other than that concerning the lost envelope at Site 2. When the cash went missing, both staff and clients were implicated, hospital security was informed, and an investigation was conducted. Distrust and a general sense of suspicion arose despite no indication that staff members were involved. Although the money was never located, new processes regarding communication about the delivery, receipt, and storage of the cash payments were then more clearly defined.

When asked directly, all three site directors said that they would participate in the same kind of study again, under similar conditions of participant remuneration.

LESSONS LEARNED

Seddon (2005) offered four key components of "good practice" with respect to payment of participants in substance abuse-related research. Not coincidently, these points coincide with most of the lessons learned in our collective experience.

The first point is to ensure effective communication about the use of the incentives with all relevant stakeholders at the start of the research. Although we prepared a brief project summary for stakeholders in order to relay information and secure letters of support for grant submission, and discussed client payments during phone conversations, we did not specifically draw attention to the issue of cash payment as an item for preproject discussion with all the site staff. So, not only should communication begin early on, but it should also occur at both manager and staff levels of the study sites. As Seddon (2005) emphasized, this early communication should cover the rationale, benefits, safeguards, and practical arrangements for the use of incentives, cash or otherwise. We would, however, expand on Seddon's point by stressing the additional challenges likely to ensue with a multisite research project in which differences are likely to arise both within and across sites. Our experience with nearly going "off the rails" on an implementation issue that was complicated by the multisite nature of the study is consistent with the challenges experienced by others in projects of this type (Dewa et al., 2002).

The second point is to be more aware of the literature on research incentives and the benefits of using cash payments. In the end, although we were sensitive to the concerns of the research "hosts," we felt a need to more thoroughly educate ourselves in order to prepare an effective response. For researchers, it is very difficult to be familiar with all the nuances of research methodology. That said, with the benefit of hindsight, we could have predicted that this would be a critical issue for the programs involved and "had our homework done" accordingly.

Third, Seddon (2005) pointed out that the cost of incentive payments should be incorporated into research proposals, because these payments offer good value for money from the perspective of research funders, inasmuch as participant payments increase the completeness and overall quality of the data. Although we had included participant payments in the original project budget, we wavered on the amount in the face of a major administrative budget cut by the funder. To better align with the wage-as-payment philosophy that was expressed in the literature, as well as with a more detailed assessment of participant time commitments, we returned to our original amount and made the required cuts in another budget line.

Finally, Seddon (2005) advocated for clear and effective arrangements for the health and safety of fieldworkers dispensing incentives, as well as arrangements for financial accountability. Although personal safety was not an issue from a physical standpoint, it took a minicrisis at one of our sites to make us realize that our procedures were not as well understood as we had thought, consequently putting staff and clients at risk of the emotional stress associated with an issue of financial accountability.

In the end, our project recruited a total of 546 participants with complete information. Both the study team and the managers and staff of the study sites agreed on the success of the collaboration and its likely contribution to evidence-based practice for people with concurrent disorders accessing substance abuse treatment.

TO READ FURTHER

Thomson, C. L., Morley, K. C., Teesson, M., Sannibale, C., & Haber, P. S. (2008). Issues with recruitment to randomized controlled trial in the drug and alcohol field: A literature review and Australian case study. *Drug and Alcohol Review, 27,* 115–122.

This article discusses a wide range of issues related to conducting randomized controlled trials. It extends the content of this chapter by placing compensation issues for research participants in a large context related to other kinds of potential barriers to participation.

Grady, C., Dicket, N., Jawetz, T., Gensler, G., & Emanuel, E. (2005). An analysis of U.S. practices of paying research participants. *Contemporary Clinical Trials, 26*, 365–375.

This article analyses the practices in the United States in paying research participants in health-related research. It helps to put payment issues in the drug research field in the larger context of health research generally. It covers the types of studies that offer payment, to what types of subjects, and how amounts are determined.

Fry, C. L., Hall, W., Ritter, A., & Jenkinson, R. (2006). The ethics of paying drug users who participate in research: A review and practical recommendations. *Journal of Empirical Research on Human Research Ethics, 1*(4), 21–36.

This article reviews the literature on payment practices and guidelines and the risks and harms that may arise from paying drug-using participants. General principles, key questions, and procedural options are highlighted and suggestions offered for an applied approach to ethical research payments.

Seddon, T. (2005). Paying drug users to take part in research: Justice, human rights and business perspectives on the use of incentive payments. *Addiction Research and Theory, 13*, 101–109.

This article explores the question of paying drug users to take part in research from the perspective of three models: justice, human rights, and business. Issues discussed include whether cash payments are appropriate, payment amounts, whether incentives jeopardize informed consent, and whether they offer good value for money for research funders.

REFERENCES

College on Problems of Drug Dependence. (1995). Human subject issues in drug abuse research. *Drug and Alcohol Dependence, 37*, 167–175.

Dewa, C. S., Durbin, J., Eastabrook, S., Ochoka, J., Boydell, K. M., Wasylenki, D., et al. (2002). Considering a multi-site study? Taking the leap and having a soft landing. *Journal of Community Psychology, 30*(3), 1–15.

Dickert, N., Emanuel, E., & Grady, C. (2002). Paying research subjects: An analysis of current policies. *Annals of Internal Medicine, 136*, 368–373.

Festinger, D. S., Marlowe, D. B., Croft, J. R., Dugosh, K. L., Mastro, N. K., Lee, P. A., et al. (2005). Do research payments precipitate drug use or coerce participation? *Drug and Alcohol Dependence, 78*, 275–281.

First, M. B., Spitzer, R. L., Gibbon, M., & Williams, J. B. W. (2002). *Structured Clinical Interview for DSM-IV Axis I Disorders, Research Version, Patient*

Edition (SCID–I/P). New York: Biometrics Research, New York State Psychiatric Institute.

Fry, C., & Dwyer, R. (2001). For love or money? An exploratory study of why injecting drug users participate in research. *Addiction, 96*, 1319–1325.

Fry, C. L., Hall, W., Ritter, A., & Jenkinson, R. (2006). The ethics of paying drug users who participate in research: A review and practical recommendations. *Journal of Empirical Research on Human Subject Ethics, 1*(4), 21–36.

Fry, C. L., Ritter, A., Baldwin, S., Bowen, K., Gardiner, P., Holt, T., et al. (2005). Paying research subjects: A study of current practices in Australia. *Journal of Medical Ethics, 31*, 542–547.

Grady, C. (2005). Payment of clinical research subjects. *Journal of Clinical Investigation, 117*, 1681–1687.

Grant, R. W., & Sugarman, J. (2004). Ethics in human subjects research: Do incentives matter? *Journal of Medicine and Philosophy, 29*, 717–738.

Health Canada. (2001). *Best practices: Concurrent mental health and substance use disorders.* Ottawa: Health Canada.

Kurlander, J. E., Simon-Dack, S. L., & Gorelick, D. A. (2006). Spending of remuneration by subjects in non-treatment drug abuse research studies. *American Journal of Drug and Alcohol Abuse, 32*, 527–540.

McCrady, B. S., & Bux, D. A. (1999). Ethical issues in informed consent with substance abusers. *Journal of Consulting and Clinical Psychology, 67*, 186–193.

Rothfleisch, J., Ronith, E., Rhoades, H., & Schmitz, J. (1999). Use of monetary reinforcers by cocaine-dependent outpatients. *Journal of Substance Abuse Treatment, 17*, 229–236.

Seddon, T. (2005). Paying drug users to take part in research: Justice, human rights and business perspectives on the use of incentive payments. *Addiction Research and Theory, 13*, 101–109.

Slomka, J., McCurdy, S., Ratiff, E. A., Timpson, S., & Williams, M. L. (2007). Perceptions of financial payment for research participation among African-American drug users in HIV studies. *Journal of General Internal Medicine, 22*, 1403–1409.

Vandrey, R., Bigelow, G. E., & Stitzer, M. (2007). Contingency management in cocaine abusers: A dose–effect comparison of goods-based versus cash-based incentives. *Experimental and Clinical Psychopharmacology, 15*, 338–343.

Wright, S., Klee, H., & Reid, P. (1998). Interviewing illicit drug users: Observations from the field. *Addiction Research, 6*, 517–535.

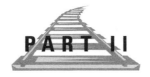

PART II

ACCESSING THE PARTICIPANTS

Once you have successfully jumped through the ethics hoop, you are ready to recruit participants. Not so fast! You have to gain access to the target population. Whoever the target population is, researchers have to obtain approval from relevant "authority" figures, often called gatekeepers (for a reason that will soon become all too obvious), to contact potential participants and recruit them into the study. Making matters worse, there are often many gatekeepers. Different groups of stakeholders in a research project can act as gatekeepers. For instance, administrators in a school district or principals at a particular school, teachers, parents, and the students themselves are stakeholders, having a say in terms of approving the project. Directors and managers of clinical programs, healthcare professionals, and members of a patient's family form a multilayered system of gatekeepers in all health institutions—in primary, acute, and long-term care settings. Leaders of geographically circumscribed (e.g., small town) or dispersed (e.g., cultural group) communities, and of advocacy groups, also serve as gatekeepers. Similarly, "guardians" of databases and/or records kept by governmental or nongovernmental agencies are equally powerful gatekeepers. What is less well known is that there are formal and informal gatekeepers. Formal gatekeepers are in an official position to grant approval to access a target population. In addition to ethics boards, formal gatekeepers consist of clinical directors of institutions participating in the study, administrators in a school, or key figures or representatives of a community. Informal gatekeepers are people who assume various positions within the recruitment sites and are seen by colleagues as spokespersons or informal leaders. They exert pressure on others and, consequently, play an important role in endorsing the study and providing access to participants. Examples of informal gatekeepers are expert professionals (often referred to as "opinion leaders") and active, outspoken members of a parent or patient association.

Researchers have to identify the formal and informal gatekeepers and obtain their "blessings" if the study is to get off the ground. Although finding out who the formal gatekeepers are may be easier than recognizing the informal ones, researchers must secure approval to access the population from both groups. As described in the next five chapters, researchers have to meet with the identified gatekeepers to explain the study, highlight its scientific value, and discuss the logistics of recruitment and/or data collection. As stated by MacLean in Chapter 7, gatekeepers can "make or break" access to participants; that is, they may endorse the study and support researchers in their endeavors, or they may deny access to the target population. Gatekeepers may misinterpret the intent of the study and become suspicious of the investigators' activities, raising questions about various aspects of the study, as described by Dos Santos in Chapter 5. As reported by Dergal Serafini (Chapter 6), even though some gatekeepers may not quite understand research and may not value its contribution to practice, they too can express concerns about the study. She also describes how gatekeepers may have their own agendas, wanting a study to go off in other directions to address questions they have. MacLean's experience (Chapter 7) powerfully illustrates the role of informal gatekeepers in this step of research and the importance of gaining their trust to achieve entry into a social system. Dhami and Souza (Chapter 8) and Veldhuizen and colleagues (Chapter 9) depict the obstacles they faced to get access to available records and datasets, respectively.

These stories clearly delineate the impact of gatekeepers' decisions on a study's integrity. In some instances, gatekeepers require researchers to follow a set of rules and regulations and/or to clarify aspects of the study prior to granting approval. The result is a delay in starting, and therefore in completing, the study (Chapters 8 and 9). On other occasions, gatekeepers who control access to the population allow researchers to approach only a specific subgroup of participants (Chapter 5), which has the potential to bias the sample. Finally, gatekeepers may interfere with the study plan. They may express their views as to whom should be investigated and how they should be recruited, as well illustrated in

Chapter 6. In that instance the gatekeepers denied access to the target population originally defined by the researcher but approved access to their selected group.

As you read more of this book, you will notice that although later chapters focus on different aspects of research, and hence are placed in different sections, many of them touch on issues of access and gatekeepers; check the matrix for other examples.

Armed with patience and clear communication skills, researchers can engage gatekeepers in meaningful negotiation to gain access to participants or to reach a compromise that all can live with.

CHAPTER 5

Frailty, Thy Name Is Macho

JOSÉ QUIRINO DOS SANTOS

BACKGROUND OF THE STUDY

The seaside city of Santos, in Brazil, is considered to be the largest port in the Southern Hemisphere, employing thousands of stevedores. The prevalence of sexually transmitted diseases, AIDS among them, rose sharply in the beginning of the 1990s. Scared and baffled by this mysterious menace, a small group of dockyard workers came to our nongovernmental organization (NGO) seeking help. At the time, I headed this NGO, where blood tests and follow-up of seropositive cases of an ever-increasing clientele kept us very busy.

We decided to keep watch on the members of this small group in their everyday activities. This approach was soon replaced by a standard qualitative research plan consisting of in-depth interviews, as well as ethnographic observations, looking for reasons for the high prevalence of HIV/AIDS. We were not interested in the mounting numbers per se, but in their occurrence—that is, the hows and whys of this situation. And at the end, we had to be able to help those seaside professionals to understand their own behavior. The research was then launched.

THE CHALLENGES AND SOLUTIONS

After training six psychologists for interviewing stevedores in their working environment, which meant 3 full days of nonstop advising on what to see, what to say, what to do, how to record an interview, how to correct mishaps, how to cope with harassment and other possible situations, I was

told that they could not start the job. The reason was that the state police
were suspicious of women entering the docks with tape recorders and cameras. This is how we discovered that we were under surveillance. So we
decided that I had to pay a courtesy visit to the chief of police and his aides
and try to smooth things out. The chief, with no previous introduction or
even a simple greeting, spit out: "You're giving syringes to those junkies!
They're behaving bad, real bad. We won't sit here and just watch this coke-
injecting party.... Shame on you, you so-called physicians! You are just
helping these scum to their means."

One of us, a social worker, said angrily, "Do you really think that
those guys are spreading AIDS to everybody, just because they share the
same syringe? No sir, they're just aping their American counterparts, who,
as you know, are forbidden to even carry a syringe on them; and there, in
that country, to share such a device is taken as some sort of companionship,
as belonging, as being part of something exclusive! You must understand
that we are not promoting drugs to those guys; they're already hooked on
coke. All we're doing is teaching them to protect themselves; even being
against drugs, as we are, you cannot stop a junkie from taking coke just
like that, out of a pompous will." The policeman ignored this interjection
and her line of reasoning, pushing the argument that not only does the pos-
session of a syringe allow a junkie to gain primacy among his peers—the
thing being exhibited like a trophy—but also that others would want to join
in, forming a group with leader and followers. At the end, he argued, everybody becomes addicted, and worse still, people who don't own a syringe
will have a chance to get a shot and eventually get hooked into an expensive
drug consumption pattern, even though not having enough money to buy
their own injection equipment. His point was that the youth from poorer
social strata can acquire richer people's bad habits out of this collective
experience, otherwise inaccessible to them.

At this point, our humiliated social worker became visibly angry and
then cut the policeman short: "Chief, those stories of rich and poor are
nonsense. Listen, I have an 11-year-old daughter at home who has been
totally blind since birth. I'll show you that even so, being a child and blind
as well, she can buy a syringe very easily, as anyone can. There are no such
things as 'showing off' syringes, being poor or whatever.... Let me use
your telephone, please." She called home and asked her daughter to buy a
syringe and call her back once this was done. A few minutes later the girl
called back. Her mother picked up the phone and repeated aloud what the
girl said, so everyone could hear: "Did you buy it, sweetie? Kind of quick,
hey? Oh, so you phoned the pharmacy and asked for delivery, hey? How
much d'you pay ... only a few cents, hey? Also including a length of rubber string ... great! Thanks." She said to the chief, "As you can see, sir,
it's very easy to buy those things in this town. Anyone can inject himself
at a very low cost. So don't blame us on this matter. It's not fair. The ques-

tion is: Those things are so cheap and easy to buy, why do people stick together to get a shot? The answer that we got out of our observations is simple. People want to stick together when they get stoned and share their experiences. For them, drug using is a good occasion to socialize; it brings togetherness."

After a number of vague accusations of this kind, followed by very to-the-point responses, we had the feeling of winning the game. A dreadful and tricky game it was, leaving a taste of fear and humiliation in our mouths. This guy was obviously not convinced, he agreed with us only in order to get rid of the newsmen who waited outside (being there because we tipped them off). After an apparently conciliatory peroration on not pushing things very far, he dismissed us, leaving us with the impression that he considered us a band of despicable outlaws receiving a big favor. Later on, in a less pessimistic mood, for then we could move quite freely at the docks, not fearing going to prison, we felt sure of having won a battle, a Lilliputian one, but a victory anyway.

Why did this absurd, aggressive, dialogue happen? At the time, the NGO for prevention of sexually transmitted diseases (STDs) and HIV/AIDS that I headed was staffed by infectious disease specialists, social workers, and psychologists. In this Brazilian harbor town, the constant arrival of foreign sailors was believed to be the main reason, if not the only one, for the soaring rates of AIDS infection. Presumably, prostitutes were infected by sailors and passed the disease on to their local clients, who would then disseminate it to their wives, other women, and so on. Surveying the communities around the port, we found that women in the trade were actually infected in great numbers. But we didn't find any positive link to supposedly contaminated foreign sailors. On the contrary, they were remarkably clean, even spontaneously wearing condoms. All kinds of wild conjectures were made, so we decided to get things straight and began a survey. On the second day of data gathering in the port, we were approached by some firemen from the fire station beside our office (they were a special battalion of the Militarized State Police). They told us about rumors concerning our presence in the harbor: They knew that our presence seemed very suspicious to the regular cops (the Civil State Police), who said we were preparing to denounce the drug market system in order to replace the local mafia. These firemen knew us, understood our purposes, but couldn't protect us, they said. We were on our own. This is why we had carefully and respectfully asked for the meeting with the chief of police. And at the end of this sharp-tongued meeting, we got a sermon on ethics, instead of being questioned about our doings at the docks.

We were disgusted and our spirits were running low, despite the tiny victory at the chief of police's office. But there was something else, the drug scene, to be dealt with. We knew that the drug gangs were much more important than the two state police forces (Civil and Militarized)

or the private harbor security corps. Behind the port administrative offi-
cers and their red tape procedures, the dealers were the real controllers of
all loading-unloading operations on cargo ships, overruling the stevedore
union's tough guys. At the beginning they ignored our open attempts to
make contact. Through some clients of our NGO, the prostitutes, those
guys made us emphatically aware of the danger of being there, doing this
"stupid thing disguised as a research," as nobody would believe it, because
what we were "really" doing there was to spy on them for some unknown
mob that would wipe them out and take their (profitable) place. This menacing interpretation of our presence at the port had to be countered, very
cautiously, for we now were in real danger. I changed the routine of my
weekly traveling to the port, choosing the bus instead of my car; my always
being in a crowd made an attack less probable. As the firemen's help was
out of the question, and the civil police decreasing their rare harbor patrols,
we had no choice. It was either negotiating with the dealers or getting out
of town to save our necks. There was no one to complain to, as the local
"authorities" formed a solid group bound by their common interests.

At that time, almost in despair, we had to decide what to do, and
despite all these insane happenings, we decided to stay and do the job. The
only person who would listen to our complaints was a reporter we knew
to be in contact with the drug system. Next day, the big drug lord agreed
to meet with us on his own premises and on his own terms: no women, no
recorders. After answering at length all his questions and those of his aides,
and having guaranteed that our presence would not interfere with any interests of the drug traffic whatsoever, he conceded to let us stay around, under
surveillance of course, in order to ask only authorized questions to people "working" at the docks and in the vicinity, obviously strolling around
under orders of the system. The traffic lights for our data gathering shifted
to green again. Once more, the situation appeared not so gloomy. Yet I had
the impression of being trained into becoming a manic–depressive person,
alternating moments of great joy and the utmost sadness.

Then, in a moment of relief and not much pessimism, we resumed
our work for the nth time. But again we were challenged. This time it was
by the union leaders, who popped onto the scene at a most unexpected
moment, given that we had obtained the agreement of the police and the
drug system, hoping to work in peace. These were the guys who controlled
the composition and distribution of the job gangs entering a ship, as well as
establishing the amounts to be paid to the stevedores as wages and benefits.
Truculent by professional need, if we may say so, the union's leaders were
simply denying us the right to speak to their people, namely, any stevedore.
Again we had to pay our sweating compliments to a big guy, this time the
tubarão (shark) who exploited the *bagrinhos* (small fry), precisely those we
wanted to interview. This shark was perhaps the worst of them all, being
vicious, extremely rude, and openly menacing.

At this point, we just couldn't pull out, each one of our team being deeply engaged in this work, so there was nothing else to do but cut a deal with the union leaders, any deal. And indeed we agreed to follow the guy's orders not to interview anyone who had not been screened by the union. In other words, this guy would designate the persons with whom we were allowed to speak, the union-trusted members, of course. Big dilemma: Would the stevedores chosen by the drug system be the same ones picked by the union? Our field of maneuver was drastically reduced. The research was now menaced by the sheer lack of persons to be interviewed (in an intact universe of 9,000 individuals). Another issue of concern was the "document of informed and agreed consent to be interviewed in the best interests of science and the bettering of health at the docks." Moreover, we had to present this document to the mob members sent to us and obtain their agreement, in an ironic inversion of roles, for it seemed that we were the ones who should get them to promise, preferably in written form, that we would remain intact and sound after the fieldwork.

We accepted this imposition. Thinking about it now, it seems that we would have accepted any imposition. Our psychologists could then enter the docks to hear from the mouths of the "chosen ones," one after the other, that life at the port was great, everything was normal, the union provided for every need of the boys and their families, the police were great, drug using was something unheard of at the docks. Data began flowing in again, through the not-so-bright spokespersons of the union who happened to be there, idle but having the approval of the system, patiently waiting to volunteer their share to science. Our diligent interviewers had to be briefed again, adapting to the delicate circumstances. Actually, they did a splendid job with this, squeezing out all the juice they could from those dockworkers carefully picked by the union, being also screened by the drug system to be "safely" put at our service. As the days went by, we began to grow suspicious of those persons, believing them to have been figuratively thrown in our way to slow us down and eventually induce us to give up the data gathering and thus make us abandon everything and go home. This suspicion proved to be true, for a couple of them cracked and spilled the scam.

There was a positive aspect, though. The interviews came out fat and rich in details, with plenty of emotional idioms that were coded and classified to form a colorful and spontaneous description of the daily life at the port and its neighborhood. One of those guys sent to us was so pitifully brutal and ignorant as to compare AIDS with other diseases by saying that cancer is much worse, because it can be seen! In cancer, he said, "small bugs" are the disease itself. A certain buddy of his "caught" cancer and went to the hospital; his family forbade any visits during the morning in this union hospital where he was a patient. One day, this guy entered his friend's room early in the morning, without knocking, and saw his friend's brother applying a raw steak to his face; at 6:00 P.M. the meat was all gone, having been eaten by the small bugs. Every day this procedure was repeated—till he died in pain. "This ... is cancer!" said he. No other disease can be so ugly, AIDS being nothing in comparison.

Some days later our work had evolved and our presence within the port premises had become a banal fact, when something happened: We were approached by some of the dockside small fry. They were responding to a demand, we were told, by their fellow stevedores, who sent this group to us, asking in a very befuddled way for an explanation of what was occurring to them—a mounting number of colleagues falling ill every month, diagnosed with AIDS. They asked us to do anything we wanted or needed, including interviewing, to help them find a way to escape this curse. They soon became the main group in terms of interviewing for our work. They believed that these interviews could help them out of that awful situation, and therefore they started to respect and help us. We shifted our daily routine to include more and more of those guys, but carefully did not dismiss the dock flies pushed by the system and the union. We then came to realize that we had struck gold, but had to pay a toll to the local groups by continuing to interview their people.

These latecomers to the research, among all participants in our work, were the ones to, unintentionally, provide us with important clues to the mysterious spread of the disease. They unknowingly put forward the main mechanism of AIDS contamination in the harbor, undeniably more logical (that later proved to be right), which practically excluded the seamen in town from the accountable infectors we had already ranked on our scale. These workers told us that when they accumulated extra pay in a single day (for working in the rain, on night shifts, or with hazardous cargos, harmful gases, etc.), the cash paid was spent in the joints near the port with women and friends. They all feasted together, drank a lot, and smoked a lot of grass; the men would go to bed with the girls from nearby hotels, not wearing condoms as a sign of mutual trust among pals (or drunken old sex friends), as well as some sort of a defying and triumphal attitude of the type "Us is us, the rest is shit." At first, we imagined the HIV/AIDS virus was passing from the women to the men, then to their wives, and through promiscuity among couples, to one another. Later we discovered with amazement that the actual contamination process was inverted. In the first place, it was the men who infected the prostitutes, who in turn infected other men, as seropositivity tests revealed. The question then was, where did the men get the virus? The answer was not an easy one for those belonging to this group, without exception, taking the embarrassing contours of a confession.

Sewing together many loose ends of several stories, what we got was that when a ship was emptied and the job was done (and the promise of a big wad of cash was in order), a strange kind of madness came over the men, making them sing aloud and smoke pot while still in the ship's hold, some taking coke as well, and as a totally mad but "natural" consequence, they had sex with one another. This last part was the difficult one to relate, for they strongly believed themselves to belong to an extremely macho society, in which more than just for pleasure, sex is an exercise of domination—women playing a passive and subordinate part, and men acting as equals (among themselves) and dominant (over the women). In a ship's hold, all these beliefs underwent an inversion of what appeared to them as a dangerously compromising assertion of selfishness needing then to be neutralized in a most disconcerting and contradictory manner—that is, through a complete abandonment of male values and letting this be shown to their true pals. What before was dominance now became subordination and deep comradeship. They insisted that not everyone in the hold would have the guts to do this, especially those who talked to us. In some cases, though, when talking about this activity, a grain of pride was visible in their disturbed look. It was as if by behaving in an antimacho way, they confirmed a higher order of manhood.

LESSONS LEARNED

In conclusion, after experiencing the pure horror of the reality to be studied, at the start of our research—a feeling that got worse every time we were contacted by go-betweens to the main foci of local power—we came eventually to understand it in a more unbiased way. Horror gave way to indifference, and then to acceptance, as the elaborate abstractions we dealt with took us to the core of this unique and intricate society existing within an extremely delicate balance of forces.

No wonder all those who had any importance in this dockside community—from big drug dealers to police bosses, from trade unionists to pimps—tried to push us away from their unmindful and somewhat innocent flock. Much more than acting just for profit, they were actually protecting a way of life, a segment of the national culture, perhaps the only one they could live with, although not having the slightest hint of what they were doing.

Little by little we came to realize that all the locally important people were not obstacles thrown in our path, but mere outsiders to our research. They belonged to the local world and—knowing it or not—they were part of our work, playing an indispensable part in it: when they interfered with our fieldwork, when they unveiled strong opinions about themselves. Without them, our work would have been incomplete, dull, and in vain. They behaved precisely as expected, namely, as counterparts to the common workers who interested us at the beginning. They were right, our research object was warped. It should have included all of them. Perhaps this was the real disaster.

Of course, the research attained its proposed ends. The extremely rich outcomes, together with the ethnographic observations, were very appropriate in the information sessions where we taught many of the stevedores. These findings, though, could be considered as an unforeseen plus. This unexpectedness, this contingency, is typical of good research dealing with unconscious social behavior taken "in the act," and "qualitatively" explored.

TO READ FURTHER

Cultural studies, to merit the name of scientific research, need two basic ingredients: a trustworthy theory, sound enough to support the erection of the research's design–analysis building, and an attentive mind, to detect particular traits where and when they briefly flicker into the established objectivity level, in the course of data gathering.

Douglas, M. (1994). *Risk and blame: Essays in cultural theory.* London: Routledge.

An extraordinary author in the cultural studies field is Mary Douglas, whose theoretical models of reality are comprehensive and useful for researchers who are deciphering cultural reality within the field of good, sound science. One of her main explorative concepts is the social group, through which she deals with AIDS and epidemics in general in a useful and practical manner.

Steward, J. (1955). *Theory of culture change.* Champaign: University of Illinois Press.

Culture change is not a new concept, being the leitmotif of the functionalist school, as even Julian Steward, an evolutionist, has shown a long time ago. He sees society as a complex web that gains coherence at the level of social groups engaged in reciprocating action, each group having its norms, each group helping the individual to attain his or her niche in society, and in there finding stimulus and comfort.

For those who wish to go still further, classic philosophers of culture can be recommended, such as Claude Lévi-Strauss, Marcel Mauss, Maurice Merleau-Ponty, and Ernst Cassirer. All are easily available on the Internet.

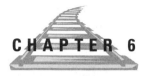

CHAPTER 6

Power in Numbers
Research with Families in Long-Term Care

JULIE M. DERGAL SERAFINI

BACKGROUND OF THE STUDY

In the last decade much research attention has focused on quality of care in nursing homes in Canada and the United States (Hilmer, Wodchis, Gill, Anderson, & Rochon, 2005; Stevenson, 2006). Yet despite this focus on nursing homes, and on staffing as one of the indicators of quality of care, there has been no discussion or research on "private companions," who have been identified as a visible group of healthcare workers within nursing homes. A private companion is defined as a person hired, managed, and paid privately by the family to provide a range of services, such as companionship and assistance with activities of daily living, to an older adult. The private companion may or may not have any relevant training or experience and either accompanies the older adult upon admission or is hired after the older adult has moved into the nursing home.

Private companions seem to be addressing a need—of the family member, the resident, or both—that is not being met by the institution. To understand more about private companions in nursing homes, a comprehensive literature search was undertaken, yet no studies were identified that examined private companions in long-term care settings. Most of our knowledge of this group is based on anecdotal evidence. Therefore, a starting point for examining this complex issue is to understand the reasons private companions are hired by family members and identify the need private companions fill in long-term care facilities.

Existing research in long-term care provides several possible reasons that may explain the presence of private companions in long-term care. First, research suggests that families have concerns about the quality of care in nursing homes, including inadequate staffing (Castle & Engberg, 2007), improvements needed in food, laundry, activities, amount of care and personalized attention (Ejaz, Noelker, Schur, Whitlach, & Looman, 2002), inadequate stimulation, inadequate cleanliness, lack of respect for the older adult's dignity, and the overuse of drugs (Wright, 2000). Despite increases in healthcare funding for long-term care, private companions may be hired to supplement the existing level of care and services provided to the older adult by the institution. Second, research suggests that the quality of care in nursing homes is a source of burden for many family members (Canadian Study on Health and Aging Working Group, 1994; Coen, Swanwick, O'Boyle, & Coakley, 1997; Cutler Riddick, Fleshner, & Kraft, 1992). Some family members of institutionalized older adults experience burden levels similar to those of family members caring for community-dwelling older adults (Bowman, Mukherjee, & Fortinsky, 1998; Dellasega, 1991), and others report higher burden levels for different domains, depending on the location of the older adult (Parris Stephens, Kinney, & Ogrocki, 1991). As a result, private companions may be hired to buffer the effects of the institutional stressors experienced by family members. Third, private companions may also act as surrogates for family members when they experience barriers to being with their relatives in nursing homes, due to factors such as geographical distance, transportation problems, poor relationships with staff, and a limited network of family and friends (Lindeman & Port, 2004).

There are many other plausible reasons that may account for the presence of private companions in nursing homes: the increased care needs of people in long-term care because of people living longer with more chronic conditions; families' and residents' greater expectations of care; family members feeling guilty either for placing their relatives in a nursing home or for not spending as much time with them as they would like, and the inclusion of private companions having become a common practice or expectation within an institution. Although these ideas are plausible reasons that private companions have appeared in long-term care facilities, there is an obvious need for research to investigate these claims. As a doctoral student, I was therefore most excited to have identified an untouched area of research with numerous possibilities to explore.

THE ORIGINAL STUDY DESIGN

The original intention was to focus on the private companions themselves. The objectives of the study were to describe who private companions were, what duties they performed, and why they were hired. Mixed methods would be used, which included a self-administered questionnaire to all private companions (n = 600), along with in-depth interviews with some of them (n = 30). When I began planning my dissertation research, the long-term care facility where I had planned to collect my data was in the process of implementing a Private Companion Program, which included mandatory 1-day training sessions, many of which were scheduled over a period of several months. What a fantastic recruitment opportunity! I knew about these planned sessions because I had been invited to sit on the steering committee for the Private Companion Program. As a result, I planned to request 30 minutes during each session to describe my study and administer the questionnaire. At the end of the questionnaire, private companions would be asked to provide their contact information if they were willing to participate in an interview. As all private companions had to complete the training, I thought recruitment would not only be easy and inexpensive, but would also be methodologically rigorous—especially as response rate is best for questionnaires administered in person. I would have access to all private companions, so I had a large recruitment pool, and I expected a good response rate, given that I would be available in person to describe the study, answer any questions, and the subjects could easily return them to me after the session. I also expected a good "buy-in" for the study because I would be supported by and working with the long-term care facility that had already received support from families for these training sessions. In addition, no identifying personal information was being requested, so the private companions' anonymity would be preserved unless they decided to participate in a future interview and provided their contact information. Finally, as many of the private companions' first language was not English, any concerns about language barriers or comprehension of the questions could be easily addressed either by me or by asking their peers. I was very pleased with the study design and so was my supervisory committee. In addition, I would be able to collect my data within a reasonable time frame. Finally, there was light at the end of the tunnel—the hope of graduating and getting a job was in sight, along with having an exciting program of research to develop—and then the bubble broke. If you thought it was too good to be true, it was.

THE CHALLENGES

Research is conducted in long-term care facilities worldwide. Apart from the most important reason for conducting long-term care research, which is to improve the care provided to older people living in these facilities, there are also logistical issues that make long-term care facilities appealing to researchers, especially students. For example, the researcher, particularly if he or she is affiliated with the facility, will have access to a convenient pool of potential study participants, access to existing data, and familiarity with the culture of how the institution operates. Frankly put, the researcher knows the ins and outs, the who's who, and what hoops need to be jumped through to make sure that the research can be implemented and conducted in a methodologically sound way. As a result, choosing a study site for my doctoral dissertation was very simple, a long-term care facility that I was already very familiar with, which would facilitate my study being conducted in a smooth and timely manner. Moreover, I had chosen a facility that prided itself on integrating research and practice, so this would be easy, or so I thought. However, there was one major factor I had not taken into account: the many families involved in the long-term care facility. Although family members have, fortunately, made enormous strides in having their voices heard in long-term care facilities to advocate for improved care and services, gaining their acceptance and support for my study was a major challenge that had to be overcome if the study was allowed to be conducted and possibly successful.

When I raised my study plans at a Private Companion Steering Committee meeting, I encountered three main challenges. The first was the issue of explaining research issues to nonresearchers. The committee was made up of the heads of various clinical, educational, and administrative departments and others who would have direct involvement with the Private Companion Program. Then there was I, the student researcher, the sole researcher on the committee, with only a few letters after my name, trying to counter and respond to what seemed like very reasonable ideas to the entire committee: Why couldn't I just put up posters around the facility asking the Private Companions to contact me if they wanted to participate? How would this research I'm doing make a difference to clinical practice? So what if we don't know anything about private companions? The families are happy and so are the residents, and the staff seem to appreciate the help. It is here where my abilities were truly tested—could I explain in lay terms the importance of sample size, response rate, having a known denominator, and the need for empirical evidence? I must have answered somewhat to the committee's satisfaction, as we then moved on to "re-creating" my research study, which was my second challenge—trying to accommodate competing interests. So after being able to convince the committee that this study was in fact worthwhile, ideas began to emerge. The nurses thought I should get the nursing staff's perspective, the social workers thought I should get the family members' perspective, and others thought it would be great to include other nursing homes and to meet with the Ministry of Health and Long-Term Care and policymakers. Yes, all of these were great ideas—but they would be my life's long work! As I sat nodding and listening to these ideas, I thought, I am only one person, with no funding, and trying to graduate. Fortunately, the committee members could appreciate that although this was an exciting area of research, the project had to be feasible. It was the last challenge that took on a life of its own—the families. I had chosen a very interesting and novel topic, but it was also a very sensitive issue. Due to the fact that private companions were hired and managed by family members, and many were new immigrants, there was a lot of heated debate and discussion about the Private Companion Program itself. Therefore, my research became highly contentious. The consensus of the committee was that my research proposal would have to be presented to and approved by the Family Council in order to proceed. I was stuck—it was the families who had the final say, and there was nothing I could say to respond. So off I went to a Family Council meeting.

It was very clear early on in the meeting that accessing the private companions would be considered outrageous and unacceptable. Somehow, family members thought that they should determine whether the private companions participated in the study, and most did not support their involvement. Being prepared for the possible resistance that I would encounter, I put forth variations of the study to attempt to obtain approval for something, anything—again, I needed to finish and graduate, so I needed to get moving. To make a long story short, there were numerous concerns about my study that arose in the Family Council meeting. Although I left quite discouraged, the bottom line was that if I didn't include private companions in my study, but focused on families instead, there was some support for this new direction. Sometimes you have to take what you can get.

OVERCOMING THE DIFFICULTIES

I therefore shifted gears and decided that my dissertation research would involve conducting a cross-sectional mailed survey with all family members of older adults in a nursing home ($n = 472$) and conducting in person interviews with 30 of them. Although this was a modification of the study population, I thought it would still be interesting to get family members' perspectives on private companions, and so I moved forward. Although I was concerned about the response rate with a mailed survey, especially given the sensitivity of the topic, I had decided to use Dillman's (2000) method, which has been used extensively to ensure a large response rate, based on a suggestion offered by the assistant vice-president of research where I was conducting my study. Dillman's method is a five-step process that requires an introductory letter, an initial mailing, a reminder postcard, another mailing, and an alternate method of contact (e.g., a phone call). Oh yes, one minor detail—where would I get the money to send out these multiple mailings? After I had pursued many avenues, including approaching the long-term care facility itself, it was one of my thesis committee members who generously offered me support through a research grant. I met with my supervisory committee, and I spent a lot of time networking with key stakeholders at the institution to obtain their support and to figure out some of the logistics to conducting the research. I developed a questionnaire using a battery of preexisting scales to tap key variables, piloted the questionnaire, made revisions, and repiloted the final questionnaire. My dissertation proposal was then accepted, my ethics proposal was approved by both the university and the long-term care facility, and I was set. Finally! Wait.... Now you see it, now you don't! I had just begun to contact the key players in the institution to let them know that the study was moving forward and to request access to the information I had previously discussed with them (e.g., using an existing mailing list with all of the families' contact information, having volunteers conduct the follow-up phone call, obtaining existing secondary data), when my ethics approval from the facility was rescinded. Two key issues were raised: privacy and Family Council approval.

The long-term care facility's ethics committee would not reinstate my approval until I had satisfied the institution's and Family Council's requests, which included expanding the number of study sites, modifying the content of the study questionnaire, eliminating several desired study variables, and altering the data collection methods. The first issue was that family members were concerned about being recognized in the course of disseminating the study results. They were therefore requesting that I find two or three other institutions that would allow me to conduct my research with their families. Through the help of my supervisor, I was able to obtain two letters of support from other facilities. Second, family members wanted me to remove and modify some of the questions in the questionnaire even though it had already been piloted and nothing was red flagged. Nevertheless, I did what was asked. I removed the questions about religion and culture, and the income questions were modified. Fortunately, however, I was able to justify keeping questions that made up standardized measures, despite their apparent obtrusiveness or awkwardness to family members. Next, because of privacy issues, there was no way the phone calls were going to happen. Only the people directly involved in the resident's circle of care could have access to family members' contact information. I tried a variety of strategies, such as suggesting that the designated volunteer on each floor could contact the families that they already knew, or that social workers who already had contact with families could assist with the phone calls. Nothing worked. It was a dead end. I had to give in or not be able to conduct the study. So I eliminated the phone calls and tried to find an alternate way of staying true to Dillman's method in order to increase my response rate. His suggestion is that the final contact be distinguished from the previous contacts either in appearance or method—the latter option was out. I decided to opt for another mailing and tried to make the presentation of the final mailing different from the others—the envelope was a different color and size, the outside had a large colored label that said, "Important

Please Read" to draw attention, and the questionnaire inside was printed on paper of a different color from that of previous mailings. These modifications were the best I could do with the resources I had, and they had to suffice. The last and final compromise was not being able to use data from an existing database that the institution had maintained. The hope was to be able to describe the older adults who had a private companion or not, in order to provide more context for the use of private companions and to see whether there was a difference in private companion use based on resident characteristics. Again, it was an issue with privacy that was raised—that the data could be used only for the purpose for which they were originally collected. This issue was a recent change in policy, necessitated by new privacy legislation in the province. Given that there was some struggle to obtain just the names and mailing addresses of family members, even though they remained anonymous to me and were accessed only by a research statistician who had signed a confidentiality agreement, it was not in my best interest to dispute the institution's position on this matter. As a result, the study moved forward and I obtained a response rate just over 60%, which was better than anticipated, given the initial resistance by family members and the sensitivity of the topic. While the in-depth interviews are ongoing, there is hope in sight of one day soon completing my dissertation, graduating, and, yes, even getting a job!

LESSONS LEARNED

Every challenge in our lives teaches us something. The following are several recommendations to consider in future research involving family members. These recommendations are based on lessons learned by working with family members of older people in long-term care and in dealing with the organizational structure of an institution and competing interests.

1. *Network, network, network.* Invest time with families and people in the institution from the very beginning to tell them about the importance and novelty of the study. Research cannot be done in isolation, and we inevitably have to rely on others. So pick and choose your battles—and be kind to those helping you! I discussed my study with many stakeholders and people from different clinical departments within the facility to obtain as much support for the study as possible.

2. *Be flexible—something is better than nothing.* Listen to families and other stakeholders; allow them to have input into your study by changing what you can without compromising the study integrity. I realized that I wasn't going to get everything I wanted in terms of accessing existing data and collecting all of the information I wanted, but I would still have valuable information—and I would still be able to get my doctorate!

3. *Balance optimism with realism and perseverance.* Do not give up on your original study plans, but be realistic in terms of time, resources, and other competing priorities about what can be accomplished. Do not lose sight of your goal, which is not to create a perfect study (as one does not exist) but to make a contribution to at least one of three areas, namely, research, policy, and practice. Let go of what you can't control and move on.

4. *Organization will save the day.* It is very important to keep all correspondence, documentation, and notes from meetings prior to and throughout the course of the study. When in doubt about what was said, or agreed upon, rely on the written word.

5. *There is power in numbers.* Despite the delays and barriers I encountered in conducting my research, it is comforting to know that families have a strong voice in long-term care and that their opinions matter. As each one of us may have a family member in long-term care someday, don't be afraid to speak up, and don't be afraid to participate in research. There is power in numbers for research too.

TO READ FURTHER

Decker, C. L., & Adamek, M. E. (2004). Meeting the challenges of social work research in long term care. *Social Work in Health Care, 38,* 47–65.

This article highlights key challenges in conducting research in long-term care, such as the institutional environment, subjects' privacy and confidentiality, family members, and methodological rigor. Issues unique to the institutional setting are presented and practical strategies are recommended to address these issues.

CIHR Privacy Advisory Committee. (2005). *CIHR best practices for protecting privacy in health research.* Ottawa: Author.

Conducting research in nursing homes using both preexisting data and new data presents some privacy challenges. This CIHR document provides a guiding framework for the researcher, using 10 elements of best practice, to appropriately protect the privacy of research participants at each phase of the research.

Dillman D. A. (2000). *Mail and internet surveys: The tailored design method* (2nd ed.). New York: Wiley.

In a long-term care setting, the use of mailed surveys allows the researcher to reach a large sample of family members who have relatives in a nursing home, while being both cost- and time-efficient. In this text, Dillman presents an empirically supported method for achieving a desirable response rate using mail and Internet surveys. He provides a step-by-step outline, with examples, of how to increase participant response throughout the data collection phase.

REFERENCES

Bowman, K. F., Mukherjee, S., & Fortinsky, R. H. (1998). Exploring strain in community and nursing home family caregivers. *Journal of Applied Gerontology, 17,* 371–393.

Canadian Study on Health and Aging Working Group. (1994). Patterns of caring for people with dementia in Canada. *Canadian Journal on Aging, 13,* 470–487.

Castle, N. G., & Engberg, J. (2007). The influence of staffing characteristics on quality of care in nursing homes. *Health Services Research, 42,* 1822–1847.

Coen, R. F., Swanwick, G. R., O'Boyle, C. A., & Coakley, D. (1997). Behaviour disturbance and other predictors of caregiver burden in Alzheimer's disease. *International Journal of Geriatric Psychiatry, 12,* 331–336.

Cutler Riddick, C., Fleshner, E., & Kraft, G. (1992). Caregiver adaptation to having a relative with dementia admitted to a nursing home. *Journal of Gerontological Social Work, 19,* 51–76.

Dellasega, C. (1991). Caregiving stress among community caregivers for the elderly: Does institutionalization make a difference? *Journal of Community Health Nursing, 8,* 197–205.

Dillman, D. A. (2000). *Mail and internet surveys: The tailored design method* (2nd ed.). New York: Wiley.

Ejaz, F. K., Noelker, L. S., Schur, D., Whitlach, C. J., & Looman, W. J. (2002). Family satisfaction with nursing home care for relatives with dementia. *Journal of Applied Gerontology, 21,* 368–384.

Hilmer, M. P., Wodchis, W. P., Gill, S. S., Anderson, G. M., & Rochon, P. A. (2005). Nursing home profit status and quality of care: Is there any evidence of an association? *Medical Care Research and Review, 62,* 139–146.

Lindeman Port, C. (2004) Identifying changeable barriers to family involvement in the nursing home for cognitively impaired residents. *The Gerontologist, 44,* 770–778.

Parris Stephens, M. A., Kinney, J. M., & Ogrocki, P. K. (1991). Stressors and well-being among caregivers to older adults with dementia: The in-home versus nursing home experience. *The Gerontologist, 31,* 217–223.

Stevenson, D. G. (2006). Nursing home consumer complaints and quality of care: A national view. *Medical Care Research and Review, 63,* 347–368.

Wright, F. (2000). The role of family care-givers for an older person resident in a care home. *British Journal of Social Work, 30,* 649–661.

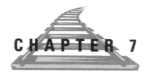

CHAPTER 7

Getting the Wrong Gatekeeper

LYNNE MACLEAN

BACKGROUND OF THE STUDY

Qualitative cross-cultural work of many types requires investigators to go to new places and speak with participants from cultures other than their own. To do this, investigators need entry into the community and access to participants, often through a gatekeeper or a community contact. The benefits of working with gatekeepers are well documented (Gallesich, 1982; Groger, Mayberry, & Straker, 1999; Munroe & Munroe, 1986). Gaining entry into a community and establishing trust are vital components of cross-cultural and ethnographic research (Morse & Field, 1995), and gatekeepers are important in this process. In fact, the access provided by gatekeepers, as well as the access denied by them, can result in biased results and "'scrounging sampling'—desperate and continuing efforts, against mounting odds, to round out the collection of individuals with relevant types of experiences we know to exist but have not been able to capture" (Groger et al., 1999, p. 830).

I relate my experience of collecting data in two remote communities, of which the second posed major challenges in recruiting participants. Because these are small communities, where people may be easily identifiable, I do not provide much information on their location, nor reference the study itself in the description of its relevant details. I had previously lived and practiced in the first community as a counseling psychologist, was well known, had friends and family there, and had little need of a gatekeeper. In the second community, I was alone, without reputation or an existing support network. I needed a supportive gatekeeper there. I knew this, but didn't realize to what extent both formal and informal gatekeepers would be required, nor what would happen if I had only formal gatekeepers from one of the two cultures I was studying. I certainly didn't think about what would happen if I got the wrong person.

In the years I had worked in the first community, I had become frustrated, as a mental health practitioner working in a different cultural setting, in applying treatment approaches that did not fit the people I was now working with. These approaches had worked well for me in previous settings in urban North America. So, after moving back to urban Canada, when I had the opportunity to do some funded research, I wanted to do something that might contribute suggestions for different ways of working in different cultural environments. I chose depression as my focus, a serious and common mental health issue that has plagued, and continues to plague, people worldwide. In 2002, the World Health Organization (WHO) estimated that 154 million people globally suffer from depression, and it is currently ranked the seventh most important cause of disease burden in low- and middle-income countries (World Health Organization, 2008).

At the time of this study, researchers were aware that the experience of depression varied culturally in its causes and symptoms; that response to different treatment approaches varied from culture to culture around the world; and, further, that reactions to depression by nondepressed people, and its meaning within a culture, also varied (MacLean, 1991). In developing treatment approaches that work in a particular culture, it is important to understand a mental health phenomenon both in terms of its commonalities with its manifestations elsewhere, and its local variations, what Berry (1980) would consider "etics and emics" of a psychological phenomenon. In working through the emic and etic process of cross-cultural research, and given the lack of knowledge at the time about this phenomenon for the cultures of concern, I chose a mixed-methods, three-stage approach, in which the first two stages were qualitative, involving interviews and theme validation from members of two linguistically different cultures each in two communities. The third stage involved construct mapping through theme sorting by mental health practitioners from both cultures.

THE CHALLENGES

The first challenge in conducting research in a new place is that of gaining entry to a community. Gaining entry involves both receiving official authorization (Munroe & Munroe, 1986) and achieving psychological entry (Gallesich, 1982). Achieving psychological entry requires becoming sufficiently trusted and accepted to be allowed access into a social system (Gallesich, 1982). It was helpful for accessing both communities that I was known as someone who had previously lived and practiced in one of the two communities, as well as in other communities similar to them. As pointed out earlier, in the first community I still had friends and family, former coworkers, and a little "street cred."

Although this reputation was somewhat helpful in the second community, it was not enough. It meant that local mental health, health, social service, and pastoral service providers were ready to hear me out and check with their clients about involvement in my research. Once I had worked my way through the pool of participants available via this group, as well as via friends and relatives of people I knew from the first community, my participant well had run dry. Furthermore, the people I was able to recruit through the professionals were primarily from only one of the two cultures of interest.

Community gatekeepers can be seen as people who, because of their formal or informal importance to the social system, can make or break your entry by providing approval or disapproval, as well as direct aid (MacLean, 1990). In small communities, word spreads very quickly. The formal gatekeepers, people with official importance, are the mayors, councilors, chiefs, or religious leaders. They may be able to point you in the direction of the informal gatekeepers. Otherwise, you must find the informal gatekeepers through judicious questioning and listening, or luck.

I knew I needed to access a supportive community gatekeeper, ideally from the culture I was not accessing. I knew I needed one who spoke the languages of both cultures. I did have names of appropriate people to contact as a result of the government and community science licensing process. This process required researchers to submit proposals after gaining letters of support from official community sources such as mayors or community councils. Such formal research authorization processes are not uncommon (Munroe & Munroe, 1986). As well as protecting communities from research they would find unduly intrusive, this process also provided the researcher with contact people once in field. Unfortunately for me, at the time I arrived in the second community, all these people were out of town at a set of major political meetings and elections. As key members of the community, they were all delegates. In hearing of my problem, one of the service providers (who was not from the culture I needed) suggested hiring a community contact person for recruitment, and she gave me the name of a person she thought was well connected and respected in the culture of interest in the community (thank goodness for grant money). Of course, this bilingual person was a member of the culture of interest and would serve as a type of gatekeeper, considering community people who might be interested, deciding whom to check for their potential interest, and then arranging interviews for (and sometimes, with) me. Munroe and Munroe (1986) suggest that such an assistant can provide aid with indigenous languages, information regarding the sociocultural system, and guidelines for navigating through the community.

What happens when the community contact/gatekeeper comes up short, with few potential participants showing interest? The contact person kept careful track of who was contacted and their responses. Very few were willing to take part. Once this contact person decided that all avenues had been explored, she suggested that we end the assistantship.

I was feeling very disheartened. I wasn't prepared for the feelings of despair coming at this time. There was a lot riding on this research for me professionally. I was far away from my husband, family, and close friends. I was boarding with a family who lived very differently than I was used to. As much as I was greatly enjoying other aspects of the research, I was wondering if anything was going to work out. At that point, I was not aware that morale problems and personal crises are not unusual for cross-cultural researchers in the field (Munroe & Munroe, 1986). Scrounging sampling (Groger et al., 1999) was starting to appear necessary.

I had thought through design issues relevant to these particular cultures, such as using completely transparent methods with no manipulation or hint of manipulation (Barnett & Dyer, 1983); a preference for qualitative, nonsurvey approaches with face-to-face contact (MacLean, 1990); a distrust of and difficulty with random selection (I. Poelzer, personal communication, February 1988); and a discovery, while there, of a community dissatisfaction with telephones, which would have made telephone approaches infeasible (MacLean, 1990). My community contact person spoke both languages, thus covering a criterion that could be important in trust building and gaining entry. I couldn't see how I might alter things to improve the response rate.

Then things got worse. The former community contact person publicly criticized my research design in a small, closed gathering of people to whom I was presenting. I had been trying to be very careful in both my research design and activities to conduct work that was respectful, in an area where colonialization and oppression still imposed heavy burdens in all aspects of life. I defended my approach as best I could, but I feared that perhaps she was right and that what I was planning to do was at best poorly designed, and at worst, disrespectful of the community. I wondered if I should just pack up and go home and limit my findings to the first community. Or should I abandon the whole project?

OVERCOMING THE DIFFICULTIES

I fell upon a successful strategy by luck. First, I confided my worries to a good friend from the cultural group of interest. Her comment: "Don't worry. Nobody listens to So-and-So. She doesn't know what she's talking about. Depression is a big problem here. Your study is good. It will help the community. Keep trying."

Second, I found a woman willing to be my community contact and main recruiter. I found my second, and wonderful, community contact after being intensively checked out and tested by another formal gatekeeper, once he returned from the political sessions. He passed along her name after we had a couple of meetings in which I and my project were thoroughly examined. His stamp of approval certainly didn't hurt, as he also offered free translation services should I need them. But the main change came with the community contact person. She was marvelous, quite interested in the topic of depression, also bilingual, and very efficient. Thanks to her, my sample became more "purposive" and "judgmental," less one of convenience, included a variety of key informants, was able to meet all demographic criteria, and gave me the flexibility to recruit new types of participants as needed during the iterative process of the project's unfolding. Because of her help, I ended up with many, many interested participants willing to discuss a very personal mental health issue that they felt it was high time to deal with. These participants included several who had turned away the initial community contact person. Although I originally had expected I might need to hire an interpreter, the hiring of a woman from that culture who was well respected in the community as a community contact was not my idea. However, I became very grateful to be able to work with this person. Having the right individual using her personal contact knowledge and skills for recruitment was a vital underpinning to the eventual success of this project.

LESSONS LEARNED

My advice is that researchers consider the following (in the absence of friends or luck):

1. Personal contact is very important. It's more important in some settings than in others, but finding the right people to support you and your work is key, particularly if you are working in culture different from your own.

2. Locate a senior gatekeeper from the cultural group. Go outside the formal professional service systems if the service providers are not from the cultures of interest. They may be able to provide you with great people for gatekeepers from their own cultures, but might be less aware of who would be sufficiently respected in other cultures.

3. Be sure to choose someone who can speak both your language and the language of the culture of interest. This could be an identifier for someone important in the community, who serves as a bridge between his or her culture and yours (and the mainstream culture). Others in the community

might wait for the bilingual person to check you out first, before agreeing to speak with you.

4. When considering gatekeepers or contact people, find out their initial degree of interest in your research area, if this is possible. This personal interest may influence their motivation to help you. This is an especially important point in working with community leaders. If they feel that what they are doing for you also benefits their community, they are probably more likely to "sell" to community participants the importance of becoming involved.

5. Change gatekeepers and community contact people if the first ones don't work out.

6. Expect to be thoroughly checked out yourself. It's only fair.

7. Remember that you become a symbolic gatekeeper/contact person for the community of researchers in the future, whether you ever meet them or not. One of my colleagues had done some work in previous years in a community I was involved with for a different study. When I met people in the community, many were willing to take part in my research because of the favorable impression of research they had been left with owing to the positive way the previous researcher had conducted herself. This conduct had included returning her research findings back to the community.

8. Persevere. You aren't the only one to have gone through times like these in the field, so don't give up. This too shall pass. The rewards will be worth the effort, not just in terms of your research work, but also in terms of the amazing people you'll meet, stories you'll hear, and friends you'll make along the way.

Now, we just have to line up all the right community gatekeepers with all the right research gatekeepers, and keep the information flowing in both directions.

ACKNOWLEDGMENT

I would like to acknowledge Alma Estable and Mechthild Meyer of the Community Health Research Unit for their very helpful comments on the chapter.

TO READ FURTHER

Berry, J. W. (1980). Introduction to methodology. In H. C. Triandis & J. W. Berry (Eds.), *Handbook of cross cultural psychology: Vol. 2. Methodology* (pp. 1–28). Boston: Allyn & Bacon.

This chapter provides a good overview of some key components of cross-cultural psychology research methods in general. The entire book is a classic in the area.

Munroe, R. L., & Munroe, R. H. (1986). Field work in cross-cultural psychology. In W. J. Lonner & J. W. Berry (Eds.), *Field methods in cross-cultural research* (pp. 112–137). Beverly Hills, CA: Sage.

Another classic, with useful information for the field researcher in particular.

REFERENCES

Barnett, D. C., & Dyer, A. J. (1983). *Research related to native people at the University of Saskatchewan 1912–1983*. Saskatoon: University of Saskatchewan.

Berry, J. W. (1980). Introduction to methodology. In H. C. Triandis & J. W. Berry (Eds.), *Handbook of cross cultural psychology: Vol. 2. Methodology* (pp. 1–28). Boston: Allyn & Bacon.

Gallesich, J. (1982). *The profession and practice of consultation: A handbook for consultants and consumers of consultation services*. San Francisco: Jossey-Bass.

Groger, L., Mayberry, P. S., & Straker, J. K. (1999). What we didn't learn because of who wouldn't talk to us. *Qualitative Health Research, 9,* 829–835.

MacLean, L. M. (1990, June 1). *Accessing samples in cross-cultural field research: Why should I talk with this nosey white researcher?* Paper presented at the annual convention of the Canadian Psychological Association. Ottawa, ON.

MacLean, L. M. (1991). *The experience of depression for Chipewyan and Euro-Canadian northern women (Canada)*. Unpublished doctoral dissertation, University of Saskatchewan, Saskatoon, SK.

Morse, J. M., & Field, P. A. (1995). *Qualitative research methods for health professionals*. London: Sage.

Munroe, R. L., & Munroe, R. H. (1986). Field work in cross-cultural psychology. In W. J. Lonner & J. W. Berry (Eds.), *Field methods in cross-cultural research* (pp. 112–137). Beverly Hills, CA: Sage.

World Health Organization. (2008). WHO fact file: Ten facts on mental health. Retrieved January 12, 2008, from *www.who.int/features/factfiles/mental_health/mental_health_facts/en/index1.html*.

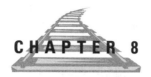

CHAPTER 8

Breaking into Court

MANDEEP K. DHAMI
KAREN A. SOUZA

BACKGROUND OF THE STUDY

In 2005 we were jointly commissioned by two organizations that have an interest in criminal justice to conduct a national research project on sentencing. This would be the largest and most comprehensive court record-based analysis of sentencing ever conducted in England and Wales. Previous court record-based research on sentencing was outdated, relatively small-scale, and methodologically limited (e.g., Flood-Page & Mackie, 1998; Hood, 1992). The main goal of our research was to determine the various multilevel factors (e.g., offender and case, judge, court, and area factors) that predict sentencing decisions on adult offenders, for specific offense types, in all types of criminal courts across the country. It was anticipated that in addition to contributing to developments in sentencing theory, the findings of this research would be useful for the development of sentencing guidelines that could support sentencers in their decision making and promote consistency and transparency in sentencing.

The proposed method was a retrospective analysis of court records of people who had been sentenced. A group of specially trained fieldworkers would extract and code information from (mostly paper) records in individual courthouses. Using a specially developed computerized data collection instrument and index to documents in court records, the fieldworkers would collect data on certain case-related factors (e.g., nature of offense, plea) and offender-related factors (e.g., race, gender), as well as the decisions made on a case at the sentencing stage (e.g., length of custodial sentence, amount of fine). (Data on judge-, court-, and area-level factors would be collected from other sources.) Fieldworkers would collect data from approximately 12,000 records of adults sentenced in the past year or so for specific types of more and less serious offenses, including violent, property, drug, and driving offenses, in a large sample of both the lower (magistrates') and higher (Crown) courts across England and Wales.

We first conducted a pilot study to assess the feasibility of this methodology and determine any improvements that could be made to facilitate data collection. The pilot study involved nine fieldworkers, who collected data on 181 records of sentenced adults in 2004 from nine courts across the country. Overall, this pilot demonstrated the feasibility of sampling court records, collecting data from court records, and managing data collection procedures. A few specific recommendations were also made to ensure the effectiveness and efficiency of data collection. However, despite the largely encouraging findings of the pilot study, we encountered a number of obstacles to gaining access to courts and court records that eventually reduced the scope of the pilot study in terms of the number of courts involved and the number of records analyzed.

THE CHALLENGES

For our research on sentencing, official "gatekeepers" controlled the formal access that we had to potential research settings such as courts and to sources of data such as records of sentenced cases in those courts (Jupp, 1989). However, because we were funded by two organizations that had strong connections to the department that oversees research access to courts, we did not anticipate encountering the types of problems that would normally be faced by researchers who do not have any formal links to their chosen research settings. Nor did we anticipate the intensity with which we experienced such problems or the negative consequences they had for the pilot study. After all, why would gatekeepers create barriers to access when the findings of our research could be of potential value to them in terms of helping the courts in their business of sentencing? Indeed, the pilot study was not explicitly designed to test the procedure of gaining access to courts and court records, but rather to test the procedure for data collection once fieldworkers were in the courts.

Court record-based research is challenging not only because it involves gaining access to largely "closed" settings, but also because it involves gaining access to highly sensitive and confidential data (Neuman & Wiegand, 2000). Therefore, in order to gain formal access to courts and court records, all research staff were required to undergo a rigorous and costly security clearance procedure. This included criminal record checks as well as counterterrorist checks. In addition, we were required to complete an access agreement that protects sensitive data under the terms of the Data

Protection Act. This involved a complex and lengthy procedure that provided highly restrictive access.

It took 16 months for the access agreement to be authorized by the department that oversees research in the courts. This setback was partly due to the fact that the access agreement required the security checks to be completed first. However, it was due mostly to the fact that the access agreement required us to identify the sample of records that we wished to study. Yet without the access agreement, we were not authorized to have access to any courts or records and so were unable to select these records. This was a Catch-22 situation.

In fact, it took 10 months from the time that the 15 recruited field-workers completed their training to when they could begin data collection for the pilot study. The lengthy delay had several negative implications. One implication was the increase in the financial cost of the pilot study. Field-workers who had initially been recruited on a temporary contract to cover the period of data collection now had to be paid for an extra 10 months while they waited to start work.

Second, regardless of being paid, fieldworkers began to lose morale and interest in the research to the point that six of them resigned or did not want their employment extended before the beginning of the pilot study. This had an adverse impact on the scope of the pilot study in terms of the number of courts that could be included and the amount of data that could be collected within the specified access period for the pilot study: Instead of sampling 15 courts and 255 records, we eventually collected data from 9 courts on 181 cases.

Finally, the lengthy delay meant that the pilot study began in mid-2007 instead of 2006, and by this point some sampled records of those sentenced in 2004 had been destroyed. This is because court policy is to destroy records after 3 years.

The access agreement was also quite restrictive in terms of the dates and duration of access to courts. The restriction was partly imposed so that the pilot study would have minimal impact on the work of court staff and on normal court business. From our experiences, we had estimated that it would take approximately 6 days for each fieldworker to collect data from the small sample of records he or she was assigned in his or her court. The access agreement provided little room for leverage in the unexpected event that a fieldworker could not attend court or could not collect data for other reasons during the specified access period. This created a problem for one fieldworker when he had to stop fieldwork owing to a family emergency and his access expired before he could complete the "reliability in data collection" part of the pilot study.

Once the appropriate security checks had been completed and the access agreement had been authorized, the fieldworkers were able to enter the chosen courts and access the sample of sentenced records therein. In these circumstances, the court managers and the court staff became "informal" gatekeepers. Thus, even when access is theoretically allowed, in practice it may still be denied (Jupp, 1989).

Fortunately, the research sponsors had sent a formal letter to each court manager, explaining the purpose and procedure of the pilot study, and had identified a member of the court staff as a liaison in each court who would assist with data collection procedures (e.g., retrieving the sampled records and providing a work space for fieldworkers). We had assigned fieldworkers to particular courts in their areas, and data collection took place in the courts holding the records. Fieldworkers were instructed to take with them to court a copy of the authorized access agreement, a letter of introduction provided by the sponsors, and a form of personal identification. Fieldworkers' entry into the courts proved smooth and efficient.

Nevertheless, there were some challenges in regard to the retrieval of sampled records. In particular, although lists of sampled records were sent to each pilot court in advance so the liaisons could retrieve them from storage prior to the fieldworkers' arrival, in one of the nine courts this did not happen. A lack of court staff was the explanation provided. The restrictive access agreement, however, did not allow fieldworkers to retrieve records themselves.

OVERCOMING THE DIFFICULTIES

We received some assistance from the research sponsors in our efforts to overcome the challenges we faced in gaining access to courts and court records for the pilot study. However, we were unable to overcome the problem of the one fieldworker whose access agreement expired before he could finish the pilot study.

As mentioned earlier, completion of the access agreement seemed an impossible task inasmuch as it required researchers to identify the records that would be studied, but access to courts and records would be given only after the access agreement was authorized. After numerous and lengthy negotiations with the department that authorizes access agreements, the research sponsors finally resolved the issue by obtaining and providing us with a database of all individuals sentenced in 2004 in England and Wales, from a different source. This was essentially a "sampling frame" that contained all the necessary information (i.e., case number, court appearance date, and offender's name and date of birth) for us to sample and identify the records that we wished to study. Clearly, researchers who are not funded by organizations with useful links to research settings and data sources probably could not intervene to overcome this first challenge.

The unanticipated costs of the security clearance checks and the costs of employing fieldworkers for an extra 10 months were fortunately met by the research sponsors. This would be unlikely if the sponsors were from a smaller organization and if the research was funded from a fixed budget. The research sponsors were also able to negotiate to speed up the process of conducting the security clearance checks. However, the sponsors were largely unsuccessful in speeding up the general process of authorizing the access agreement. Again, less influential sponsors would not necessarily have been able to facilitate these processes.

We tried to counteract the negative impact that the delay with the access agreement had on fieldworkers by developing and providing additional training modules to help them use their time productively, such as asking them to familiarize themselves with the computerized data collection instrument and practice coding information using fictitious records, as well as visiting courts to sit in the public gallery for observation. In addition, we continually reassured them that the pilot study would eventually start and reminded them of the important implications that the research could have for sentencing theory, policy, and practice. The research sponsors also sent the fieldworkers a letter to thank them for their patience.

In order to minimize the adverse implications for the scope of the pilot study that were due to six fieldworkers leaving the research project before the pilot study began, we arranged for others to "cover for them" as much as possible. Thus, one of the remaining fieldworkers collected data in two (instead of one) courts, and one fieldworker collected extra data in her assigned court. A member of the research team also stepped in to act as a fieldworker for the pilot study.

When we realized that several of the sampled court records from 2004 had been destroyed, we used the database provided by the research sponsors to promptly resample records and sent the list to fieldworkers and their court liaisons before access expired. In fact, we had originally oversampled court records by 10% to be prepared in the event of attrition (e.g., if records could not be located because they were misplaced), and so the situation was not as severe as it could have been. It is worth pointing out that such resampling would not have been possible without the database.

Finally, the fieldworker who was faced with the situation where the court liaison did not provide her with the sampled records had to retrieve them from the archives herself, although this was contrary to the access agreement. The fieldworker spent 1½ days tracking and retrieving records, and although this significantly reduced the very limited time available for data collection, she did manage to complete data collection within the specified time frame.

Despite finding ways to cope with the challenges of gaining access to courts and court records, the problems we faced did ultimately have a negative impact on the scope of the pilot study. However, we believe that we managed to successfully minimize these negative implications. Unfortunately, this cannot be said of other attempts to conduct court-based research, or research in criminal justice settings more generally (Jupp, 1989).

LESSONS LEARNED

The pilot study demonstrated the effectiveness of our chosen methodology for conducting research on sentencing. Although we had not anticipated the challenges to gaining access to courts and court records, we did find solutions so that the pilot study was completed. Furthermore, we (and the research sponsors) have learned several lessons that will be useful.

Beyond this, we recognize that several of our assumptions about gatekeeping and gaining access need to be revised accordingly. Therefore, we conclude that:

- Researchers who are funded by organizations that have links to research settings and sources of data cannot necessarily be guaranteed access (at least in a timely manner).
- Gatekeepers who have a potential positive stake in the research findings do not necessarily have to support the research process and allow access.
- Even when formal gatekeepers allow access, informal gatekeepers may not.

A final twist in the tale of our research on sentencing is that since the pilot study was completed, one of the organizations that sponsored the research has now merged with the department that oversees research in the courts and authorizes the access agreements. Hence, the gatekeepers have now unwittingly become one of the research sponsors.

TO READ FURTHER

Broadhead, R. S., & Rist, R. C. (1976). Gatekeepers and the social control of social research. *Social Problems, 23,* 325–336.

This article discusses the impact that gatekeepers have on the research process from limiting entry to restricting publication.

Feldman, M. S., Bell, J., & Berger, M. (Eds.). (2003). *Gaining access: A practical and theoretical guide for qualitative researchers.* Lanham, MD: Altamira Press.

This book provides prescriptive advice on how to enter field settings in order to collect observational and interview data.

REFERENCES

Flood-Page, C., & Mackie, A. (1998). *Sentencing practice: An examination of decisions in magistrates' courts and the Crown court in the mid-1990s.* HORS No. 180. London: Home Office.

Hood, R. (1992). *Race and sentencing.* Oxford, UK: Clarendon Press.

Jupp, V. (1989). *Methods of criminological research.* London: Routledge.

Neuman, W. L., & Wiegand, B. (2000). *Criminal justice research methods.* London: Allyn & Bacon.

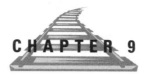

CHAPTER 9

The RDC Archipelago

SCOTT VELDHUIZEN
JOHN CAIRNEY
DAVID L. STREINER

BACKGROUND OF THE STUDY

Secondary data analysis is popular and necessary in the social sciences and in public health research. Necessary, because very few researchers have the resources to collect representative data on a national or international scale. Popular, because the choice between collecting one's own data and not collecting one's own data is, for experienced researchers, really a terribly easy one. Secondary data analysis is common in disciplines such as economics, sociology, and epidemiology and has been used to answer many important, and countless unimportant, questions in those fields.

Canada's national statistical agency, Statistics Canada, regularly conducts public health and labor force surveys with sample sizes in the tens of thousands. It is one of the few organizations in the country with the resources and the expertise—to say nothing of the institutional stability and the collective attention span—to collect this type of data. Surveys of this kind are among the largest and highest-quality sources of data available on a range of public health issues.

After their agents have wedged their feet in the doors of thousands of Canadian households, the selected citizens have answered hundreds of prying questions, and results have been checked for joke names and entered into databases, however, Statistics Canada still faces the problem of ensuring that all this information is put to some sort of use. Some results are reported to various levels of government. The agency itself publishes summaries and notifies an eager press and a celebrating nation that another survey has been completed. Comparatively little actual analysis, however, will actually have been done by this stage. The solution the agency has adopted is to set out the results in a carefully controlled setting and allow academic researchers to swarm in and pick over them.

In view of the need to preserve respondents' privacy, the agency has chosen to implement a system of a kind increasingly popular with the custodians of large research datasets. The master data files, stripped of identifying information, are made available at locked-down facilities known as Research Data Centres (RDCs), which are located on university campuses across the country. Aleksandr Solzhenitsyn (1968) and his fellow *zeks* were forced to slave away in the gulag archipelago, an environment he compared to the first circle of hell. The RDC archipelago was our own "first circle" (and one located in an equally inhospitable environment).

Our research team has frequently used the RDC system to do epidemiological research. In 2002, Statistics Canada conducted the first national mental health survey of Canadians, a survey that included information on six major mental disorders, as well as a host of other data on service use, medication use, and the usual suspects in community surveys (demographic information, socioeconomic status, etc.), all on an impressive sample of about 37,000 Canadians (Gravel & Béland, 2005). Although we could quibble about what was not included, or bemoan the strange ways in which some sections of the questionnaire were constructed, this survey remains an important data source that can be (and in some cases has been) used to conduct worthwhile research on the epidemiology of mental disorders in Canada. Our own efforts have produced a number of articles, including work on the epidemiology of social phobia (Cairney et al., 2007a), the association between age and disorder (Streiner, Cairney, & Veldhuizen, 2006), the screening potential of a brief measure of psychological distress (Cairney, Veldhuizen, Wade, Kurdyak, & Streiner, 2007b), and the geographical distribution of problem substance use in Canada (Veldhuizen, Urbanoski, & Cairney, 2007). These represent a vanishingly small proportion of the work turned out by RDC users in various fields in the past several years (Statistics Canada, 2008).

We have benefited from the work Statistics Canada does and have even built careers—of a kind—in part on the data it has provided, but we have also experienced frustrations with the current system of data access. We are not alone in this (e.g., Philp, 2005). Although there are other documents that should be consulted by researchers seeking to understand the RDC system (Statistics Canada, 2005; Kafka, 1926/1930), we offer here an overview drawn from firsthand experience. Although we have not been involved in any true catastrophes, akin to running off the rails into the side of a mountain and detonating, there have been projects that have simply run late, broken down, stopped at every village along the line for no good reason, or hit bumps that have caused us to spill coffee on ourselves and swear loudly in front of a carriage full of elderly nuns. We describe a number of problems and inconveniences. Where we have drawn lessons from these episodes, we attempt to offer constructive advice. Where we have not, we complain about them anyway. For reasons of space, we pass over problems caused by our own incompetence and focus on the bureaucratic hurdles that complicate the research process.

Although we describe Statistics Canada's data access system, many of our experiences are likely to be, we believe, familiar to users of secondary data elsewhere. Where they are not, the proliferation of RDC-like systems internationally leads us to think they soon will be. In the United States, the Census Bureau and the National Center for Health Statistics operate similar facilities. These are known as "Research Data Centers," and appear to differ from Statistics Canada's system mostly in the word "Center," which is spelled in the quaint American manner. The Institute for Clinical and Evaluative Sciences in Ontario operates a heavily restricted system for access to the government's administrative health data that, as far as security is concerned, is to an RDC what Fort Knox is to Microsoft Windows. The age of relatively unfettered access to government data for researchers seems to be drawing to a close worldwide.

THE CHALLENGES

Infiltration

Access to the RDC is not outrageously difficult to obtain, but the process demands patience. (See Chapter 34 for another description of this challenge.) Although it is possible to substitute apathy or weary resignation, patience is best, and researchers planning to work with databases controlled by government institutions should either possess it or be willing to acquire it, whether through religion, philosophy, or psychosurgery.

The first step is the preparation of a research proposal, a document that outlines the work planned and justifies the use of the master files. Public use files are available without the administrative hassles, but they do not contain complete information and it is not possible when using them to adjust properly for the surveys' complex designs. This interposition of yet another proposal requirement between the researcher, who has already often written a grant and a document for ethics review, and his or her research is the first instance in which a serene general outlook will pay dividends. It should be noted that merely receiving approval (and funding) from a peer-review federal granting agency does not give access to the data, even when Statistics Canada itself is a partner in the review process.

In our case, the Canadian Institutes of Health Research (CIHR; the Canadian equivalent of the National Institutes of Health in the United

States) and Statistics Canada released a call for a limited number of proposals. These were then peer-reviewed by an independent committee of scientists. Despite the fact that the reviewers had considered both scientific merit and need for detailed survey data, we discovered an unpleasant fact: Access to Statistics Canada data is controlled by a different federal research granting body, the Social Sciences and Humanities Research Council (SSHRC, pronounced "shirk"). So we had to submit our proposal again, on a different form, and with a completely different format for our curricula vitae (CVs). This was not only an incredible pain in our seating area, it engendered a 6-month delay after CIHR approval. Were we approved yet? Not really. Although we now had been granted the seal of approval by two research boards, the project still had to be approved by Statistics Canada itself.

Before Statistics Canada issues such an approval, the first-time RDC researcher faces a background check intended to weed out identity thieves, blackmailers, and serial parking offenders (however, to our knowledge, no one has ever actually failed this check). At this stage, the process passes out of the hands of Statistics Canada and into those of the Royal Canadian Mounted Police (RCMP). The length of the security check is highly variable, possibly because some at the RCMP find it hard to accept that the agency has no higher priority than combing through the arrest records of social scientists and graduate students. One of us (S. V.) waited 8 months (admittedly a record, as far as we know), despite a past containing nothing more sinister than a speeding ticket, a lost passport, and a teenage misunderstanding with a record of the month club. A delay of this kind is awkward in research, inasmuch as it is long enough for grants to expire, contracts to lapse, research assistants to come to their senses, and senior collaborators to forget who you (or they) are. Should the security check be passed—or, presumably, if it fails spectacularly enough—the final stage of the clearance process may include fingerprinting. Being fingerprinted by the government can be unsettling, but it represents almost the final hurdle in gaining RDC access.

The end result of this process is Enhanced Reliability status. This level of clearance is required of government employees, or "deemed employees," who have access to sensitive materials. It provides (we have made inquiries) no access to documents on UFO coverups or secret government research into the supernatural and comes with no license to commit any sort of violent crime without consequences. It does, however, provide, at last, an entrée into one of the RDCs themselves.

Indoctrination

Should the original research proposal still seem like a good idea (and the investigators have not retired or lapsed into genteel dementia), the next stage is to swear the "Oath or Affirmation of Office and Secrecy" and sign a contract with Statistics Canada and the Queen of England agreeing to become a deemed employee of the agency and to perform the work originally proposed. This is followed by a short training session in which new researchers are issued a pass card that allows access to the RDC and are introduced to the rules of that institution. Although it would suit the parallel we have (fitfully) been trying to draw to paint this process as some sort of sinister ritual, honesty—and a law code that is far too draconian, in our view, on matters of libel—obliges us to admit that it is brief, friendly, and professional. The lights are fluorescent and fixed in the ceiling, not swinging naked at the end of a wire or shone uncomfortably into your face; the pipes are hidden within the walls, not exposed and dripping; and any rodents you may see will have been brought in by yourself for reasons only you could possibly understand.

The rules of the RDC are few and simple. Every piece of information a researcher wishes to take out of the RDC must be examined by a Statistics Canada employee for possible disclosure risk. This means that any results based on a very small number of respondents will not be released, for fear that specific individuals could be identified. Results, except perhaps for overall sample sizes, should ordinarily be bootstrapped, or at least weighted. Saturated models and the carrying of edged weapons are discouraged.

Survival

The first, and often most important, of the difficulties with using Statistics Canada's master data files is that one needs to be physically present at the RDC in order to do so. The seriousness of this problem varies with one's location relative to the RDC, the weather, and one's native apathy. Setting aside whole days to work in the RDC is a scheduling challenge for researchers who attend many meetings or have teaching commitments, and going for shorter periods during the day means an extra commute. The ideal solution for many researchers is to use a low-ranking research support worker or graduate student who has no alternative outside of productive labor in the private sector. For faculty members (i.e., the ones who actually dreamed up the research), the challenge of achieving this physical presence is frequently insurmountable.

The RDC we use is a large, windowless room filled with rows of carrels. The design stresses beige and pale yellow. It is warm, and oxygen levels are low. Fluorescent lights and computers hum compelling electronic lullabies. If it were not for the adrenaline-boosting, pulse-quickening nature of statistical analysis, a degree of willpower might be required to maintain full alertness. Workstations, fortunately, are fast and include a good selection of statistical software (although rarely the specific package that we want). The open working area, however, can present another difficulty to scientists unused to sharing a room with other researchers, in that some of the latter will have some of the same irritating habits—eating chips with their mouths open, having loud and inane conversations on cell phones, high-fiving or chest bumping whenever a model converges—as themselves.

Results from the surveys stored at the RDC are generally expected to be bootstrapped using a set of weights supplied by Statistics Canada. Depending on the size of the dataset, the nature of the model, and the software used, this process can be relatively quick or agonizingly slow. Bootstrapping also requires the development of specialized skills on the part of the researcher, including solitaire playing or juggling, giving reviewers the impression that one understands the statistical theory underpinning the bootstrap, and composing short notes that will persuade other researchers not to turn off machines that have been locked and left on overnight.

If something should result from a spell in the RDC that seems worth bringing out into the wider world, it must, as we have mentioned, be examined by a Statistics Canada analyst for possible "disclosure risk." (The RDC is otherwise something like Las Vegas, in this one respect only: Things that happen there, stay there.) The vetting process can occasionally be a tense one, inasmuch as the analysts are mandated to err on the side of caution, whereas researchers are mandated to err on the side of publishing any set of numbers that falls to hand alongside claims that they represent a critically important contribution to the field (but that further research is necessary). With some types of output, such as regression results, there is rarely any trouble. In other situations, both parties can find the going difficult. In one of our projects we used geographic information system software to produce a set of maps of the prevalence of substance-related problems. To us, it was inconceivable that anyone could look at one of these and worry that some individual somewhere might be identifiable. From the analyst's perspective, however, it was equally difficult, at first, to look at such a thing and be sure that disclosure really was impossible. Although this difficulty was successfully brazened out, we had more trouble when trying to take results from a spatial cluster scan out of the RDC. Staff members pointed out—probably correctly, annoyingly—that this could result in the identification of some of the clusters used in designing the survey itself. In other cases, though, the logic of release concerns is less obvious. Removing covariance matrices from the RDC, for example, would make it possible to do some types of analyses (such as structural equation modeling) from the relative comfort of our offices, but we have had requests of this kind denied on grounds that they may represent a risk to respondents' privacy. Although we have stared long and hard at covariance matrices—and, to be honest, interesting images have sometimes emerged (much like those computer generated 3-D art posters so popular a few years back)—we have yet to see the face of one of the respondents to these surveys.

LESSONS LEARNED

Slowly and reluctantly, we learned several things about the use of government data in a restricted setting. The first is that it's not something we would pursue as a hobby. More usefully, the vetting process taught us to think carefully about possible disclosure risk. We also discovered the importance of keeping output as simple as possible. We were in the habit of working with results while waiting for other models to finish bootstrapping, but we cut this out after realizing—and it took no more than five or six similar experiences for us to spot this pattern—that every number we calculated from the results, every chart we drew, and every bit of interpretation we scrawled in a margin would be subjected to the same scrutiny. Taking results out of the RDC can be like going through the border security of a country not very friendly with your own; the wisest thing to do is to pack lightly and leave behind anything that could be difficult to explain.

Statistics Canada analysts are also instructed to look for the possibility of "residual disclosure," which is the risk that emerges when two or more very similar sets of results are released. This may happen if a group definition is changed very slightly, so that a small number of cases migrate from one cell to another. The problem in this situation is that someone with both definitions, both sets of results, certain additional information, advanced training in statistics, a tremendous amount of time on his or her hands, and either a motive we can't guess at or an incredibly eccentric idea about what constitutes a good time, could conceivably infer something about individual respondents. This level of caution can seem paranoid to researchers, mostly because they're not the ones who would be liable legally or be pilloried in the media should something like this happen. It remains, however, a good reason to get things more or less right with the first set of results.

Another reason that not having a complete and detailed analysis plan can make the RDC experience a painful one is that the vetting process is not instantaneous. It may take several days to receive the results, depending on staff scheduling and the volume of other requests. If your colleagues are in the habit of cross-tabulating every variable in enormous public health surveys with every other and you have failed to budget for a gang of thugs to discourage this sort of behavior on their part, your own project can be delayed. A more common problem—common, at least in projects we have been involved in—is that it is almost inevitable that one uninteresting but necessary-for-publication test statistic will be forgotten. In normal circumstances, this is not a serious problem; the oversight can be blamed on the research assistant and the test rerun. When working at an RDC, however, a new request for disclosure will have to be prepared and the entire project will be delayed while the missing number works its way through the system. Should this happen several times consecutively—and it has—schedules can become stretched and indeed seriously damaged.

Although we may—do—find aspects of the RDC system unpleasant, we are also prepared to admit that it may have its virtues. It succeeds, for example, in providing access to detailed survey data while safeguarding respondents' privacy. As unwelcome as the additional requirements are, they could also be said to formalize the research process in such a way that projects that are well planned and methodologically sound suffer least. Instead of viewing it as the first circle of hell, it may be more appropriate to see the RDC system as a kind of purgatory where researchers are purified of bad research practices. People who fail to come up with clear research questions and analytical plans, who needlessly run large numbers of statistical tests, who agree to work with coauthors who respond to every analytical decision with a shrug and a glib "let's try it both ways"—it is these, or at least their graduate students, who suffer in a Sisyphean cycle of revision, bootstrapping, and vetting.

Although we have often wondered what life would be like if researchers, once approved, could use RDC datasets for long periods without justifying every project, even the proposal process could be said to serve a useful function. Although restricting access in this way means that some important questions will go unanswered, it also means that some foolish questions will go unasked. A freer system of access could, arguably, result in a certain amount of uncontrolled data mining. By requiring a level of commitment and some sort of a priori rationale for the research project—actual theoretical frameworks and plausible hypotheses have been sighted in these documents—the RDC bottleneck may limit the number of spurious or confounded associations that find their way into the literature.

One of the surprisingly numerous ways in which the RDC system is actually quite unlike a network of Siberian prison camps is that leaving it behind is relatively simple. Access to data is on a time-limited contract. When the contract expires, and the analysts are tired of giving you extensions because you consistently forget to request all the results you need, the pass cards are returned and the legal association between the researcher, Statistics Canada, and the Queen is dissolved. As much as the three of you may continue to see each other socially (e.g., at poker nights or motocross races), your formal obligations to one another are over. The courteous, legal, and usually forgotten final step is to provide Statistics Canada with a copy of any published work that may have resulted from an RDC project.

TO READ FURTHER

Most countries make at least some data available via remote access or through universities. For researchers determined to have the RDC experience, the best places to start are the websites of the organizations responsible for providing access to them. These include:

Statistics Canada's "Research Data Centre" program (*www.statcan.gc.ca/
rdc-cdr/index-eng.htm*)

U.S. Census Bureau's "Research Data Center" network (*www.ces.census.
gov/index.php/ces/researchprogram*)

U.S. Center for Disease Control and Prevention's "Research Data Center"
(*www.cdc.gov/nchs/r&d/rdc.htm*)

Australian Bureau of Statistics' "ABS Site Data Laboratory" (*www.abs.gov.
au*)

A good general guide to the location and analysis of health survey data is:

Boslaugh, S. (2007). *Secondary data sources for public health: A practical guide.*
New York: Cambridge University Press.

This handy book provides an overview of general issues related to secondary
data analysis and describes a number of specific, mostly American, data sources.

REFERENCES

Cairney, J., McCabe, L., Veldhuizen, S., Corna, L., Streiner, D. L., & Herrmann,
N. (2007a). Epidemiology of social phobia in later life. *American Journal of
Geriatric Psychiatry, 15,* 224–233.

Cairney, J., Veldhuizen, S., Wade, T. J., Kurdyak, P., & Streiner, D. L. (2007b).
Evaluation of two measures of psychological distress as screeners for current
depression in the general population. *Canadian Journal of Psychiatry, 52,*
111–120.

Gravel, R., & Béland, Y. (2005). The Canadian Community Health Survey: Mental Health and Well-Being. *Canadian Journal of Psychiatry, 50,* 573–579.

Kafka, F. (1926/1930). *The castle* (W. Muir & E. Muir, Trans.). New York:
Knopf.

Philp, M. (2005, February 10). Statscan locks up treasure-trove of data on childhood. *The Globe and Mail.*

Solzhenitsyn, A. (1968). *The first circle* (T. P. Whitney, Trans.). Evanston, IL:
Northwest University Press.

Statistics Canada. (2005). *Guide for researchers under agreement with Statistics
Canada.* Ottawa: Author.

Statistics Canada. (2008). *Studies from the RDCs.* Retrieved January 19, 2008,
from *www.statcan.ca/ english/rdc/pubs publications.htm.*

Streiner, D. L., Cairney, J., & Veldhuizen, S. (2006). The epidemiology of psychological problems in the elderly. *Canadian Journal of Psychiatry, 51,* 185–
191.

Veldhuizen, S., Urbanoski, K., & Cairney, J. (2007). Geographical variation in the
prevalence of substance-related problems in Canada. *Canadian Journal of
Psychiatry, 52,* 426–433.

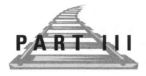

PART III

RECRUITMENT AND RETENTION

Obviously, you can't do a study unless you have willing participants (don't bother to read this section if you use pigeons, white rats, or college sophomores). You have to enroll enough of them to have adequate power for your statistical tests and, in many situations, they have to be a nonbiased sample of the population.

Once you are working outside the university, there are a number of recruitment strategies you can use to make people aware of the study— advertising in the local media, having gatekeepers refer participants, sending a prenotification letter, using list servers of relevant groups, and so on. Ideally, the strategies should enable you to reach a wide segment of the population in order to make the sample as representative as possible. Whenever possible, the number of people invited to participate should be larger than the required sample size to account for those who refuse or drop out and to increase the likelihood of obtaining the needed number of participants. However, problems can arise. Factors that can interfere with recruitment relate to the nature of the strategies used, the sociopolitical context within the recruitment sites, the characteristics of the population, and the research topic itself, such as its interest and salience to the target population. The following nine chapters illustrate the contribution of these factors on recruitment in studies targeting different populations and using different designs.

1. *The nature of strategies.* Koch and Tabor (Chapter 10) discuss the advantages and limitations of using paper and web-based sign-up forms and reminders for recruiting psychology students into survey and experimental studies. Sidani and colleagues (Chapter 11) address the advantages of using a group format for recruiting staff in long-term care settings; it generates peer pressure that increases enrollment. Random or probability sampling techniques require the availability of a sampling frame—that is, a list of potential participants. Montoro-Rodriguez and Smith (Chapter 15) describe alternative sampling strategies that can be used when a comprehensive and accurate list of participants does not exist, as in the case of a geographically dispersed and "rare" population.

2. *The sociopolitical context in the recruitment sites.* Recruitment sites often are independent entities characterized by features that may serve as barriers to recruitment. Sidani and colleagues (Chapter 11) and Joyce (Chapter 14) started recruitment at a time when the staff members at the respective sites were experiencing distress, which contributed to low recruitment rates. Policies limiting staff's role in recruitment and the staff's lack of interest in the research topic, as described by Piercy (Chapter 12), demand a search for alternative recruitment strategies.

3. *Characteristics of the target population.* Barrette (Chapter 13) illustrates the influence of the group's characteristics not only on recruitment but also on the research topic. Key stakeholders in housing projects mistrusted the researchers' motives and allowed entry and access to the population only after the research topic was modified to meet their needs. (Our placement of the various chapters was somewhat arbitrary.) Van Reekum (Chapter 16) brings to light a problem frequently encountered in clinical trials, that of specifying a very stringent set of eligibility criteria, and demonstrates its impact on enrollment.

4. *Characteristics of the treatment.* The nature of the treatment being evaluated may be a deterrent to enrollment in randomized clinical trials. Concern about safety was deemed to be the reason for declining participation by 80% of eligible individuals recruited by van Reekam (Chapter 16). Concern with randomizing patients to different treatment options is another factor that can affect recruitment, as explained by Joyce (Chapter 14).

Retention strategies are necessary to keep participants interested and engaged in a project. In longitudinal studies aimed at looking at changes over time, participants may discontinue completing the measures, for various reasons. These relate to the characteristics of the participants (e.g., loss of interest in the study) and of the study (e.g., demanding protocol leading to response burden), as well as uncontrollable events such as illness. At-risk populations that are economically disadvantaged and ethnically diverse present with unique characteristics that contribute to a high attrition rate. In Chapter 17, Goncy and colleagues identify specific features of these populations that interfere with timely and complete data collection. The participants' mistrust of research led them to question the intent of the study and to refuse further participation. Their economic status resulted in frequent moves and working outside the usual business hours, making contact at the preset times more difficult. The consequence of attrition, particularly in at-risk or disadvantaged populations, is that the final sample may be too small and not representative of the larger group; this occurs when those who complete the study differ on key characteristics from those who dropped out. In interventional studies, the nature of the treatment is another reason for attrition. In Keller and colleagues' study (Chapter 18), participants considered the intervention to be unacceptable because it was not consistent with their cultural norms, beliefs, and values. As a result, they did not adhere to it and ultimately dropped out of the study.

As illustrated in the following chapters, researchers should incorporate multiple recruitment and retention strategies to obtain a representative sample of an adequate size. The strategies need to be carefully selected and tailored to the characteristics of the target population.

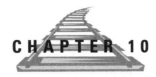

CHAPTER 10

Small Colleges and Small *n*'s

CHRISTOPHER KOCH
ANNA TABOR

BACKGROUND OF THE STUDY

When one of us (C. K.) was in graduate school at a large state university, we had a room in the psychology department dedicated for research sign-ups. The room was filled with study descriptions and sign-up sheets. Students would go to that room to sign up for research opportunities to fulfill their research participation requirements. The number of studies was monitored by a graduate assistant who made sure there were enough research opportunities to accommodate the number of students enrolled in the introductory psychology courses. Professors were not involved in the process, and all sign-ups took place outside class time. The system was relatively efficient but impersonal.

One of the advantages often mentioned about attending a small school is the personal contact with professors. This level of contact is related to relatively small class sizes, which place the instructors and students in close proximity to each other. The small class sizes also allow for more interaction among students and professors. Indeed, professors are frequently on a first-name basis with their students. Within this type of setting, it is common to discuss research opportunities during class time. This was the practice at the small school I taught at after graduate school.

Although mentioning a new research opportunity may only take a few minutes, passing around sign-up sheets can be disruptive and take 5 to 10 minutes of class time to fully circulate. This approach, however, seemed to be an effective method, at least in theory. Our sign-up sheets had a column with time slots for students to select from, with corresponding tear-off reminder slips. Therefore, the researcher had a record of student participants and the students had reminder cards for their selected time slots, giving them information about when and where to show up for the study as well as contact information to use in case they were not able to keep their appointments.

THE CHALLENGES

Despite the strengths of the system, it was not without its flaws. Apart from the time it took in class to distribute the sign-up list within a class period, it also took time to distribute the list across classes. In order to avoid multiple sign-ups for a particular time slot, only one sign-up list was used. This list had to go from instructor to instructor between classes. At minimum, this was a 2-day process. If an instructor forgot to distribute the list during a class period, it would take longer for students to volunteer for a study. Another problem was that students often misplaced the reminder slips and, as a result, they often forgot their research appointments. This became problematic for timely completion of research projects when the no-show rate rose to 30–40%.

OVERCOMING THE DIFFICULTIES

In an effort to expedite the sign-up process and reduce the no-show rate, we decided to pursue an alternative method for obtaining research volunteers. In addition, with the widespread use of Moodle (a course-management system) on campus, we wanted a web-based solution because students were used to finding course-related material online. As a result, we adopted Experimentrak (and later Sona's Experiment Management System) as a subject pool management system. Research management software, such as Experimentrak, is designed to help recruit research participants, track research participation, send e-mail reminders to participants, and automatically assign research participation credit. Students are required to register within the system. Once they confirm their registration, students are able to sign up for experiments. E-mails are automatically sent to the students, reminding them of the scheduled research appointments. After completing an experiment, research credit is automatically posted so that instructors are able to access an updated list of participation hours at all times. In addition, students are able to check the number of participation hours/points they have earned at any time. The system also helps manage rooms so that a particular lab or other research-designated room is never double booked.

Another feature that we have found extremely helpful is the ability to mass e-mail all registered students about upcoming or newly posted studies.

With the mass e-mail announcements and online sign-up process, we have seen our needed participation pool fill within hours instead of days. In addition, the automatic e-mail reminders have helped reduce our no-show rate to less than 5%. Instructors have also appreciated the ability to check on participation credit throughout the semester.

The system also allows for the design and administration of online questionnaires. Again, students receive an e-mail about the study being posted online, and they have the ability to go directly to the questionnaire from the sign-up page. Once they complete the questionnaire, their accounts are updated so that they are credited with participation time for their responses. Data are downloadable as an Excel file to eliminate the need for data entry.

We took advantage of the questionnaire function to create a screening instrument that students completed upon registering for the system. The screening instrument included measures of visual acuity and color vision for perception research, personality measures for individual difference research, and so on. There are at least two benefits of having the screening responses. First, students completing the measures before participating in an experiment saved time. Second, the responses could be used to screen participants. For example, in one study we wanted to limit some sign-up times to males and other times to females. Because sex was asked in the screening instrument, we were able to have the system screen participants so that only males were allowed to sign up for the male-designated times and only females for female-designated times.

Finally, we were able to customize our FAQ sheet for the system so that we could address the questions common among our own students. Furthermore, we were able to edit the user manual for the system. In fact, we customized two manuals. One manual was made available online as a pdf and focused on student use of the system. The second manual was made available to researchers so that they knew how to use the system for their own research projects.

LESSONS LEARNED

Despite the numerous benefits we experienced with the online research management system, there are a number of considerations that need to be addressed. Under our old paper system, responsibility for soliciting participation and awarding research credit was distributed across faculty in the department. With the new online system, however, one faculty member is responsible for managing studies. Although this relieves the majority of faculty members from some of the responsibility, it also increases the time demand placed on the individual who manages the system. That individual must also respond to technical questions about the system and other questions students have about the system, as well as the individual studies, because the manager is often the main contact person for questions. Therefore, there are some administrative issues unique to the software-based approach that we did not have to deal with using our paper-based approach.

In addition, the ease with which online questionnaires can be created and completed can present potential problems. Studies using online questionnaires are easy and convenient to participate in. Thus, given the choice between an experiment conducted at another location and a survey conducted online, students generally select the online study over the lab-based study. Horvath, Pury, and Johnson (2006) noted that having a greater number of online studies than in person studies can make access to participants difficult for those doing laboratory experiments or even in-person correlational studies. Horvath, Pury, and Johnson further note that online studies can be associated with ethical violations due to missing or poor debriefing and reduced educational value for the participants (cf., Sieber & Saks, 1989; McCord, 1991; also see American Psychological Association, 2002). Thus, it is important for the department to establish guidelines for using the research management system that protect against these potential problems. For instance, we limit the number of questionnaire studies available to students until the end of the semester to encourage participation in in-person studies. We also hold a research symposium at the end of each semester so that participants can learn more about the studies in which they participated and the results associated with them.

In summary, we found that switching to an online research management system was an effective strategy for efficiently managing research participation. It provided an effective tool for gaining research volunteers and assigning research credit. However, it is important to account for potential problems when using such a system in order to eliminate possible ethical and external validity concerns.

TO READ FURTHER

Johnson, R. W. (1973). The obtaining of experimental subjects. *Canadian Psychologist, 14,* 208–211.

Research management systems are relatively new. Therefore, the literature associated with research management systems is currently underdeveloped. However, Johnson offers several suggestions on how to manage a research pool to minimize unrestricted volunteering and coerced participation that are consistent with the capabilities of research management systems.

REFERENCES

American Psychological Association (2002). Ethical principles of psychologists and code of conduct. *American Psychologist, 57,* 1060–1073.

Horvath, M., Pury, C. L. S., & Johnson, J. (2006). Online surveys in participation pools: Implications for students, researchers, and participant pool managers. *Teaching of Psychology, 33,* 273–275.

McCord, D. M. (1991). Ethics-sensitive management of the university human subject pool. *American Psychologist, 46,* 151.

Sieber, J. E., & Saks, M. J. (1989). A census of subject pool characteristics and policies. *American Psychologist, 44,* 1053–1061.

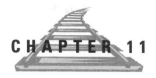

CHAPTER 11

Mitigating the Impact
of External Forces

SOURAYA SIDANI
DAVID L. STREINER
CHANTALE MARIE LECLERC

BACKGROUND OF THE STUDY

The importance of recruitment is well recognized. It is the step in a research study that contributes to the accrual of the sample size required to achieve statistical power and the full exploration of the research questions through the collection of rich qualitative data. The timing and the strategies for recruitment can influence potential participants' decision to enroll in a study, as we encountered in a study designed to evaluate the effects of an intervention in long-term care facilities.

What we were looking at was an intervention called "abilities-focused morning care" (AFMC), which is an approach that nursing staff can use when providing personal care to people with dementia. A large proportion of personal care is provided in the morning. Persons with moderate to severe dementia have a decreased ability to participate in their personal care and may exhibit challenging behaviors such as aggression or agitation during this episode of care. The AFMC approach entails individualizing personal care in a way that is responsive to the retained abilities of persons with dementia, with the goal of maximizing what they can do themselves and reducing the behaviors that caregivers find difficult. The AFMC approach consists of selecting and implementing specific interventions that are consistent with the persons' retained abilities.

The study took place in long-term care facilities. A quasi-experimental wait-list control group design was planned, whereby nursing staff members on the experimental units would receive instructions on the nature and implementation of the AFMC approach immediately after we collected the pretest data, and those on the comparison units would receive the same instructions after completion of the posttest data collection. Outcome data were obtained at pretest, posttest, and 3-month follow-up.

Outcome data included nursing staff's perception and use of the AFMC specific interventions when providing morning care to persons with dementia. Two methods were used to collect data: self-report and observation. The self-report instrument asked about the staff members' views on the utility and ease of implementation of the AFMC interventions, as well as whether or not they applied these interventions when providing morning care, in order to determine the extent to which the staff could integrate the interventions into day-to-day practice. Because of our concerns about self-report bias, research assistants (RAs) observed the staff members while they were providing morning care to persons with dementia. The RAs served as nonparticipant observers, noting and documenting the staff's use of the AFMC interventions. The RAs carried out the observations with minimal intrusion, while respecting the privacy of the persons with dementia. At each measurement time (i.e., pretest, posttest, and follow-up), each staff member was to be observed while providing morning care to the same person with dementia, on 2 separate days. This was done to minimize random irrelevancies, which could negatively influence the reliability of the observations.

THE CHALLENGES

After we had obtained ethics approval and administrative support for the study, the RAs began to recruit nursing staff. They arranged with the unit manager to introduce the study to nursing staff members at a regularly scheduled unit staff meeting. The RAs used a standard script to explain the study's purpose and protocol, the research activities in which the nursing staff would participate, the risks and benefits of participation, the voluntary nature of the nursing staff's participation, and the staff members' rights as research participants. In addition, each staff member was provided with a letter that covered the information given during the meeting. The letter also contained the telephone numbers of the RA and the principal investigator, to be used if staff members had any questions or concerns.

At the end of the meeting, the RAs recorded the names and initial reactions (i.e., expressed interest in the study) of the nursing staff members in attendance. The RAs posted a flyer on the unit's bulletin board to tell the staff about the study and the anticipated research activities. The poster served to alert members of the nursing staff who did not attend the introductory meeting and to remind those who did attend about the upcoming study. The RAs then made arrangements to meet individually with the staff members who expressed an interest in the study. During these meetings, the RAs further clarified aspects of the study, answered any questions, obtained written consent, and planned for pretest data collection.

The recruitment plan conformed to ethical guidelines and was consistent with recommendations to use different strategies to reach the full range of subgroups constituting the target population (Baines, 1984). So, what went wrong? In retrospect, two factors may have contributed to the recruitment challenges we encountered: the timing when we started recruitment and the influence of peers.

Timing

At the time recruitment for the study began, a major provincial report on the quality of care in long-term care facilities and nursing homes was receiving extensive media attention, culminating in the presentation of a documentary on local television stations. The documentary depicted instances of nursing staff members abusing people living in such facilities, captured by hidden cameras placed in the rooms by concerned family members. The documentary was aired about a week before recruitment began. The staff members whom we approached to participate in the study were aware of the report and documentary. In the introductory recruitment meeting, they questioned the nature and purpose of the study. In particular, they questioned the "real" intent of the observation aspect of data collection. They were concerned that the study had a "hidden agenda" and was linked to "investigations of abuse" of persons residing in long-term care and nursing homes by the staff. Most of them were apprehensive about the study and highly concerned that the researchers and/or RAs would interpret and report some of their behaviors in providing personal morning care as "abuse." This state of mind led some staff members to decline enrollment in the study because they did not "want to be observed."

In addition to the report and documentary, there were other events at the time of recruiting nursing staff on some units. These units were housed in teaching facilities, where research was also being conducted by other investigators. When the RAs approached the nursing staff members on these units to participate in our study, some refused because they were either engaged in or had just finished being in another study. They said that their involvement in research-related activities increased their workload, which in the presence of staff shortages, especially in long-term care, interferes with providing care. They worked hard to maintain a balance of research and practice demands. They needed time to "recover" from this experience before starting with yet another research project.

Influence of Peers

As we described earlier, one of the recruitment strategies used in the study involved an introductory meeting with the nursing staff. This introduction was held as part of a regularly scheduled meeting attended by all staff members assigned to the unit. This recruitment strategy was considered efficient because it facilitated reaching a large number of potential participants. However, the RAs observed that in such group meetings, the initial reaction or response of a few staff members affected the effectiveness of recruitment. In some instances, a few staff members expressed interest and gave verbal agreement to enroll in the study once the RA introduced the study. This initial positive response encouraged the remaining staff members in attendance to take part in the study. Crosby, Ventura, Finnick, Lohr, and Feldman (1991) reported this type of peer pressure during recruitment. In other instances, a few nursing staff members voiced negative comments about the study (e.g., questioning the utility of the AFMC interventions, concern about the observation of staff members, or a perception that involvement in an intervention study would result in more work) and publicly declined to participate. This initial reaction discouraged other staff members from enrolling in the study. Young and Dombrowski (1990) reported a similar negative influence of group meetings on recruitment.

OVERCOMING THE DIFFICULTIES

Understanding the influence of external factors is critical to the success of a research study. To circumvent some of the challenges we experienced, we used a number of strategies.

The documentary aired on local stations intensified the nursing staff members' concern about the intent of the observation aspect of the study. To address this concern, the investigators and RAs clarified the purpose of the study in the introductory meeting. They reassured the staff that the intent was to determine the effectiveness of the AFMC interventions in reducing agitation shown by persons with dementia during personal care. They emphasized that the observations did not aim to evaluate their individual performances. The RAs reiterated these points during individual meetings with members of the nursing staff and reinforced the nonevaluative nature of the study by pointing to relevant statements in the consent form. Effective communication has been recommended as a strategy to address potential participants' misunderstanding of research protocols (Connolly, Schneider, & Hill, 2004). Effective communication is characterized by listening to and respecting participants' concerns and clarifying the purpose and nature of the research-related activities in which participants will be involved, and the way in which the results will be used, while using clear, simple, and nontechnical terms. This strategy worked to some degree and alleviated the concerns of some staff members.

What could be done to overcome the nursing staff's feeling overwhelmed with multiple research demands? There is no easy, straightforward answer to this question. When dealing with staff members who explicitly reported this feeling, the RAs showed they understood the situation and discussed with them alternative times for recruitment activities. These alternative times represented a compromise to accommodate the needs of the staff and the demands of the research study. Postponing the time of recruitment for a few weeks until the other research studies' activities were completed was well received and effective. The staff members appreciated the RAs' understanding and flexibility and decided to enroll in our study when approached to participate at a later time. Such flexibility on the part of the research team, if affordable, can contribute to staff members' positive experiences with research (e.g., reduced the sense of competing research and practice demands and burnout; feeling that the researchers understood their pressures), which can facilitate recruitment and participation in future research endeavors. Investigators conducting studies in healthcare facilities rely on staff members to implement various aspects of a research study.

How could we overcome the initial negative responses that a few staff members expressed in the introductory meeting? Getting over this barrier was achieved by using two recruitment strategies. Following the introductory meeting with the unit staff, the RAs made arrangements to meet with staff members individually. The purpose of the individual meetings was to discuss study participation away from peer pressure. The RAs explored the staff members' reluctance and addressed any concerns. The individual contact was effective in reversing the initial reluctance of several members of the staff who subsequently agreed to enroll in the study.

LESSONS LEARNED

Recruitment of nursing staff for participation in the intervention evaluation study presented some challenges. The timing of the study and peer pressure served as barriers to enrollment. The research team, including the investigators and RAs, worked collaboratively to devise and implement strategies to overcome the barriers that were encountered.

Providing comprehensive information about the study and its purpose, as well as the research activities in which the nursing staff are expected to engage, is a requirement to meet ethical standards and to address any misconceptions about the study. The information must be presented in simple terms and should be clarified on repeated occasions. Explanations of the study requirements at each contact with potential participants and repeated clarifications of the demands on time, amount of effort needed, and potential personal benefits have been mentioned as strategies to enhance recruitment (Connolly et al., 2004; Pruitt & Privette, 2001; Steinke, 2004). Emphasizing that the nursing staff's performance is *not* subject to evaluation (when staff members suspect that it is) can alleviate fear and concern about participation in the research.

Demonstrating respect and flexibility is critical for enhancing enrollment when approaching potential participants. Researchers must convey a sense of compassion by treating them as "human beings" with needs and interests, and not just as experimental subjects. Acknowledging and addressing concerns about the study can promote a sense of respect and trust between researchers and potential participants (Grant & DePew, 1997). Respect is also conveyed when researchers show flexibility in the study implementation by accommodating the study activities to potential participants' routine (Pruitt & Privette, 2001). Flexibility requires seeking potential participants' input in planning for the most appropriate way and time to carry out the research activities while meeting the study requirements.

The use of more than one strategy or format for recruiting study participants is effective in increasing enrollment. The group format (e.g., unit staff meeting) is efficient in reaching a large number of potential participants but is subject to peer pressure, both positive and negative. Therefore, it should be followed with individual meetings during which the RAs tailor the recruitment efforts to the participants' characteristics and concerns.

It also helps to seek the assistance of persons who know and understand the population of interest in order to carefully plan the timing and nature of recruitment activities. For instance, strategies could be adapted to reach informal leaders or those with a large sphere of influence.

Finally, it would be prudent for researchers to account for the up-front work that needs to be done to get a study started in a given setting, within the timeline for the study's completion, by not underestimating this very critical facet of the research endeavor. Building in sufficient time to use all the strategies we have discussed to enroll participants into the research plan would help to avoid the need to ask funders and study sites for additional time to complete the study. A rule of thumb that we have found fairly accurate is to make your most pessimistic estimate of how long it will take to get the project off the ground—and then multiply by 3!

The strategies we used to address the challenges were effective. Our recruitment efforts resulted in a larger than anticipated sample of nursing staff: 133 staff members took part in the study when 78 were required, as based on power analysis. Of course, we had approval for a no-cost extension.

TO READ FURTHER

Connolly, N. B., Schneider, D., & Hill, A. M. (2004). Improving enrollment in cancer clinical trials. *Oncology Nursing Forum, 31*, 610–614.

This article reports results of three approaches used to identify successful recruitment strategies used by research staff in cancer clinical trials. The findings pointed to factors influencing individuals' decisions to enroll in the trials and suggested specific techniques that can facilitate participation. The approaches may be applied with other populations to guide development and/or refinement of recruitment efforts.

REFERENCES

Baines, C. J. (1984). Impediments to recruitment in the Canadian National Breast Screening Study: Response and resolution. *Controlled Clinical Trials, 5*, 129–140.

Connolly, N. B., Schneider, D., & Hill, A. M. (2004). Improving enrollment in cancer clinical trials. *Oncology Nursing Forum, 31*, 610–614.

Crosby, F., Ventura, M. R., Finnick, M., Lohr, G., & Feldman, M. J. (1991). Enhancing subject recruitment for nursing research. *Clinical Nurse Specialist, 5*, 25–30.

Grant, J. S., & DePew, D. D. (1999). Recruiting and retaining research participants for a clinical intervention study. *Journal of Neuroscience Nursing, 31*, 357–362.

Pruitt, R. H., & Privette, A. B. (2001). Planning strategies for the avoidance of pitfalls in intervention research. *Journal of Advanced Nursing, 35*, 514–520.

Steinke, E. E. (2004). Research ethics, informed consent, and participant recruitment. *Clinical Nurse Specialist, 18*, 88–97.

Young, C. L., & Dombrowski, M. (1990). Psychosocial influences on research subject recruitment, enrollment and retention. *Social Work in Health Care, 14*, 43–57.

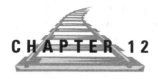

CHAPTER 12

A Trip to the School of Hard Knocks
Recruiting Participants from Health Service Agencies for Qualitative Studies of Aging

KATHLEEN W. PIERCY

BACKGROUND OF THE STUDY

I tackled my second research project as an assistant professor with great enthusiasm. Quickly I assembled a research team of three graduate students and one undergraduate student, chosen for their potential to contribute to the study and high level of motivation to learn the research process. Our study would examine how well the family caregivers of elderly relatives receiving home- and community-based services understood their choices for providing long-term care, and how such care was currently being provided and financed. Because we sought the views of family caregivers for several complex issues related to family-based home care, we selected a qualitative methodology for our study. The goal was to conduct in-depth interviews with family caregivers because their detailed descriptions of care provision issues were the best means of capturing both unique experiences as well as those common to elder care provision.

When seeking samples for qualitative studies of healthcare issues, researchers usually need to make several levels of contacts to succeed at locating and recruiting participants. In my previous study, several home health agencies had given me access to their staff, and once the staff members understood the study, they discussed it with their clients in such a way that recruiting clients and their caregivers went smoothly. I sought to duplicate this process in the new study.

Because my university is located in a town with a modest, homogeneous population, I planned to recruit my sample of 30 caregivers from a part of the state with a larger and more diverse population. As I laid the groundwork for recruiting a sample, the odyssey began.

At the outset, I pitched the study to an urban county agency that provides many services to older adults, including home care and adult day services. The agency director agreed to participate in the study. To get access to this agency, the project needed approval by the state's Institutional Review Board (IRB), a process that took a couple of months. After the study was accepted, a staff meeting was arranged. A few days before this meeting I received a letter from the agency's director that included the statement, "We, of course, do not have the resources to recruit for you for your project." Because I was too excited about the prospect of getting the project started, I glossed over this statement, failing to grasp the magnitude of what this would mean for my study.

THE CHALLENGES

At the meeting, the staff members seemed genuinely excited about the project as I described it to them. Then the director dropped what felt like a bomb. I could not use agency staff members to help me directly in any way to recruit from the agency's clientele. It would put posters and flyers about the study in senior centers. That was all; the agency would do nothing else. No mailings to eligible clients, no meetings with staff who provided home-based services, nothing. I felt stymied: People who need home care or adult day services do not attend senior centers nor do most of their caregivers. Essentially, my efforts to work with this agency ended before they began.

After recovering from this blow, I sought out private home health agencies again. First I contacted one with offices around the state. I presented the study to this agency's staff members at their annual meeting and several of them talked with me afterward, but no referrals were made. I tried another agency; it agreed to participate, but never referred anyone to me. A second county agency was contacted; again, there was interest but no referrals. I was getting panicky. I had student assistance and funding for 1 year, and it was now 4 months into the project with no sample identified or data collected.

OVERCOMING THE DIFFICULTIES

I convened a meeting of my research team to troubleshoot the problem. These four bright women were not only sympathetic, they also brainstormed what ultimately became the solution to our problem. First, they suggested that I drop the notion of working with people who didn't know our university very well and proposed that we work with several local agencies to get our sample. Second, they suggested that we ask students in my class on aging to refer family members or friends. Third, one of them had moved to a suburban county about an hour away and offered to meet with the agency director there. I left the meeting feeling somewhat encouraged for the first time in weeks.

All of these ideas ultimately paid off. Students eagerly referred their parents, in-laws, aunts, or neighbors who were caregivers, and many of these participants actually lived in the county I had initially targeted for recruitment. Two local county agencies referred people of diverse financial backgrounds. And the agency director in the suburban county was very supportive of the project and gave us access to staff members, who ultimately linked us to clients and their caregivers. From this last source, some minority group participation was obtained. Each of these strategies won us about a third of our participants. What was interesting was that without deliberately setting a goal of obtaining a sample diverse in its financial holdings, we obtained one through these methods. For a study on financing long-term care, this outcome was quite fortuitous.

LESSONS LEARNED

I learned several important lessons from these experiences. Chief among those lessons was that my assumption that my earlier successes in recruiting from selected organizations would be replicated with minimal effort was very naïve. Efforts that I should have made, and that I recommend to anyone trying to recruit from healthcare agencies, are presented in the following paragraphs.

Get to Know the Target Organizations

The large urban organization with which I began my recruitment efforts was more than 10 times larger than the local county agency with which I had worked on a previous study. In addition, its geographical area of service coverage was huge. Had I spent more time learning about the organization and discussing with its director the nature of successful recruitment for qualitative research studies, I might have understood early in the process why their organization couldn't help me more with recruitment. The director might have encouraged me to work with a smaller agency, possibly facilitating that process. I then might have avoided the loss of the 2 months it took to get through the state IRB process, as well as wasting resources on flyers and posters in senior centers that got no response.

My advice is to take time to introduce yourself and your work and to get to know the organizational structure and culture of agencies with which you wish to work. One or two meetings may not be enough exposure for this process to occur. Sandfort (2003) suggests investing a considerable amount of concentrated time in learning organizational contexts before asking organizations to participate in field research. In healthcare settings, such learning can occur through informational telephone interviews with agency directors, spending time in agencies observing meetings and informally interviewing key managers and staff members, and shadowing staff members as they go about daily routines. Such groundwork can legitimize one's presence (Sandfort, 2003) and open access to agency clientele through a process of building trust and rapport with staff members while demonstrating respect for organizational boundaries. Alternately, through this process, it may become apparent that one must move on to other prospective recruitment sources if a given organization is unreceptive to outsiders or plagued by conditions, such as chronic overwork and high staff turnover, that severely constrain its ability to assist researchers with recruitment efforts.

Educate Agency Staff about the Research Process and Outcomes

We academics sometimes assume that practitioners view research as inherently beneficial and worthy of their participation. Although most practitioners are exposed to research findings in their education, they may have little personal experience with the research process. They likely will have questions, often unspoken, about the research process and its products or outcomes. Both agency management and staff members should be briefed thoroughly on the purpose of the research project, as well as given access to a copy of the interview questions that the researcher plans to ask study participants. It may be wise to invite staff or management members to assist with question development and wording. Members of management may be more likely to approve a research project that addresses, at least in part, concerns of theirs that are relevant to the project's purpose. Thus, adding a couple of questions to the qualitative interview that speak to those concerns may result in approved research that is seen as directly benefiting the agency and not just the research institution.

Similarly, agency staff members may worry that clients may reveal information about service provision that would place them in an unflattering light. In-depth interviews usually address a wide range of topics and concerns, and some participants may stray from focal topics to share information they deem relevant to the study. How issues of confidentiality and anonymity will be handled should be explained to agency staff before projects are approved and researchers enter the field. In reports made to agencies, as well as publications derived from the study, great care must be taken to present and summarize qualitative data in ways that do not reveal specific identities of either staff members or participating clients.

Giving Back to Organizations That Assist in Recruitment

Assisting researchers with recruitment of study participants is no small task, and agencies that do so should be rewarded in some tangible way for their efforts. There are several forms these rewards can take. First, send the agencies the articles and other materials that you publish from your work (Ginger, 2003). Second, whenever possible, consider conducting a workshop or in-service training in your area of expertise for agency staff. Before leaving the field, discuss and select a topic for presentation that may be useful in improving service provision. Finally, ask members of management for suggestions on how you might reward their staff members for their hard work in supporting your research project. As a rule, managers have good ideas of what their staff members most appreciate in the way of thanks for their assistance.

CONCLUSION

I concluded this study a much wiser researcher than when I began it. I learned that there is no time to nurse a bruised ego when there is research to be done; to succeed, you pick yourself up quickly, learn from your mistakes and missteps, and like a salesperson, accept rejection and prepare yourself to pursue a new target. I shall forever be grateful to the four research assistants who rallied to help me find participants when I was nearly certain there were none to be found.

The intensive interview process used in qualitative research is less familiar to healthcare service practitioners than traditional survey methods of research, and sample recruitment is far more labor-intensive in qualitative research projects. Thus, considerable sustained effort is essential to educate and woo agency personnel in asking them to invite their clientele and staff to participate in such research. However, the rich contextual findings of qualitative studies of aging make the recruitment challenges well worth the effort expended.

TO READ FURTHER

Butera, K. J. (2006). Manhunt: The challenge of enticing men to participate in a study on friendship. *Qualitative Inquiry, 12,* 1262–1282.

In her study of gender and friendship, Butera encountered severe difficulties in recruiting adult male participants. In this article, she describes the various problems she encountered in recruiting men, discusses reasons for their reluctance to participate in her study, and offers several useful strategies for dealing with these recruitment challenges. She emphasizes the need to "sell" the study as critical to researchers' success in attracting wary populations. She also stresses the need to involve a male co-researcher, a strategy that can be applied to other situations in which the principal investigator does not possess "insider" status.

Eide, P., & Allen, C. B. (2005). Recruiting transcultural qualitative research participants: A conceptual model. *International Journal of Qualitative Methods, 4*(2), 44–56.

The purpose of this article is to describe successful ways of recruiting persons of cultural backgrounds other than those of the researchers. The authors focus on three concepts—cultural context, trust, and knowing the person—that must be negotiated for recruitment and data collection to proceed. They note that researchers' humility and caring behaviors contribute to building "a bridge of trust" that facilitates the development of relationships needed before research can be conducted. The authors also present a conceptual model of intercultural recruitment that may be useful to those planning to study persons from various cultural backgrounds.

REFERENCES

Ginger, C. (2003). Access and participation in a government agency. In M. S. Feldman, J. Bell, & M. T. Berger (Eds.), *Gaining access: A practical and theoretical guide for qualitative researchers* (pp. 154–159). Walnut Creek, CA: Altamira Press.

Sandfort, J. (2003). Accessing multiple human service organizations for field-based research. In M. S. Feldman, J. Bell, & M. T. Berger (Eds.), *Gaining access: A practical and theoretical guide for qualitative researchers* (pp. 110–115). Walnut Creek, CA: Altamira Press.

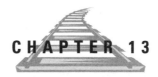

CHAPTER 13

All Aboard!

Using Community Leaders
to Keep Clinical Researchers on Track

PHILIPPE A. BARRETTE

BACKGROUND OF THE STUDY

The early 1970s were marked by the emergence of community health centers to provide social and psychiatric services to poor and disadvantaged persons. Awareness of the need for services was increasing (Beaupre, 1974). In many ways, not much has changed. There has always been and will always be an interest by the nonpoor to address the needs of the poor.

Based at an eastern Canadian psychiatric hospital in the 1970s, my colleagues and I shared the goal of improving access to treatment for low-income families. Our team was multidisciplinary, representing psychiatry, psychology, and social work. My own professional training focused on intrapsychic struggles, the role of the unconscious, and understanding the implications of Freud's drive theories. In my field, the poor were acknowledged but, as a rule, they did not come for psychotherapy twice a week. At our community teaching hospital they were significantly underrepresented, with less than 4% of their anticipated numbers seeking help.

Community interventions have two key stakeholders: the intervener and the recipient. These roles are different but entwined. One role is to deliver, whereas the other is to receive, but "there's many a slip between the cup and the lip." In our effort to bring forth a community intervention to improve the life quality of working-poor children, there were indeed "many slips." It was not a smooth process. We were faced with several ethical, political, and program delivery research problems, some of which were unexpected, causing delays and increasing costs. What began as a 3-year intervention escalated to more than 7 years of study before the intervention could be launched. This is the story of the evolving relationship between the investigators and the study participants and how the success of the community intervention rose and fell over the course of that relationship. Five of the more difficult challenges we faced and the lessons we learned from them are discussed.

THE CHALLENGES

Choosing the Study and Control Groups: Design Issues and the Ethics of Choosing One Underserved Population for Intervention over Another

After nearly 2 years of planning by our research team, which included developing a working relationship with the local university's Department of Epidemiology Community Research Department, we contacted the municipal housing authority in a city of 250,000. This organization was responsible for housing approximately 3,150 working-poor and welfare families and their 7,000 children residing in 26 housing projects. We introduced ourselves to the chief administrator and explained our seemingly simple goal: to assess the mental health and well-being of children of poor families, specifically, their tenants' children. The housing authority was quick to deny us permission. All decisions affecting the residents had to go through the tenants' association and each public housing project had its own.

This was unexpected information and our first major obstacle. Previously, we had believed that we could gain access to this community through the housing authority alone. Now, we would have to contact each of the 26 different tenants' associations in as many housing complexes in order to determine the experimental group and gain permission to work with one of them. That is, we would have to collect data to determine the nature and specific characteristics of each housing project such as children's ages, numbers, and quality of life, in order to find a suitable pairing of experimental and control housing projects. That approach had several problems. One was that it could upset people in communities who would not be selected for the experimental group and therefore possibly benefit from the interventions meant to improve life quality. We would be asking for their cooperation to collect data without providing anything in return. Meeting the potential identified needs of those families residing in 26 housing projects was beyond our scope. Another concern was that those in the selected experimental group might not agree to participate.

Our solution was to choose the study and control groups first, before requesting permission from the various tenants' associations to work with their communities. With this approach, randomization precedes consent

(Snowdon, Elbourne, & Garcia, 1999; Zelen, 1979) and those participants who are offered the intervention can either decline or accept (Homer, 2002). The control group remains unaware that randomization has taken place, thus avoiding potential disappointment at not being included in the first place. By using this method, our selection could occur without alarming or upsetting the community unnecessarily. The task seemed impossible. How do you study a population without having direct contact with them? The answer lay in the use of unobtrusive data, a relatively uncommon methodology at the time.

Unobtrusive data (Webb, Campbell, Schwartz, & Sechrest, 1966) are gained from information available in public records or personal observations. By definition, information is retrieved through secondary data sources, without requiring direct contact with participants. (e.g., number of fire hydrants per housing project). The advantage of using unobtrusive measures as a prelude to a community intervention is that it allows a comparison of each housing project's base level quality of life without transgressing the tenants' right to privacy. These measures are obtained without alerting, identifying, or affecting either the experimental or control group. Further, unobtrusive data can be more objective than subjective data, which are based on opinions alone.

The major disadvantage of using unobtrusive measures is that although the intervention may be effective in improving the life quality of the experimental group, any gains may be difficult to illustrate. This is due to the potential major baseline differences between the intervention and control groups that could not be captured at the outset (Webb et al., 1966). Nonetheless, whatever bias is caused by surmising the quality of life in one project will be reflected no less in analyzing the second housing development.

To find our experimental and study groups among all 26 housing projects in the city, we initially applied two selection criteria: the number of units and the number of children by age groups. This allowed us to identify the sites having the most children. We hoped that identifying and targeting larger sites would offset complications arising from losing children from the sample owing to their families' mobility (moving out of the project).

This gave us six comparable housing projects. We then applied two sets of unobtrusive measures to these sites: physical traces and archival. The physical traces measures referred to physical characteristics of the housing sites—that is, the age and condition of the built environment, on-site visual analysis, architectural design, building type and mix (high-, medium-, or low-rise), number and type of bedrooms, unit size, density, land site design, age of project, and population count. The archival measures were aggregate data procured from social, public, and civil agencies. The information was retrieved from various sources and included number of psychiatric admissions, number of police calls, number of fires or false alarms, mobility rate both within the housing project and externally, numbers and types of incidents reported by police for adult and youth liaison divisions, security reports from the housing authority, the housing authority's rating of housing projects according to management difficulty, rent arrears, numbers and causes of psychiatric admissions to children's inpatient/outpatient and adult inpatient/outpatient units, the number of active cases and children in the care of the Children's Aid Society, and the numbers of mother-led single-parent families and father-led single-parent families. The archival measures were useful, as it was necessary to select housing projects that had comparable socioeconomic profiles (Offord & Jones, 1983).

To get these sensitive data meant networking with our community contacts. For example, the housing authority referred us to the fire department chief. Having one major political arm of the local government in support of our request for information made it easier for another to give us permission. When it came to approaching the police, the awareness that their colleagues in the fire department were on board made their participation and cooperation almost automatic. Although the information was considered public, in order to actually retrieve the fire department data meant sitting in the back room of a fire hall, sifting through logs and logs of fire reports that covered a large geographic area serviced by various stations. The police department was slightly easier, in that it provided reams of paper with printouts for 6 months regarding incidents in a general catchment area. From this output, specific study group site areas could be combed out.

Ultimately, the unobtrusive profile exercise gave us an opportunity to compare six housing projects on a variety of cultural, quality-of-life, social, demographic, and psychological factors. We decided to use a conservative model, that is, to select what would be considered the two most disadvantaged and comparable housing projects. The thinking was that if we could make a difference and improve the most difficult social housing environment, perhaps we could then help other less stressed communities. The model was conservative in the sense that we were trying to create a positive change against the most difficult odds. The housing projects themselves were considered to be the experimental or control groups, rather than specific children, parents, or families occupying these projects.

Although we were aware that the two housing projects were in equal need of services and interventions, by definition, we had to choose one as a control group in order to proceed with the research. This was our ethical dilemma: knowing that one project would not be accessing badly needed help and services. The control group would simply continue to take advantage of the community resources they were already naturally receiving. Regarding the intervention group, the decision was that if a need was identified, services and crisis interventions would be offered immediately, rather than waiting for the outcome of a report months or perhaps years later.

Because of the time required to do a proper literature survey, meet with the community leaders, agencies, government departments and school boards, develop a bilingual mental health survey (English and French), and undertake the unobtrusive community profile, it took 2 years after our research team had been formed before we were able to comfortably identify and select the two study groups.

Gaining Access to the Designated Experimental (Intervention) Population

The group chosen for intervention was composed of 517 children ages 3–15 from 477 families. Family economic characteristics included 51% (or 245) working-poor families, 35% (or 166) families receiving mother's allowance, and 14% (or 66) families on welfare assistance. The control group was matched in a similar way but scored more favorably overall on the unobtrusive profile, that is, less mobility, less crime, fewer fires or false alarms, and a younger built environment. It was time to meet members of the experimental group, who as it turned out, lived less than a mile from our hospital research base. Some might even say they were in our hospital's patient catchment area, except that we rarely made "house calls."

With eager anticipation, our psychiatric research team went out one evening to the experimental group's community hall to introduce ourselves to the tenants' association. The association was composed of several mothers from the housing development who often had to live in a hostile environment, raising families on their own. They had endured years of dealing with social workers, agencies, rules, and nosy professionals and appeared somewhat hardened by all these experiences. They seemed distrustful of our motives. When we shared with them our intention to assess their children's mental health and school performance in order to provide them with skill development opportunities, they reacted protectively, with suspicion and indignation. "What gives you the right to assume our children need your help anyway?" "What are you implying, that our children are below average?" "Are you saying that we (parents) are deficient?" "That we are crazy parents?" In fact, that *had* been part of our operating middle-class thesis, belief system, and bias. We thought we were being helpful (because we thought they needed help) and were somewhat taken aback by what appeared to be a lack of gratitude on their part. "We hope you don't think you are coming in here to do another one of those damn surveys, do you?" they added. (Well, actually, we had a pretty nifty one that we had developed in conjunction with the local university's community epidemiology department and piloted over the past year, but we would be happy to park it.)

In truth, this population, like many other target groups, had become survey weary, with some residents describing themselves as "researched to death." Historically, students, from high school to the post-graduate level, often look to the poor to support their need to "write a paper" or do a study. This request puts demands on the residents for their time and personal data and exposes them to student scrutiny. In the end, a student might receive an A on his or her paper, or a graduate student a grant, but the population studied does not necessarily benefit, nor are its members always informed of the results of their participation. This particular low-income population had simply become exhausted by the middle-class student/investigator.

Okay, now what? We had spent nearly 2 years writing and developing this project, meeting with several community organizations, some of which were also suspicious of our motives (e.g., "What is a psychiatric hospital doing out in the community on our turf anyway?"). We had also spent several hours educating our outpatient hospital administrator that the definition of community psychiatry in 1975 meant that one had to actually leave the hospital to provide service. Further, we had done all this work to create an unobtrusive profile, and now the tenants were telling us that they didn't want our help. How could that be? What about all our good intentions? We weren't prepared for the hostility, the rejection, or the impasse. The research team felt derailed.

To the reader, it may seem terribly obvious, but at the time, it took some silence and desperate thinking before one of us asked, "So, what would you like us to do? Is there anything you need that we could help you with?" After a moment, a response came from one of the residents: "Well, as a matter of fact, there is ... our kid's teeth." Teeth? An awkward silence enveloped the research team. My own thoughts quickly reverted to my training in Freud, recalling his preoccupation with the oral stage, but I couldn't remember him writing much about teeth!

According to social exchange theory, everyone needs to get something in exchange for giving up something. Here we were asking parents to open their families and lifestyle to us, but for what, in return? Up to this point, we felt we were doing the tenants a big favor. In truth, *they* were the ones doing *us* a big favor: We needed them and their children but they did not need us.

Our train had come to a halt, and the community had taken on the role of a caboose. Historically, a railway caboose had several functions. It was usually the last car in a train, which conductors used as a place to sleep, write their reports, and give directions to the engineer. However, and more important, it carried lights in order to warn any unsuspecting train approaching from the rear and thereby avoid a collision. Ignoring the functional and proactive role of the caboose could lead to unintended, and sometimes dire, consequences. The community residents had begun to act as if they were the conductor giving the engineer (the researchers) directions, telling what speed to take and where to get off. More to the point, we were being told to get onto a different track altogether.

New Directions and Uncharted Track

Okay, so teeth it was. Where do you begin to help public housing tenants with their children's teeth? This was unknown territory for our psychiatric team. We began by introducing ourselves to the local dental health unit and its director. He assigned one of his staff hygienists who, in conjunction with a retired dentist who volunteered his time, assessed 500 children's teeth. In addition, we exchanged our mental health survey for a newly designed one to capture the dental habits and level of care for this population. Six months later, the results were in. Children from this low-income population had a utilization rate (i.e., visited a dentist in the past 12 months), and a level of dental health comparable to those of other Canadian children, but were likely to be older before their first visit to see a dentist. The children who had yet to visit a dentist had teeth that were four times superior to those children who had visited a dentist (Barrette, Lynch, Wu, Offord, & Last, 1981). Who knew? The common uninformed assumption had been that poor children must mean poor dental health. Not so. This was to be the first of many lessons taught by the mothers and learned by the investigators.

"My Dentures Don't Fit": Offering Emergency Help and Intervention While Waiting for the Study Results

As the dental assessment unfolded, it became readily apparent that the parents' dental health was in much more serious state than their children's. Many adults had ill-fitting, broken, or missing dentures as well as periodontal disease. Few, if any, could afford a dentist. Our original focus as a psychiatrically based children's research team had been to look at children's mental health. We were now visibly distracted by their parents' dental health and social stress. To meet their immediate needs, we liaised with the local dental and public health units, which organized free dental assessments and referrals for the adults. In some cases we were able to initiate subsidies from social services and the Red Cross for more advanced treatment. With a few telephone calls to the community, a cadre of dentists organized themselves to provide free services for these adults. In addition, while the survey interviewers were in the residents' homes, other problems were soon identified. In one case, parents who were physically handicapped were referred to and given assistance by the Visiting Homemakers Association for services and help with day-to-day household cleaning. All in all, emergency dental care was arranged for 40 adults, plus immediate medical and psychiatric care for another dozen tenants. The need was there. Our original research mandate was expanding.

Quite pleased with ourselves in a restrained academic way, we thought it was now our turn. We were ready to conduct our still nifty mental health survey, and a bilingual one at that. "Not so fast," came the response. "Before you start going into our children's schools, we need you to look into their physical health." It felt like another delay and more new track. This time we knew how to respond, and a physical health survey was designed, translated, pretested, and conducted. As in the dental results, no evidence was found to support the idea that physical health, including physician utilization, was an area of deficit among children of poverty (Offord & Jones, 1983). This was another victory for the mothers, who continued to educate and surprise the clinical research investigators with the results. With each successive survey telling the researchers that their children were "average" and "okay," the message from the participants was that perhaps they were "pretty good" mothers after all.

During our work with the tenants' association, we created a bilingual newsletter, the "blue flyer," to announce upcoming joint efforts by our research group and the association. Results of the first survey were conveyed through the flyer to every household in the community, as were the results of the second survey. We soon became known as the "blue flyer people." By dealing with the tenants' association, communicating with all the community residents via flyers, providing crisis intervention, social services assistance, and feedback of both survey results as they were completed, we reduced the stigma associated with our intervention (we were the people from the "crazy hospital"). No doubt this had an impact on the residents' involvement, with an incredible 85% and 92%, respectively, participating in these two surveys.

Merging Track

Following the second survey, we approached the tenants' association with much care and caution. Looking for guidance and direction, this time we asked its members what *they* wanted to do. In doing so, we had moved our "caboose" to the front of the train, calling it our Tenants' Advisory Council. At this juncture, the members shared their concern regarding their children's behavior problems and school performance and the lack of recreational facilities or opportunities for skill development. After 4 years of planning, an unobtrusive profile, and two surveys, we were now able to return to our original agenda.

One year later, the results from the educational, emotional, and skill development survey were in. The poor children were found to be disadvantaged as compared with their middle-class peers in all three areas. As compared with middle-class controls, they were significantly more likely to have repeated a grade, to be considered conduct problems, or to be placed in a special education class, and were perceived by their teachers as hyperactive almost four times as often. Similarly, nonschool skills, such as swimming, were less developed and the children had significantly fewer opportunities to receive instruction in music, hockey, or swimming (Offord, Last, & Barrette, 1985). The participation rate for this survey was 98%.

As a result of these latest findings and in combination with the results from the previous dental and physical surveys, our clinical research group was in a position to propose a Skill Development Program to the experimental community. This child-directed intervention would provide recreational (nonschool) activities, including all costs and equipment, in both sport (e.g., swimming and hockey) and nonsport skills (e.g., guitar and ballet) over a 3-year period. The housing tenants' association, which also acted as our advisory council, had gradually become a major advocate of our work. In a subsequent grant submission for this Skill Development Program, we were able to attach the following:

> We are happy to hear of your group's intentions to provide improved recreational and skill development resources for our children from low income families. We would like to fully endorse and support any grant application.... As you have recently found out for yourselves, our children do not benefit from the same advantages as middle class children. We look forward with enthusiasm to working closely with you on this important effort.
> (*Signed*) Tenants Council, April 1979

It was a long way from "*We hope you don't think you are coming in here to do another one of those damn surveys, do you?*" The original target group and stakeholders of our intervention had become our co-investigators and our biggest ally. The caboose, laden with internal community consultants and resources, had been moved to its rightful place at the front of the research train (by then, there was less chance of a collision). Seven years after our initial formation of a community research team, we were now in a position to actually to do what we had originally intended: to advance the life quality of children residing in a low-income community (Offord & Jones, 1983). The train was finally leaving the station.

LESSONS LEARNED

1. It is a prerequisite to be engaged with the local residents from the outset and to regard them as an equal partner. Having community residents form an advisory group can significantly improve participation rates and sustain the life of, if not add new life to, the project. In our study, the tenants were instrumental in helping us achieve rare participation rates of 85%, 92%, and 98% in the three surveys, respectively. At the outset, colleagues and others had predicted that we would be lucky if we obtained a 50% participation rate with this specific population.

2. It is essential to be flexible and willing to share the role of expert. Any researcher's intention "to do good" may not be perceived as such by the recipient. Our progress was tempered, measured, monitored, and governed by the housing tenants' association. Instead of giving direction, we took direction. In the end, the counsel received from the advisory group, coupled with our role adaptation, set a stable groundwork that allowed for the project's ultimate success.

3. Be patient with the process, as *not all trains run on time*. Expand the timetable to accommodate the community's priorities and to allow for a period of building trust and problem solving. Problem solving (intervention) is based on trust; trust is based on listening accurately.

4. Offer real help and intervene when needed, rather than when the study results emerge. This serves to build trust and a working relationship with the participants. It is also more just.

5. "Laying new track" brings with it unexpected expenses. Each yearly delay and additional unplanned survey meant new costs for interviewers' salaries and translation costs for the subsequent interview manuals. In addition, extra efforts had to be initiated to protect hospital-based research staff in their positions for their ongoing dedication to this project. The time frame had ballooned from the 4 years that we had negotiated with our hospital administrator (who had a great sense of humor) to 7 years before we actually began the intervention.

6. Community work provides a wonderful training ground for professionals to learn humility, patience, teamwork, and a respect for process.

ACKNOWLEDGMENTS

The original community research team consisted of Philippe Barrette, MSW, PhD; Lyse Burgess, PhD; Claire Fair, BA; Marshall Jones, PhD; John Last, MD; Sharon Lazar, MSW; Joan Mclean, MSW; Dan Offord, MD; and Xavier Plaus, PhD.

TO READ FURTHER

To better understand and be more sensitive to the cultural differences between the middle-class investigator and his low-income population, the reader may want to review the following:

Adams, P. L., & McDonald, N. F. (1968). Clinical cooling out of poor people. *American Journal of Orthopsychiatry, 38*, 457–463.

This article speaks to a subtle societal process in which the poor are simultaneously rebuffed and consoled. They are shunted between services that are inaccessible, and over time, they lose heart and hope. The poor are "cooled out" and then they drop out.

Freire, P. (1970). *Pedagogy of the oppressed*. New York: Continuum.

Freire identifies the education system as a middle class vehicle specifically designed to lull the disadvantaged into accepting what they are given without question. He encourages the poor to be in a state of "conscientizaçao"—that is, to learn to perceive social, political, and economic contradictions and to take action against these oppressive elements.

Alinsky, S. D. (1971). *Rules for radicals: A pragmatic primer for realistic radicals.* New York: Random House.

Alinsky takes a more proactive approach. His remedy is to generate conflict as a way of mobilizing the poor in their own communities. His writings and activity in community organization in Chicago housing projects have inspired President Barack Obama and served as the subject of Hillary Clinton's senior thesis.

Berne, E. (1964). *Games people play.* New York: Grove.

Adams and McDonald (1968) refer to Berne's work to partly explain the historical relationship pattern between the oppressor and the oppressed. Berne describes the ritual "I'm only trying to help you." In a version of this "game," the poor are treated as though "they need fixing" without letting them have the requisite tools or resources "to be fixed."

REFERENCES

Barrette, P. A., Lynch, G. W., Wu, A. S. M., Offord, D. R., & Last, J. (1981). Dental utilization and dental health status of children from a rent-to-income housing complex. *Canadian Journal of Public Health, 72,* 105–110.

Beaupre, L. (1974). Local centre of community care means: Accessibility, continuity and participation. *Canadian Association of Social Workers, 4,* 4–6.

Homer, C. S. (2002). Using the Zelen design in randomized controlled trials: Debates and controversies. *Journal of Advanced Nursing, 38,* 200–207.

Offord, D. R., & Jones, M. B. (1983). Skill development: An intervention program for the prevention of antisocial behaviour. In S. B. Guze, F. J. Earls, & J. E. Barrett (Eds.), *Childhood psychopathology and development* (pp. 165–188). New York: Raven Press.

Offord, D. R., Last, J., & Barrette, P. A. (1985). A comparison of the school performance, emotional adjustment and skill development of poor and middle-class children. *Canadian Journal of Public Health, 76,* 174–178.

Snowdon C., Elbourne D., & Garcia, J. (1999). Zelen randomization: Attitudes of parents participating in a neonatal clinical trial. *Controlled Clinical Trials, 20,* 149–171.

Webb, E. J., Campbell, D. T., Schwartz, R. D., & Sechrest, L. (1966). *Unobtrusive measures: Non-reactive research in the social sciences.* Chicago: Rand-McNally.

Zelen, M. (1979). A new design for clinical trials. *New England Journal of Medicine, 300,* 1242–1245.

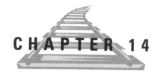

CHAPTER 14

Changing Horses in Midstream
Transforming a Study to Address Recruitment Problems

ANTHONY S. JOYCE

BACKGROUND OF THE STUDY

My work environment is the outpatient service of a university-based department of psychiatry. I am the coordinator of the Psychotherapy Research and Evaluation Unit, which is regarded as one component of the service and is closely affiliated with an assessment and treatment clinic and two partial hospitalization programs. Our research group has been quite invested in a particular approach to short-term, time-limited (20-session) individual psychotherapy, having studied and refined a manualized form of the treatment since 1985 (see Piper, Joyce, McCallum, Azim, & Ogrodniczuk, 2001). The therapy orientation is psychodynamic, making the model somewhat unique in a practice and research era dominated by the cognitive-behavioral approach. We have presented evidence for the therapy's effectiveness, based on a controlled clinical trial (Piper, Azim, McCallum, & Joyce, 1990) and a comparative trial of two versions (interpretive, supportive) of the approach (Piper, Joyce, McCallum, & Azim, 1998) with samples of mixed-diagnosis psychiatric outpatients. With the latest iteration of our model, we were interested in a more rigorous test and therefore decided to target a specific patient group, that is, patients who present with a recurrent major depressive illness.

Recurrent depression is associated with more pronounced symptoms and dysfunction than acute conditions, and patients with this diagnosis make a disproportionate demand on mental health treatment resources

(Coryell & Winokur, 1992; Dunner, 2001). The literature has also featured a considerable debate about the limited impact of antidepressant medications for these patients, in terms of both the areas of functioning positively affected (e.g., quality of interpersonal relationships) and the prevention of recurrence over the long term (Antonuccio, Danton, DeNelsky, Greenberg, & Gordon, 1999). Combination treatments have consequently been recommended for patients with this condition (Thase, 1997). Initially, then, our interest was in the relative benefit of combining our psychotherapy and medication treatment, over medication alone, in the treatment of patients with recurrent depression seen at our university hospital outpatient clinic.

We proposed the use of a clinical trial approach in the "horse race" of these two treatment conditions. Patients would be randomly assigned to a condition and our outcome assessors would be blind to this assignment. Response to treatment would be evaluated on multiple occasions, using a comprehensive battery of self-report and interview measures, as patients were followed for the recommended period of 2 years. We were confident that we had addressed all the details of our clinical research plan—submitting four grant applications before securing any funding had meant heavy use of the fine-tooth comb—and naturally assumed that our clinicians and clinical service would again be up to the task. We were mistaken.

THE CHALLENGES

Unanticipated problems with the recruitment of patients emerged almost immediately after the study received ethics and administrative approval and was implemented. Two core problems could be identified, and both appeared to be associated with issues among our cohort of clinic therapists. The first was a degree of therapist "satiation," even burnout, with the clinical research process. Our staff has seen very little turnover since the 1980s (its members have been around as long as I), and during this span they had been involved with six large-scale clinical trial studies, each requiring 3 to 5 years to reach completion. In retrospect, it is possible that we took for granted that we'd enjoy the kind of enthusiasm and energy the therapists had brought to our previous research projects. Instead, we were faced with a degree of apathy and dearth of interest that we had not encountered previously.

The second issue was more procedural. Often, a therapist completed the initial assessment and concluded that he or she had an appropriate patient for psychotherapy. The therapist would then balk at making the referral, however, knowing that the patient had only a 50–50 chance of receiving the desired treatment (i.e., the combination). In these instances the therapist would choose to retain the patient and provide therapy him-

or herself, rather than supply the project with an appropriate recruit. There were also occasions when the patient made a similar decision after being introduced to and possibly even assessed for the study; at some juncture, the patient would be unwilling to "roll the die" and perhaps not be assigned to the treatment condition he or she wanted. The irony was inescapable: Here were appropriate patients, savvy about psychotherapy and interested in engaging in treatment, but our offer of the project was putting them off. The study had stumbled out of the gate and we needed to do something.

OVERCOMING THE DIFFICULTIES

After putting the entire project on hold—not hard to do, given the flow of patients we had to contend with—we addressed the recruitment problem on two fronts. First, we engaged the clinical staff in a series of group discussions, aimed at an airing of attitudes toward the study and involvement in clinical research more generally. The therapists' concern that their patients would get the treatment for which they were best suited came through loud and clear. Other, deeper issues also emerged. One therapist, A, mentioned feeling inhibited about the referral of a "difficult" patient, apprehensive that a colleague would be assigned to provide the therapy for this patient and resent her, A, for the referral. A reality check on the mechanics of patient assignment—patients would be randomized to therapists but with attention to the level of the therapist's caseload—emphasized that referred patients would be spread equally across the pool of therapists.

A particularly painful admission occupied all members of the discussion. In the previous comparative study of two versions of the therapy model, one therapist, B, consistently dazzled us with her skillful competence and achieved impressive outcomes with all her patients. The wife of another key therapist and a close friend of many of the staff, B had been a central figure in the study and for the clinic as a whole. Sometime after that study concluded, B received a diagnosis of metastatic colon cancer. The staff was devastated. All were profoundly moved by how B managed the short time remaining with calm and acceptance. Our shared grief had become submerged after a year without B, and it was at this time that the new project was implemented. For many, engaging in the activities associated with the research—case discussions in our clinical research seminar, for example—was simply too poignant a reminder of B's absence, often leading to feelings of ambivalence about the study. The expression of these often difficult emotions was beneficial and promoted a sense of group cohesiveness—it was resolved that B would have wanted to see us proceed with the kind of work we had excelled in during her time with us.

As a second approach to the problem, the study protocol was completely revamped. The clinical trial, aimed at comparing the effectiveness of two treatment strategies, became a naturalistic "follow-along" study. In the revised plan, *all* recruited patients were to receive psychotherapy as a first-line intervention—no more deciding on the patient's treatment fate with a coin toss. Once therapy had started, the patient's progress was to be monitored closely. If progress was not as expected at certain "critical evaluations," the patient was scheduled to meet with a project psychiatrist for consideration of the need to augment the therapy with antidepressant treatment. Continued nonresponse at subsequent critical evaluations would prompt successively more assertive pharmacological interventions, in line with the standardized medications protocol we had developed in the planning stages. In a sense, we were banking on the demonstrated effectiveness of our therapy to do the job alone. Moreover, the research focus shifted from a "horse race" between two treatment strategies to an effort to identify the patient variables that were associated with the need for more assertive treatment in order to achieve recovery from depression. We continued to address the treatment of outpatients with recurrent depression, and the measurement strategies developed in the initial proposal were still being employed. The shift in focus and the potential implications of the study for practice, however, proved to be of greater interest to our clinicians, and they were able to provide unequivocal support for the revamped project. After the necessary negotiations with the funding agency and the faculty's Research Ethics Board (REB), the study was "restarted."

LESSONS LEARNED

One lesson had been learned previously but was emphatically reinforced by this experience: The clinicians involved in your project are an integral part of the investigative team, and their input is often critical to the health and success of the endeavor. As we found out, it can result in a shock to take for granted that the clinicians will be enthusiastic, cooperative, and interested in the objectives of your study. It's likely much better to ask them about the project in the planning stages rather than finding that things are not as expected when implementation is attempted. Feedback on the research plan from the clinicians' perspective can often highlight design flaws or inconsistencies the investigators have overlooked (a "forest for the trees" effect). And, of course, it's also important to attend to the "care and feeding" of your clinician group as the study progresses.

Second, as a researcher, you are not wedded to your initial research plan. Once a proposal has received approval (and perhaps, by God, funding!), it is not set in stone—you always have options for changes, whether minor or, as in our case, major. We discovered that our revised protocol was much more in line with what was of most interest: Who are the patients who require more than psychotherapy for recovery from recurrent depression? Who are the patients for whom the initial treatment combination (therapy plus the psychiatrist's first choice of antidepressant) proves insufficient in terms of treatment response and recovery? Answers to these questions would have been much harder to come by with our original study design. The revised design had the advantage of greater clinical relevance, both to the investigative team *and* to the therapists. Allowing for the evolution of your research objectives is important for the development of a program of studies, but it can also be critical in the conduct of a single investigation.

Were our efforts to address the recruitment problem successful? Yes and no. The patient flow into the restarted project increased substantially over what it had been but was still far below the estimates for accrual we had used in our grant application(s). Once again, the research team was forced into an admission that heretofore we had ignored or even denied: The population served by our clinic had changed considerably over the years since our previous study, and cases appropriate for psychotherapy now made up a much smaller proportion than before. To attain the target sample size we had originally specified in our proposal would likely mean quadrupling the duration of the recruitment period—I'd be retired before the study was completed if that course of action were taken! More practically, we lowered our expectations and reduced our target sample size so the study could be completed within the time window of our funding. This, of course, also meant taking another look at our plans for data analysis to ensure that we could still address our hypotheses with reasonable statistical power.

As the study progressed (or, when perceived through the lens of our original expectations, *limped along*), the rate of recruitment again declined—not precipitously, but enough to underscore that our therapist cohort is in a very different space than was the case in decades past. Back then, the therapists were with us, and we collectively felt that we could have an impact on the field—we were passionate about what we were doing. At this point, with the therapists moving into the latter stages of their career trajectories, their priorities have definitely shifted more toward their outside lives and their families, as they should be. Although I could acknowledge a similar shift, I nonetheless retain a passion for the work we've been doing and continue to do. Greater creativity may, however, be required; if the large-scale clinical trial studies simply are no longer possible, what other investigative paths might we take? We have considered taking greater advantage of the datasets established in our earlier studies, making use of our therapy session recording libraries to investigate the therapy change process at the microlevel, or taking more of an individual differences focus and studying risk and protective factors in subgroups of our patient population. Our experience with the current study suggests that there are always novel ways to address problems such as these—and to continue doing the work we love.

ACKNOWLEDGMENT

This work was supported by the Health Research Fund of the Alberta Heritage Foundation for Medical Research.

TO READ FURTHER

Mapstone, J., Elbourne, D., & Roberts, I. G. (2007). Strategies to improve recruitment to research studies (review). *Cochrane Database of Systematic Reviews 2007*, Issue 2. Art. No. MR000013.

This is a systematic review of 15 studies that tried to improve recruitment into clinical trials by various means.

REFERENCES

Antonuccio, D. O., Danton, W. G., DeNelsky, G. Y., Greenberg, R. P., & Gordon, J. S. (1999). Raising questions about antidepressants. *Psychotherapy and Psychosomatics, 68,* 3–14.

Coryell, W., & Winokur, G. (1992). Course and outcome. In E. S. Paykel (Ed.), *Handbook of affective disorders* (2nd ed., pp. 89–98). New York: Guilford Press.

Dunner, D. L. (2001). Acute and maintenance treatment of chronic depression. *Journal of Clinical Psychiatry, 62,* 10–16.

Piper, W. E., Azim, H. F. A., McCallum, M., & Joyce, A. S. (1990). Patient suitability and outcome in short-term individual psychotherapy. *Journal of Consulting and Clinical Psychology, 58,* 383–389.

Piper, W. E., Joyce, A. S., McCallum, M., & Azim, H. F. A. (1998). Interpretive and supportive forms of psychotherapy and patient personality variables. *Journal of Consulting and Clinical Psychology, 66,* 558–567.

Piper, W. E., Joyce, A. S., McCallum, M., Azim, H. F. A., & Ogrodniczuk, J. S. (2001). *Interpretive and supportive psychotherapies: Matching therapy and patient personality.* Washington, DC: American Psychological Association Press.

Thase, M. E. (1997). Integrating psychotherapy and pharmacotherapy for treatment of major depressive disorder: Current status and future considerations. *Journal of Psychotherapy Practice and Research, 6,* 300–306.

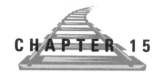

CHAPTER 15

When Cost Meets Efficiency
Rethinking Ways to Sample a Rare Population

JULIAN MONTORO-RODRIGUEZ
GREGORY C. SMITH

BACKGROUND OF THE STUDY

Grandparent caregivers, defined by the U.S. Census Bureau as people who have primary responsibility for their coresident grandchildren younger than 18, are a target population that has received increasing research attention over the past decade (Hayslip & Kaminski, 2005). However, because extant studies have chiefly involved convenience samples that are biased and unrepresentative of this unique category of family caregivers (Pruchno & Johnson, 1996; Casper & Bryson, 1998; Szinovacz, 1998), there is a need to identify techniques for obtaining population-based samples. A major obstacle to achieving this goal, however, is that grandparent caregivers are a rare subgroup of the general population and designing effective sampling methods for rare populations in general is difficult and costly (Sudman & Kalton, 1986). In fact, only about 1.5% (or 2.4 million) of the total population of people ages 30 and older living in households within the United States falls within the U.S. Census Bureau's classification of grandparents responsible for their own grandchildren under age 18 (Simmons & Dye, 2003).

Adding to the complexities of sampling this particular rare population is that the overall population of grandparent caregivers encompasses various subgroups whose degree of rarity varies sharply (Casper & Bryson, 1998). For example, estimates based on 1997 U.S. Census data are that about 63% (1.5 million) of the 2.4 million households maintained by a grandparent had at least one parent of the grandchild also residing in the home. In contrast, those households maintained by grandparents with no parents at all in residence were estimated to comprise approximately 37% (904,000) of the 2.4 million grandparent-maintained households. Caregiver grandparents of the latter type, who are commonly referred to as either "skipped generation" or "custodial" grandparents, are of particular interest to family researchers because they usually assume sole responsibility for raising a grandchild younger than age 18.

In this chapter we first describe the special challenges associated with obtaining population-based samples of rare populations in general. This discussion is followed by a description of the specific difficulties that we encountered in attempting to recruit a nationally representative sample of the very rare population of custodial grandparents, using random digit dialing (RDD) as a population-based sampling procedure. We then present alternative sampling strategies that we ended up using to offset these difficulties, and discuss their worth with respect to efficiency and cost in sampling rare populations.

THE CHALLENGE: SAMPLING RARE POPULATIONS

Two key factors affecting the sample design for any target population are the availability of funds and the existence of an adequate list (or sampling frame) for that population (Frankel, 1983). Probability sampling dictates that a "list" be available from which to select randomly so that the probability of an element's appearing in the sample is known (Levy & Lemeshow, 1999). Thus, in sampling a rare population (i.e., one constituting a small fraction of the general population) the researcher must first determine if a good list exists from which to sample (Sudman & Blair, 1999). If so, then randomly selecting respondents from that list is a straightforward procedure (Lepkowski, 1991; Sudman & Kalton, 1986). For most rare populations, however, no preestablished list is available. Consequently, extensive screening is often required to identify members of the rare population from within a random sample of the general population (Kalton & Anderson, 1989). As one might imagine, this process is often prohibitively expensive, and sampling becomes a "matter of finding needles in a haystack" (Wells, Petralia, DeVaus, & Kendig, 2003). The cost of such screening typically depends on (1) the size of the rare population, (2) the difficulty in identifying members of the population, and (3) the methodologies used in the screening process (Kalton & Anderson, 1986).

Although there are various techniques for obtaining probability samples of rare populations (see, for discussion, Kalton & Anderson, 1989; Sudman, 1972; Sudman & Kalton, 1986; Sudman, Sirken & Cowan, 1988), one of the most preferred approaches involves some form of RDD whereby households with phones are randomly selected from general population lists and screened to determine if a member of the rare population is present. The main shortcomings of RDD as a useful and efficient sampling strategy have to do with the lack of telephone ownership among certain population segments and nonresponse bias (Cummings, 1979), the small size of the rare population relative to the total population (Psaty et al., 1991), and, most important, the inclusion of numbers belonging to either nonworking or nonresidential households (Cummings, 1979; Sudman & Blair, 1999). A common approach for offsetting the last problem is to use a "list-assisted" design, which includes directory information as a source of auxiliary data for sampling from the telephone numbers generated by strict RDD (see, for details, Lepkowski, 1988). Commercial firms market such lists with minimal coverage bias (Brick, Waksberg, Kulp, & Starer, 1995; Sudman & Blair, 1999).

Various procedures have been recommended to increase sampling efficiency and reduce the costs of screening for rare populations. For example, if many geographical clusters contain few or no members of the rare population, then major efficiencies can be accomplished if these "zero segments" are eliminated or undersampled (Sudman & Blair, 1999). One drawback, though, is the bias that results from excluding those not living in highly concentrated areas (Gibson & Herzog, 1984). For example, although the U.S. Census data show considerable regional and state differences in percentages of grandparent-grandchildren coresidence across the entire United States (Simmons & Dye, 2003), those grandparent caregivers residing in low concentration areas would be excluded if a researcher decided to sample from just the more highly concentrated geographical regions of the country. This technique is also inappropriate for sampling extremely rare populations because even those areas with known concentrations of the target population are likely to contain insufficient numbers of the target group to render this method efficient (see, for discussion, Sudman, 1972).

Yet another form of disproportionate sampling is to try to separate a small special stratum containing most of the rare population, from a larger stratum containing many fewer members of the rare population (Kalton & Anderson, 1989). Then the resulting special list or stratum is sampled in disproportionately high rates (Kish, 1965; Lihr, 1999). For example, if a researcher wanted to sample randomly from the rare population of older adults who own personal computers, then narrowing the stratum to only households known to contain residents ages 65 and older might be a useful approach.

Another way to improve the efficiency of screening for rare populations is through network (or multiplicity) sampling whereby randomly selected respondents from the general population are asked if members of their social network (e.g., relatives, neighbors, coworkers) belong to the rare population (Sirken, 1970; Sudman & Blair, 1999; Sudman & Freeman, 1988; Sudman et al., 1988). The aim is to increase the amount of information obtained during a screening interview so that the number of screening contacts is reduced (Sudman & Kalton, 1986). Network sampling is especially productive in yielding samples of rare populations, such as grandparent caregivers, that have high concentrations of African Americans (see Rothbart, Fine, & Sudman, 1982). Factors affecting the efficiency of network sampling include the informants' ability to report accurately and provide contact information, the visibility of screening characteristics, and the added questions, which increase survey cost (Sudman et al., 1988).

Although in this chapter we have described each of the aforementioned techniques for sampling rare populations separately, in reality they are often used in combination (Kalton & Anderson, 1986; Lepkowski, 1991). The use of multiple techniques is illustrated in the following discussion of our attempts to sample custodial grandparents.

Problems Encountered in Recruiting and Screening Custodial Grandparents

The initial strategy of our study was to obtain a population-based sample of custodial grandmothers, using list-assisted RDD in which numbers belonging to either nonworking or nonresidential households were excluded. The overall aim of the study was to examine stress and coping among a sample of 700 U.S. households with "custodial grandmothers" who provide full-time care for 3 months or more to at least one grandchild between ages 4 and 17 in absence of the child's parents. Thus, our inclusion criteria reflected a specific target population that was geographically dispersed and even more rare than the entire population of custodial grandparent households. The latter more broadly includes households with grandchildren from birth to age 18, as well as approximately 152,000 households maintained by grandfathers only. To increase screening efficiency, a multiplicity (or network) sampling procedure was used in combination with list-assisted sampling. If a randomly called household did not include an eligible grandmother, the respondent was then asked if anyone in his or her broad social network fit the study inclusion criteria. Our assumption was that using list-assisted RDD in conjunction with multiplicity sampling would be effective in yielding sufficient numbers of eligible households.

A pilot study was conducted to test the overall efficiency of this sampling design. Of 1,503 randomly contacted households throughout the 48 contiguous states, only four qualified respondents emerged from the screening process, at a yield rate of only 0.27%. Although 14 referrals resulted from the network sampling component, just 1 yielded a qualified respondent. These results suggested that an estimated 263,025 numbers (many involving repeated callbacks) would be required to obtain the intended sample of 700 households. Obviously, this would fast become an extremely time-consuming and expensive endeavor.

The Revised Sampling Plan

Because of our ill-fated pilot results, major revisions were made to the original sampling plan. First, we switched from list-assisted RDD to a randomized mail recruitment strategy in which potentially eligible U.S. households were sent an advanced recruitment letter and asked to contact us by either e-mail or a toll-free number if the household included a custodial grandmother. Respondents were then called back and screened for study eligibility. There were several reasons for making these changes:

1. Mail surveys yield high cooperation and good response rates among special populations, especially if the topic is intrinsically interesting (Sudman & Blair, 1999; Sudman & Kalton, 1986; Traugott, Groves, & Lepkowski, 1987).
2. Letters sent from an authoritative source (e.g., on university letterhead) can automatically legitimize the survey request (Groves & Lyberg, 1988).
3. Letters avoid current problems confronting telephone screening such as telemarketing, cell phones, and call rejecting devices (Lavrakas, 1998; Link & Oldendick, 1999; Oldendick & Link, 1994; Sudman & Blair, 1999).
4. Noneligible respondents screen themselves out, thereby increasing efficiency.
5. Letters give respondents more time to contemplate participation.
6. Letters permit clearer explanation of study incentives.

A second major change from our initial sampling plan was to sample disproportionately from the approximately 38 million households containing children age 18 or younger versus sampling from the much larger stratum of 106 million total U.S. households. Such targeted lists are relatively unbiased and can be purchased from commercial firms (Lepkowski, 1988; Psaty et al., 1991). The logic of this method is based on the assumption that virtually all custodial grandmothers meeting our inclusion criteria would fall within the smaller stratum of 38 million households with children age 18 or younger, and that they would be identified with a much higher probability when using this reduced stratum as opposed to the total stratum of all U.S. households (about 106 million) estimated to exist at the time of our study. Thus, the probability of a letter reaching a household with custodial grandparents was reduced from about 1/140 to 1/50 by using this approach. Such use of disproportionate random sampling can be very powerful because small reductions in probability rates for rare populations can yield huge savings in screening costs (see, for example, Picot, Samonte, Tierney, Connor, & Powel, 2001). Multiplicity (or network) sampling was also included in the revised sampling plan by requesting ineligible households to forward recruitment letters to associates who were custodial grandparents.

TABLE 15.1. Results of Revised Sampling Plan

Outcome	N	% of total contact (yield rate)
Recruitment letters mailed	36,000	
Undeliverable letters	1,829	
Estimated contacts	34,171	
Respondents meeting study screening criteria	331	1.00
Direct hits	251	.74
Network sampling	80	.24

The results of the revised sampling plan are summarized in Table 15.1. A total of 36,000 recruitment letters were sent at random to U.S. households containing children age 18 or younger. An estimated 34,171 households were contacted after subtracting 1,829 letters that were undeliverable. These 34,171 contacts generated 331 replies from custodial grandparents who met the specific inclusion criteria specified for our study. Of these, 251 were "direct hits" and 80 arose from network sampling. It is noteworthy that the network sampling component yielded about one-fourth of the eligible respondents. In summary, the revised sampling plan resulted in a much higher yield rate or eligible households (1.0%) than did our initial use of RDD (0.27 %).

Response Rate and Cost Factors

The response rate and cost associated with any sampling plan are obviously of paramount importance to researchers (Lavrakas, 1998). As noted earlier, a straightforward random selection (e.g., every 10th person) is not possible if a comprehensive listing of the target population does not exist. In turn, investigators who face this situation are unable to calculate precise response rates and thus can only derive estimates. For example, in our study, using the ratio of the estimated number of eligible households receiving the letter over the actual yield, we calculated that the estimated response rate to our mail recruitment strategy was approximately 48.5%.

It is important to note that we also pilot tested the revised disproportionate sampling procedure, using RDD instead of a recruitment letter to determine if the improved results would similarly occur with RDD. Of 1,100 screening calls made with RDD involving the revised disproportionate sampling procedure, none produced an eligible respondent. In terms of the various recruitment and screening costs shown in Table 15.2, the average recruitment and screening cost per eligible respondent was estimated to be $108.00. One might reasonably expect such costs to rise in proportion to the rareness of the target population. In addition, it should be noted that

TABLE 15.2. Breakdown of Screening Costs to Identify Eligible Custodial Grandmothers

Cost categories	Expenditures[a]
List of 36,000 random households	$10,500
Postage	$9,600
Stationery (envelopes + letters)	$1,620
Telephone (maintenance + long-distance calls)	$1,020
Personnel	$9,817
Subtotal	$32,557
10% indirect costs	+ $3,256
Total costs	$35,813

Average cost per eligible respondent = $35,813/331 = $108.00

[a]Expenditures were incurred during the years 2002–2003.

the costs shown in Table 15.2 do not include the subsequent interviews conducted with eligible respondents.

LESSONS LEARNED

Several important points are exemplified by the experiences we encountered in our study. First, investigators must be aware that achieving a probability sample of a very rare population is likely to be both costly and difficult. Moreover, a single simple solution to sampling rare populations sample does not exist. Instead, there are multiple and often very complicated solutions that must be used in combination (Lepkowski, 1991). Nevertheless, there are two key reasons why investigators must be willing to confront the many daunting challenges that are associated with obtaining population-based samples of very rare populations: (1) If studies using nonprobability methods require multiple replications to increase their validity, then the cost of a single population-based study may ultimately be comparable if not less (Lepkowski, 1991), and (2) rare populations deserve policy and interventions formulated on sound data, not just the most conveniently obtained data.

Observations from our study also raise the question, "When is a sample good enough?" Many known threats to survey error (e.g., nonresponse, coverage bias, refusals) that are not discussed in this chapter can become even more pronounced when researchers attempt to sample rare populations. Accordingly, survey experts have conceded that deviations from pure sampling theory are tolerable with respect to rare populations. For example, one recommended technique is to develop a sampling frame for the target population whereby each person interviewed may be asked to suggest additional people for interviewing ("snowball sampling") such that respondents can be randomly selected from that frame (see, for discussion, Sudman & Kalton, 1986). Yet no clear standards exist in the literature for determining the overall quality of samples achieved by such methods.

It is also important to note that despite the improvements resulting from our revised sampling plan, we were ultimately unable to achieve our intended sample of 700 custodial grandmothers entirely through a population-based approach because of cost and time limitations. Thus, approximately half of our final sample was recruited by means of convenience sampling (e.g., mass media appeals, grandparent support groups, and social service agencies). Consequently, we have compared our convenience and population-based samples in all subsequent analyses involving data from this study (see, for example, Smith & Palmieri, 2007).

Finally, our experience with this study suggested that a *Zeitgeist* phenomenon involving changes in communication technology may now confront survey sampling. For example, recent complaints regarding telemarketing have led to increased use of call rejection devices, and we frequently encountered such devices in our initial attempt to rely on RDD. In retrospect, we believe these aftereffects of telemarketing strongly affected the initial RDD sampling plan. Another unexpected occurrence involving today's technology was that many households that received our recruitment letter decided, on their own, to post it on various websites. As a result, our callback screening procedure had to be adjusted to account for the resulting snowball contacts. Investigators should also be aware that many of today's recommended techniques for sampling rare populations are becoming outdated as the survey methodology field evolves over time, such as with the predicted replacement of telephone and mail survey procedures with online surveys (Dillman, 2000; Sudman & Blair, 1999).

In conclusion, we recommend that it is essential to pilot test any proposed method for obtaining a probability sample of a rare population. Our experience suggests that even the best of sampling plans are likely to require substantial modifications and adjustments if the project is to stay on course. In short, the sampling of rare populations demands a great deal of creativity, flexibility, and diligence on the part of investigators.

ACKNOWLEDGMENT

Work on this chapter was funded in part by National Institute of Mental Health Grant No. RO1 R01 MH66851-01 awarded to Gregory C. Smith.

TO READ FURTHER

Lepkowski, J. M. (1991). Sampling the difficult to sample. *Journal of Nutrition,* 121, 416–423.

This article provides a definition of the difficult-to-sample populations as rare populations or populations that are rare to locate, enumerate, or interview. It also reviews probability and nonprobability methods to sample rare and elusive populations and includes an illustration for sampling one of such populations, homeless people.

Picot, S. J. F., Samonte, J., Tierney, J. A., Connor, J., & Powel, L. L. (2001). Effective sampling of rare population elements. *Research on Aging, 23,* 694–712.

The purpose of this article is to describe and evaluate a step-by-step methodological approach for sampling rare populations (e.g., black female caregivers and noncaregivers). It discusses the efficiency in sampling methodology, including strategies such as having potential participants respond to an open-ended question regarding their understanding of the study participation, providing agencies with detailed specifications of requested lists, and not allowing the obtained list to age. This article provides a roadmap for sampling rare populations.

Psaty, B. M., Cheadlem, A., Curry, S., McKenna, T., Koepsell, T. D., Wickizer, T., et al. (1991). Sampling elderly in the community: A comparison of commercial telemarketing lists and random digit dialing techniques for assessing health behaviors and health status. *American Journal of Epidemiology, 134,* 96–106.

This article compares two methods of sampling elderly respondents for a telephone interview: use of Polk telemarketing lists and the method of random digit dialing. The authors conclude that sampling from commercial telemarketing lists was an efficient method of identifying elderly respondents and that the estimates of health behaviors and health status were comparable with those obtained by random dom digit dialing techniques.

REFERENCES

Brick, M. J., Waksberg, J., Kulp, D., & Starer, A. (1995). Bias in list-assisted telephone samples. *Public Opinion Quarterly, 59,* 218–235.

Casper, L. M., & Bryson, K. R. (1998). *Co-resident grandparents and their grandchildren: Grandparent maintained families.* Population Division Working Paper No. 6. Washington, DC: U.S. Bureau of the Census

Cummings, K. M. (1979). Random digit dialing: A sampling technique for telephone surveys. *Public Opinion Quarterly, 43,* 233–244.

Dillman, D. A. (2000). *Mail and internet surveys: The tailored design method* (2nd ed.). New York: Wiley.

Frankel, M. (1983). Sampling theory. In P. H. Rossi, J. D. Wright, & A. B. Anderson (Eds.), *Handbook of survey research* (pp. 21–67). New York: Academic Press.

Gibson, R., & Herzog, A. (1984). Rare element telephone screening (RETS): A procedure for augmenting the number of black elderly in national samples. *The Gerontologist, 24,* 477–482.

Groves, R. M., & Lyberg, L. E. (1988). An overview of nonresponse issues in telephone surveys. In R. M. Groves, P. P. Biemer, J. T. Massey, W. L. Nichols, & J. Waksberg (Eds.), *Telephone survey methodology* (pp. 191–212). New York: Wiley.

Hayslip, B., & Kaminski, P. L. (2005). Grandparents raising their grandchildren: A review of the literature and suggestions for practice. *The Gerontologist, 45*, 262–269.

Kalton, G., & Anderson, D. (1986). Sampling rare populations. *Journal of the Royal Statistical Society, Series A, 149*, 65–82.

Kalton, G., & Anderson, D. W. (1989). Sampling rare populations. In M. P. Lawton & A. R. Herzog (Eds.), *Special research methods for gerontology* (pp. 7–30). Amityville, NY: Baywood.

Kish, L. (1965). *Survey sampling.* New York: Wiley.

Lavrakas, P. J. (1998). Methods for sampling and interviewing in telephone surveys. In L. Bickman & D. J. Rog (Eds.), *Handbook of applied social research methods* (pp. 429–472). Thousand Oaks, CA: Sage

Lepkowski, J. M. (1988). Telephone sampling methods in the US. In R. M. Groves, P. P. Biemer, J. T. Massey, W. L. Nichols, & J. Waksberg (Eds.), *Telephone survey methodology* (pp. 73–98). New York: Wiley.

Lepkowski, J. M. (1991). Sampling the difficult to sample. *Journal of Nutrition, 121*, 416–423.

Levy, P. S., & Lemeshow, S. (1999). *Sampling of populations: Methods and applications* (3rd ed.). New York: Wiley.

Lihr, S. L. (1999). *Sampling: Design and analysis.* Pacific Grave CA: Duxbury.

Link, M. W., & Oldendick, R. W. (1999). Call screening: Is it really a problem for survey research? *Public Opinion Quarterly, 63*, 577–589.

Oldendick, R. W., & Link, M. W. (1994). The answering machine generation: Who are they and what problems do they pose for survey research? *Public Opinion Quarterly, 58*, 264–273.

Picot, S. J. F., Samonte, J., Tierney, J. A., Connor, J., & Powel, L. L. (2001). Effective sampling of rare population elements. *Research on Aging, 23*, 694–712.

Pruchno, R. A., & Johnson, K. W. (1996). Research on grandparenting: Current studies and future needs. *Generations, 20*, 65–70.

Psaty, B. M., Cheadlem, A., Curry, S., McKenna, T., Koepsell, T. D., Wickizer, T., et al. (1991). Sampling elderly in the community: A comparison of commercial telemarketing lists and random digit dialing techniques for assessing health behaviors and health status. *American Journal of Epidemiology, 134*, 96–106.

Rothbart, G. S., Fine, M., & Sudman, S. (1982). On finding and interviewing the needles in the haystack: The use of multiplicity sampling. *Public Opinion Quarterly, 46*, 408–421.

Simmons, T., & Dye, J. L. (2003). *Grandparents living with grandchildren: 2000.* Retrieved December 28, 2007, from *www.census.gov/prod/2003pubs/c2kbr-31.pdf.*

Sirken, M. G. (1970). Household surveys with multiplicity. *Journal of the American Statistical Association, 65*, 257–266.

Smith, G. C., & Palmieri, P. A. (2007). Risk for psychological difficulties in children raised by custodial grandparents. *Psychiatric Services, 58*, 1303–1310.

Sudman, S. (1972). On sampling of very rare populations. *Journal of the American Statistical Association, 67,* 335–339.

Sudman, S., & Blair, E. (1999). Sampling in the twenty-first century. *Journal of the Academy of Marketing Science, 27,* 269–277.

Sudman, S., & Freeman, H. (1988). The use of network sampling for locating the seriously ill. *Medical Care, 26,* 992–999.

Sudman, S., & Kalton, G. (1986). New developments in the sampling of special populations. *American Review of Sociology, 12,* 401–429.

Sudman, S., Sirken, M. G., & Cowan, C. D. (1988). Sampling rare and elusive populations. *Science, 240,* 991–996.

Szinovacz, M. E. (Ed.). (1998). *Handbook on grandparenthood.* Westport, CT: Greenwood Press.

Traugott, M. W., Groves, R. M., & Lepkowski, J. M. (1987). Using dual frame designs to reduce nonresponse in telephone surveys. *Public Opinion Quarterly, 51,* 522–539.

Wells, Y., Petralia, W., DeVaus, D., & Kendig, H. (2003). Recruitment for a panel study of Australian retirees: Issues in recruiting from rare and nonenumerated populations. *Research on Aging, 25,* 36–65.

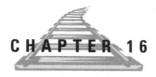

CHAPTER 16

The Story Is in the Numbers

ROBERT VAN REEKUM

BACKGROUND OF THE STUDY

We conducted a randomized controlled trial (RCT) of a type of drug called a cholinesterase inhibitor (CI) in a sample of persons who had suffered a traumatic brain injury (TBI) causing persistent cognitive impairment. CIs had previously been shown to be efficacious in the treatment of cognitive impairments arising from Alzheimer's disease, but there were no medications that have been shown to be efficacious in TBI. Given the high incidence rate for TBI in the United States. and Canada, and the high rate of persistent cognitive impairment causing handicap in this population, the RCT appeared to be greatly needed. We had some confidence in the hypothesis that the medication would be more efficacious than placebo, on the basis of some preliminary data and a solid biological rationale. Although we anticipated some significant issues with recruitment, we also expected that many individuals suffering with problematic cognitive impairment post-TBI would be eager to participate in our study and therefore that we would be able to meet the study's recruitment requirements.

THE CHALLENGES

We calculated, on the basis of our primary hypothesis, that we would need to study 40 participants per group (active and placebo) to be able to achieve an acceptable level of confidence in our results. We anticipated a 15% drop-out rate, so we estimated that we would need to recruit 46 participants per group. To find the sample, we had three major clinical/academic outpatient

TBI rehabilitation clinics on board (with motivated and conscientious co-investigators for each site). These clinics collectively see thousands of TBI cases annually.

We approached 678 potential participants over the 3 years of the study, of whom we could not contact 277. Of the 401 participants whom we were able to contact, 210 did not meet the eligibility criteria, leaving 191 eligible and available participants. Of this subgroup, 155 declined participation, leaving 36 eligible, available, and willing participants (all of whom consented to participate in the study). This group was randomized to one of the two treatment arms of the study. Fifteen were randomized to receive placebo, and 1 of these did not complete adequate outcome assessments over the course of the 6-month study and was therefore excluded from the analysis of efficacy. Twenty-one were randomized to receive active treatment; of these, 2 were excluded from the analyses as they had missed too many doses of the medication, 4 dropped out because of nausea (a common side effect of the medication), and 1 dropped out at the family physician's recommendation (because of gastrointestinal symptoms). Overall, then, of the 678 potential participants we first set out to recruit, we were able to successfully study only 14 participants per group (a total of 28) for the full duration of the 6-month study. Notably, though, our problem with the numbers related primarily to the recruitment phase rather than to retention, medication tolerability/safety, or compliance issues, which collectively had only a very minor impact on the overall numbers. Here I briefly discuss some of the issues we confronted at the recruitment stage.

We were unable to contact more than 40% (277/678) of the potential participants identified from the TBI outpatient clinic records and/or staff. Although we did not complete systematic data collection related to the reasons for our failure to establish contact, it is likely that there were many reasons for it. Individuals in the patient sample may have been unavailable at their listed addresses or phone numbers (for example, having suffered a TBI, a person may have been receiving support at a family member's home or inpatient rehabilitation, perhaps living a transient lifestyle, perhaps gave incorrect information when registering at the clinic, etc.). Although we made attempts to overcome this difficulty, there were constraints, such as limited staff time available to us, on what we could do. We were limited to an initial letter and follow-up phone calls. Ethical considerations also placed limits on our mode of approach to potential participants, including, in particular, mandating that clinic staff not recruit for the research study, given the potential for a conflict of interest between clinical care and research participation. This issue is clearly valid; however, it is also the case that the rule translates into having patients (who have suffered an injury and may be feeling particularly vulnerable) receive an invitation to participate in a study from a group of researchers whom they do not know and whom they were not seeking out, and this clearly does not create a firm basis for trust in the first instance. It may well have been the case that our failure to contact many individuals was due to this issue, in the sense that potential participants simply chose to refuse to participate by not replying to our invitations. Whatever the reasons were (and it is likely that other reasons contributed), our failure to contact more than 40% of potential participants obviously had a significant impact on our ability to recruit. From the point of view of the potential participants, this failure to establish contact also meant that they were unable to be made aware of the potential benefits associated with the study.

More than 50% (210/401) of the potential participants whom we were able to contact did not meet the eligibility criteria, which were as follows. At a screening visit, the potential participant was given a short assessment, with a commonly used test, to confirm attention or short-term memory impairment, which was an inclusion criterion. At the screening assessment, we also used standardized measures to exclude potential participants who displayed traits of ongoing posttraumatic amnesia, malingering, mania, depression or a recent psychotic episode. Additional inclusion criteria included the patient's having a diagnosis of TBI (an acceleration-deceleration event with loss of consciousness, or posttraumatic amnesia, or abnormal computerized tomography findings), being age 18–55 years, being an outpatient at one of the three TBI clinics a minimum of 6 months post-TBI, and the availability of a second-person informant for reporting of behavioral changes. Additional exclusion criteria included a history of any other central nervous system illness or insult, study medication contraindications, pregnancy risk without contraception, current substance abuse, language or physical impairments precluding testing, current use of one of the medications in the class of medication being studied, and current use of benzodiazepines or antipsychotic or anticholinergic or antiseizure or stimulant medications. Clearly, this was a long list of inclusion and exclusion criteria, and we expected a high rate of attrition at this stage of the recruitment process. From the point of view of recruiting, and as well related to generalizability of the results, it is clear that lowering the restrictions created by inclusion and exclusion criteria would be advantageous. In terms of our study, though, and given the goals of the study (early study of efficacy) and the current state of our knowledge (limited data regarding safety of the medication in nonadults or in particular patient groups), we felt that all of the inclusion and exclusion criteria that we used were essential. We felt that it was important to ensure that we were studying persons who had suffered a clinically significant TBI causing ongoing cognitive impairment, to ensure that we could adequately assess their responses to the intervention, to minimize risk to our participants, to avoid co-intervention (i.e., receiving other treatments for the condition) and contamination (patients in the placebo group getting the treatment medication from some other prescriber, such as the family physician), to avoid potential drug interactions, and to avoid potentially treating comorbid conditions that have been shown to respond to the active medication being studied (e.g., comorbid Alzheimer's disease, as might have been seen had we recruited elderly persons; the age greater than 55 years restriction was actually mandated to us, for this reason, by the reviewers at the Canadian Institutes for Health Research [CIHR], which funded the study). Each of the inclusion and exclusion criteria was carefully chosen to address these areas of concern with the study, and, regrettably, there was not much that we could (or would) do to alter them. We simply needed to understand that we were faced with a large attrition rate at this stage of recruitment, and, of course, that our (limited) budget would be further stretched by the need to assess so many potential participants.

Despite our difficulties with contacting potential participants and our stringent inclusion and exclusion criteria, we were still able to identify 191 eligible and available potential participants. Of this subgroup, however, more than 80% (155) declined participation. There were, of course, many reasons for this, including various feasibility issues. However, I believe that the main underlying reason for the majority of the refusals to participate related to the concern for safety and well-being (e.g., risk of treatment side effects, risks related to the need for multiple assessments, etc.) of the potential participant. Clearly, this reason is completely valid, particularly when one considers that these persons had all suffered a clinically significant injury (the TBI) that was causing them ongoing impairment (at least, but often not limited to, cognitive impairment), and we were now inviting them to participate in a study with a medication that had not had much prior study in this population and whose safety we could not guarantee (or even provide much in the way of data about).

(NOT) OVERCOMING THE DIFFICULTIES

Ultimately, we were unable to overcome the difficulties posed during our recruitment phase (we eventually ran out of time, and funding), and our study remains limited by its low statistical power in its ability to answer the questions we hoped it might.

LESSONS LEARNED

1. Ensure adequate funding for the extensive amounts of time and effort that will be required to recruit participants for some types of clinical research.

2. Work with ethics committees to carefully examine the risk versus benefit of constraints placed on modes of contacting potential participants. Although some modes of contacting potential participants are more "inva-

sive," or unethical for other reasons, than are others, it is also the case that not being able to establish contact has potential negative consequences not only for the study, but also for the participants (e.g., they may have wished to participate for any of a number of reasons, but did not learn about the study and hence never had the option). Note that we now live in an era when access to all of us is nearly automatic (e.g., phone, e-mails, faxes, mail, knocks on the door, etc.), that most of us are contacted by someone whom we did not invite to do so daily (typically when we are at our busiest, it seems!), and, finally, that it appears to be "ethical" for almost everyone (politicians, salespersons, bean counters, etc.) to initiate unsolicited requests of us (for contributions, political support, purchases, etc.). Our current social reality may require ethical reassessment related to limitations to access for activities (such as health-related research) that are aimed not for profit or the like, but rather for improved health and hence a secondary positive impact on the individual, his or her family, and society.

3. Carefully examine all inclusion and exclusion criteria and "exclude" those criteria that are not essential.

4. Provide support and understanding/acceptance to those potential participants who are concerned about risks related to study participation. Ultimately, it will be difficult to provide much reassurance in populations that have not had much in the way of preliminary study (e.g., as with the use of our study medication in the TBI population), and so, again, it is important to prepare adequately (get a really big grant!) for a high attrition rate if this issue applies to your intended research.

TO READ FURTHER

Campbell, M. K., Snowdon, C., Francis, D., Elbourne, D., McDonald, A. M., Knight, R., et al. (2007). Recruitment to randomised trials: Strategies for trial enrollment and participation study. The STEPS study. *Health Technology Assessment, 11,* 1–126.

This review found that of 114 trials, fewer than one-third recruited their original sample size within their time frame. The authors review practices that foster or inhibit successful recruitment.

Steinhauser, K. E., Clipp, E. C., Hays, J. C., Olsen, M., Arnold, R., Christakis, N. A., et al. (2006). Identifying, recruiting, and retaining seriously-ill patients and their caregivers in longitudinal research. *Palliative Medicine, 20,* 745–754.

This literature review and study found factors that increase enrollment in longitudinal studies, including recruitment letters sent by the personal physician, small monetary incentives, and the specific content of the letter and information brochure.

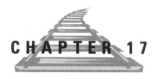

CHAPTER 17

Strategies for Retaining Participants in Longitudinal Research with Economically Disadvantaged and Ethnically Diverse Samples

ELIZABETH A. GONCY
MICHELLE E. ROLEY
MANFRED H. M. VAN DULMEN

BACKGROUND OF THE STUDY

Attrition is a common problem in longitudinal studies. It leads to several issues, including threats to internal and external validity, systematic bias of the results due to disproportionate groups, and the loss of statistical power. Both the internal and external validity are compromised when attrition occurs, which ultimately reduces the results' generalizability. The greater the attrition in a study, the less confidence researchers can have in their conclusions. Attrition also creates bias when it occurs more in some groups than in others, such as among delinquents (e.g., Farrington, Gallagher, Morley, St. Ledger, & West, 1990) or minority or low-income participants (e.g., Green, Navratil, Loeber, & Lahey, 1994). This type of selective attrition leads to problems, such as the presence of fewer people in specific conditions (e.g., treatment groups) and a loss of statistical power to examine group differences (Prinz et al., 2001).

Recent statistical advances in dealing with missing data, particularly imputation procedures that are relatively easily to implement with software packages (e.g., McKnight, McKnight, Sidani, & Figueredo, 2007), may have reduced concern about retention. These imputation procedures, however, perform optimally when the percentage of missing data is relatively small (e.g., < 20%; Schafer & Graham, 2002) and when the reason that the data are missing is not related to the intervention (for a more detailed description, see Buhi, Goodson, & Neilands, 2008). So, even though these imputation procedures may be helpful in many situations, it is still essential to minimize the amount of attrition and the potential bias it can create.

Focusing research efforts on populations with known risk factors for later psychopathology (referred to as "at-risk" participants), including low socioeconomic or ethnic minority status, is essential in order to understand the mechanisms underlying the development of psychopathology (e.g., Sroufe & Rutter, 1984). In longitudinal research with at-risk populations, selective attrition becomes even more problematic. Extenuating circumstances, such as chronic illness, in addition to other known pathology risk factors, may make longitudinal studies of these populations much more difficult than longitudinal studies with other groups.

Our longitudinal study, entitled the Northeast Ohio Study of Continuity and Change during Early Adolescence (NCCEA), looked at continuity and change in behavior problems during early adolescence. Our main aim was to investigate and systematically model change in these problems over 1 year. Typically, most projects studying continuity and change during childhood and adolescence assess behavior problems at either annual or biannual intervals (for a review of studies using group-based modeling techniques, see van Dulmen, Goncy, Vest, & Flannery, 2009). Previous research findings, however, indicate substantial heterogeneity in the course of conduct problems, such as stealing or physically fighting (Moffitt, 2007), and that adolescents who have a large number of conduct problems may change more rapidly (Lahey et al., 1995). The studies that evaluate adolescents every 6 or 12 months may not capture what happens between assessments. This is particularly important during early and middle adolescence, when trajectories of conduct problems start to diverge (see, for a recent overview, Moffitt, 2007). Therefore, the NCCEA aimed to model behavior problem changes within 3-month intervals. We also investigated whether individual variations in the course of antisocial behavior were related to the initial starting level of the problems and how family and peer processes affect changes in antisocial behavior over 1 year.

The NCCEA recruited 106 adolescents between the ages of 10 and 14 and their primary caregivers through a rolling enrollment procedure over the course of 2 years. Families were recruited in the waiting rooms of two pediatricians' offices in a midsized suburban area. Assessments included an initial in-person assessment and follow-up telephone calls 3, 6, and 9 months later. At the initial assessment, both groups of participants (i.e., adolescents and caregivers) completed a variety of measures, described in the following paragraph. Families also provided detailed contact information, granting us permission to recontact them for future assessments. This contact information included name, address, phone number, and the same information for two family members or friends who would know their current living arrangements should they move throughout the following year. Participants were not compensated for the initial assessment but received a $50 check for their participation in the follow-up assessments.

At the initial assessment, the primary caregivers completed a short demographic questionnaire, the Eyberg Child Behavior Inventory (ECBI; Eyberg & Pincus, 1999), the Center for Epidemiological Study—Depression scale (CES-D; Radloff, 1977), the Family Assessment Device—General Functioning (FAD-G; Epstein, Baldwin, & Bishop, 1983), and the Parent's Report on Close Friends (CF-P; Conduct Problems Prevention Research Group, 1990). The adolescent completed a short demographic questionnaire, the FAD-G, the Inventory of Parent and Peer Attachment (IPPA; Armsden & Greenberg, 1987), and a substance use questionnaire based on questions from the National Longitudinal Study of Adolescent Health (Harris et al., 2003). At the 3-, 6-, and 9-month follow-ups, the primary caregiver completed the ECBI via the telephone.

THE CHALLENGES

The difficulty of attrition can be intensified in longitudinal studies of economically disadvantaged and ethnically diverse populations because of additional challenges, such as frequent relocation or mistrust of research studies. Owing to the nature of the population we were studying, we encountered several challenges in retaining our participants.

The loss of telephone services, due to moving or nonpayment of bills, and change of telephone numbers were some of our biggest challenges. We lost 7 participants throughout the study because of disconnected phones, and 9 participants did not provide phone numbers at the initial assessment. Despite occasionally receiving an updated phone number via telephone company recordings, more frequently no new phone number was provided. Another common difficulty with contacting our participants by phone was reaching our participants at convenient times. Many families were from low-income households, with participants typically not working during the usual business hours.

Throughout the study, trust was also a major issue for several participants. On six occasions, participants stated they were unsure of the research project's intentions and felt that it might be exploiting their children or family. Because participants were recruited in pediatricians' offices, some children were dealing with chronic illnesses (e.g., port wine stain, leukemia), and primary caregivers were often unsure about continuing participation in the project because of these unique, stressful situations. Another challenge that was magnified in our sample of at-risk families included handling issues related to divorce and remarriage and child custody changes.

OVERCOMING THE DIFFICULTIES

When telephone numbers were lost, we used several strategies for locating the families, including the use of online searches (e.g., *switchboard. com*, *411.com*) and telephone or mail contact with the provided friend or relative for updated contact information. However, in several situations, a new phone was not listed online, or friends and relatives were reluctant to share contact information. In one particular case, a participant's recontact person had not seen or heard from the participant in more than a year, a time longer than had elapsed since we had initially recruited the participant. Unfortunately, in these situations, we lost these participants unless they contacted us.

For two reasons, we reminded participants of their participation in the study by sending them letters approximately 2 weeks before their follow-up dates. First, we asked participants to notify us if their telephone number had changed. And, if the participants had moved, the post office would either forward the letter to the family's new home or, typical to our area, return the letter to us with an updated address. These letters not only provided a second form of contact with the participants, but also allowed us to gather information on families that might have moved.

Our research staff often had to make accommodations to reach participants who worked alternate shifts or who might be sleeping during normal business hours. Research assistants (RAs) were scheduled to recontact participants at several different times throughout the week, including early morning, afternoon, evening, and weekend hours. If a work or cell phone number was provided at the initial assessment or a subsequent follow-up assessment, the RAs were also instructed to attempt to reach participants at these alternate numbers. In order to successfully complete these follow-up assessments, we also allowed a large window (2 weeks) around the target assessment date to help ensure recontact with all participants. So the RAs often made several calls (at times, as many as 20) to a target household before finally reaching the participant or passing the allocated window for follow-up.

Although relocation of participants is often a challenge to longitudinal researchers, several strategies have improved the ability to maintain contact with participants. Many studies use detailed recontact sheets to collect information for follow-up waves. Others (e.g., Krohn & Thornberry, 1999; Stouthamer-Loeber, van Kammen, & Loeber, 1992) also initially ask participants if they plan to move and encourage them to contact the researchers if they do. Other means of finding participants again may be more time-consuming and expensive, but are often necessary, including gathering contact information (e.g., names, phone numbers, addresses, Social Security numbers, driver's license numbers) and searching through public records and social agencies (e.g., Krohn & Thornberry, 1999). You may also want to try online databases (e.g., *switchboard.com*; Cotter, Burke, Loeber, & Navratil, 2002), e-mails, instant messaging systems, and online social networks to remain in contact with participants.

In cases where participants were mistrustful of the study, we reassured them of the confidential nature of the study and the importance of their continued participation. However, some of these people chose to end their participation despite the added reassurance. Before starting a study, it's essential to consider the population, and particularly to understand the participants' culture. Maintaining trust includes sustaining confidentiality and holding a reputable position within the participants' community, particularly within populations that value community support. It can be beneficial to create community advisory groups that can provide feedback, based on the goals of the study, to improve retention. For example, a community advisory group may provide the community with a reputable rationale for its members' participation in a particular study (Hudson, Leventhal, Contrada, Leventhal, & Brownlee, 2000). Further, providing diversity training or hiring researchers of a culture similar to that of the target population can improve retention (Adubato, Alper, Heenehan, Rodriquez-Mayor, & Elsafty, 2003; Spoth, Kavanagh, & Dishion, 2002; McCurdy, Gannon, & Daro, 2003; Strycker, Duncan, Duncan, He, & Desai, 2006). You can also build trust by scheduling appointments at convenient times and places (Adubato et al., 2003; Spoth, Goldberg, & Redmond, 1999) and quickly rescheduling missed appointments (Capaldi & Patterson, 1987), with staff members who have previously established trust with the participants (Armistead et al., 2004).

Because we were specifically interested in following changes in behavior problems as reported by the same caregiver, custody changes or changes in the family structure could be substantial confounding variables. To document these problems, we used a detailed computer database to record such changes. These changes in family structure often meant that relocation of the family was imminent, and therefore we relied on previous phone numbers and friends and family members to help relocate the family.

Another strategy used to reduce attrition is to provide incentives to the participants. In many cases these incentives are monetary, with different levels of compensation depending on the model of inducement (e.g., the market model, the wage-payment model, or the reimbursement model; for a complete discussion, see Dickert & Grady, 1999). In addition, bonuses for continued (Capaldi & Patterson, 1987) or timely (Armistead et al., 2004; Stouthamer-Loeber et al., 1992) participation help increase retention. Other studies (Adubato et al., 2003; Brown, 2003; Spoth et al., 1999) have used nonmonetary incentives, such as social services, food or needed household items, and babysitting services. However, it's best to avoid undue inducement, which is important to avoid ethical dilemmas of coercion and exploitation (Emanuel, 2004).

Finally, to encourage continued participation in our study, research personnel sent participants handwritten birthday and holiday cards to thank them for their continued participation and provide contact information for the project staff. We also sent two newsletters with preliminary findings and study conclusions to both thank the participants and demonstrate the importance of their participation in this study. (These contacts also had the added bonus of alerting us to address changes.)

LESSONS LEARNED

This project demonstrated several useful retention strategies, as well as the need for other ones. Our participants described the use of reminder letters, special occasion cards, newsletters, and personal phone calls as thoughtful and useful. Many of them remarked that they enjoyed hearing how their participation benefited the community. They also reported having positive feelings toward the research team because of these personal connections. This reaction reinforced the importance of maintaining a research team to help build rapport with participants throughout the study. In addition, having a project coordinator to maintain contact information and to immediately handle problems or questions from the participants was vital. Finally, the project's recontact information sheet, supplemented with a computer database, was invaluable in keeping in contact with a majority of our participants. Using these tactics, our retention rate was 76% at the first follow-up assessment phase, 70% at the second, and 77% at the completion of the study.

Some researchers have noted the benefits of various recruitment strategies to maximize retention. Capaldi and Patterson (1987) explicitly state that the greatest loss of participants occurs during recruitment. Making personal contact with participants during the recruitment process leaves a lasting impression, and participants are more likely to be retained (Armistead et al., 2004; Hudson et al., 2000). This personal contact at recruitment requires proper training, in both the community culture and the research protocol, which stresses the importance of honoring privacy and confidentiality. In our study, we used undergraduate RAs to recruit families in pediatricians' waiting rooms. Although some were very successful in recruiting families, this strategy proved to be less than optimal. A better trained, full-time in-person contact at the initial assessment may have provided the families with more information about the follow-up assessments and reassured families of the purpose of these assessments, which may have helped prevent withdrawal throughout the study.

RECOMMENDATIONS

On the basis of the review of previous retention strategies and our own experiences, we would make two recommendations. First, hiring a good project coordinator who is organized and detail-oriented is crucial. This person needs to remain in continued contact with participants and to appropriately follow up with them through reminder letters, special occasion cards, telephone updates, and assessment follow-ups. Furthermore, the project coordinator needs to be prepared to handle problems that may be encountered with participants throughout the course of the study.

Building rapport with participants, starting at initial recruitment and continuing through the entirety of the project, is also critical. This rapport helps participants feel comfortable with their participation and the study and allows them to ask pointed questions so that they can comfortably address their concerns about the project. Finally, quick and appropriate follow-through concerning any problems, concerns, or compensation is important for maintaining such rapport. Although the case study presented here was far from perfect, we learned several lessons that we could incorporate into future longitudinal studies, particularly with at-risk populations. In the initial planning stages of a longitudinal study, careful consideration of methods to reduce attrition can allow for successful retention of participants.

TO READ FURTHER

Capaldi, D., & Patterson, G. R. (1987). An approach to the problem of recruitment and retention rates for longitudinal research. *Behavioral Assessment, 9,* 169–177.

This article reviews problems related to recruitment and attrition in longitudinal research. The article focuses on biased sampling, recruitment, and retention, as well as providing an overview of techniques used in a 5-year study of delinquent males.

· Stouthamer-Loeber, M., van Kammen, W., & Loeber, R. (1992). The nuts and bolts of implementing large-scale longitudinal studies. *Violence and Victims, 7,* 63–78.

This article provides valuable insight for executing a longitudinal study. Areas discussed include planning the study, hiring staff, interviewer/assessor training and supervision, data collection validation, subject recruitment and retention, and data processing.

REFERENCES

Adubato, S., Alper, R., Heenehan, M., Rodriguez-Mayor, L., & Elsafty, M. (2003). Successful ways to increase retention in a longitudinal study of lead-exposed children. *Health and Social Work, 28,* 312–315.

Armistead, L. P., Clark, H., Barber, C. N., Dorsey, S., Hughley, J., Favors, M., et al. (2004). Participant retention in the Parents Matter! Program: Strategies and outcome. *Journal of Child and Family Studies, 13,* 67–80.

Armsden, G. C., & Greenberg, T. (1987). The Inventory of Parent and Peer Attachment: Individual differences and their relationship to psychological well-being in adolescence. *Journal of Youth and Adolescence, 16,* 427–454.

Brown, E. J. (2003). Double whammy: Accessing, recruiting, and retaining the hidden of the hidden. *Journal of Ethnicity in Substance Abuse, 2,* 43–51.

Buhi, E. R., Goodson, P., & Neilands, T. B. (2008). Out of sight, not out of mind: Strategies for handling missing data. *American Journal of Health Behavior, 32,* 83–92.

Capaldi, D., & Patterson, G. R. (1987). An approach to the problem of recruitment and retention rates for longitudinal research. *Behavioral Assessment, 9,* 169–177.

Conduct Problems Prevention Research Group (CPPRG). (1990). *Parent Report on Child's Close Friends.* Available at *www.fasttrackproject.org.*

Cotter, R. B., Burke, J. D., Loeber, R., & Navratil, J. L. (2002). Innovative retention methods in longitudinal research: A case study of the Developmental Trends Study. *Journal of Child and Family Studies, 11,* 485–498.

Dickert, N., & Grady, C. (1999). What's the price of a research subject? Approaches to payment for research participation. *New England Journal of Medicine, 15,* 198–203.

Emanuel, E. J. (2004). Ending concerns about undue inducement. *Journal of Law, Medicine, and Ethics, 32,* 100–105.

Epstein, N. B., Baldwin, L. M., & Bishop, D. S. (1983). The McMaster Family Assessment Device. *Journal of Marital and Family Therapy, 9,* 171–180.

Eyberg, S., & Pincus, D. (1999). *Eyberg Child Behavior Inventory and Sutter-Eyberg Student Behavior Inventory—Revised.* Odessa, FL: Psychological Assessment Resources.

Farrington, D. P., Gallagher, B., Morley, L., St. Ledger, R. J., & West, D. J. (1990). Minimizing attrition in longitudinal research: Methods of tracing and securing cooperation in a 24-year follow-up study. In D. Magnusson & L. R. Bergman (Eds.), *Data quality on longitudinal research* (pp. 122–147). New York: Cambridge University Press.

Green, S. M., Navratil, J. L., Loeber, R., & Lahey, B. B. (1994). Potential dropouts in a longitudinal study: Prevalence, stability, and associated characteristics. *Journal of Child and Family Studies, 3,* 69–87.

Harris, K. M., Florey, F., Tabor, J., Bearman, P. S., Jones, J., & Udry, J. R. (2003).

National Longitudinal Study of Adolescent Health: Research Design. Available at *www.cpc.unc.edu/projects/addhealth/design.*

Hudson, S. N., Leventhal, H., Contrada, R., Leventhal, E. A., & Brownlee, S. (2000). Predicting retention for older African Americans in a community study and a clinical study: Does anything work? *Journal of Mental Health and Aging, 6,* 67–78.

Krohn, M. D., & Thornberry, T. P. (1999). Retention of minority populations in panel studies of drug use. *Drugs and Society, 14,* 185–207.

Lahey, B. B., Loeber, R., Hart, E. L., Frick, P. J., Applegate, B., Zhang, Q., et al. (1995). Four-year longitudinal study of conduct disorder in boys: Patterns and predictors of persistence. *Journal of Abnormal Psychology, 104,* 83–93.

McCurdy, K., Gannon, R. A., & Daro, D. (2003). Participation patterns in home-based family support programs: Ethnic variations. *Family Relations, 52,* 3–11.

McKnight, P. E., McKnight, K. M., Sidani, S., & Figueredo, A. J. (2007). *Missing data: A gentle introduction.* New York: Guilford Press.

Moffitt, T. E. (2007). A review of research on the taxonomy of life-course persistent versus adolescence-limited antisocial behavior. In D. J. Flannery, A. T. Vazsonyi, & I. D. Waldman (Eds.), *The Cambridge handbook of violent behavior and aggression* (pp. 49–74). New York: Cambridge University Press.

Prinz, R. J., Smith, E. P., Dumas, J. E., Laughlin, J. E., White, D. W., & Barron, R. (2001). Recruitment and retention of participants in prevention trials involving family-based interventions. *American Journal of Preventative Medicine, 20,* 31–37.

Radloff, L. S. (1977). The CES-D Scale: A self-report depression scale for research in the general population. *Applied Psychological Measurement, 1,* 385–401.

Schafer, J. L., & Graham, W. (2002). Missing data: Our view of the state of the art. *Psychological Methods, 7,* 147–177.

Spoth, R. L., Goldberg, C., & Redmond, C. (1999). Engaging families in longitudinal preventive intervention research: Discrete-time survival analysis of socioeconomic and social-emotional risk factors. *Journal of Consulting and Clinical Psychology, 67,* 157–163.

Spoth, R. L., Kavanagh, K. A., & Dishion, T. J. (2002). Family-centered preventive intervention science: Toward benefits to larger populations of children, youth and families. *Prevention Science, 3,* 145–152.

Sroufe, L. A., & Rutter, M. (1984). The domain of developmental psychopathology. *Child Development, 55,* 17–29.

Stouthamer-Loeber, M., van Kammen, W., & Loeber, R. (1992). The nuts and bolts of implementing large-scale longitudinal studies. *Violence and Victims, 7,* 63–78.

Strycker, L. A., Duncan, S. C., Duncan, T. E., He, H., & Desai, N. (2006). Retention of African-American and white youth in a longitudinal substance use study. *Journal of Ethnicity in Substance Abuse, 5,* 119–131.

van Dulmen, M. H. M., Goncy, E. A., Vest, A., & Flannery, D. J. (2009). Group-based trajectory modeling of externalizing behavior problems from childhood through adolescence: Exploring discrepancies in the empirical findings. In J. Savage (Ed.), *The development of persistent criminality* (pp. 288–314). Oxford, UK: Oxford University Press.

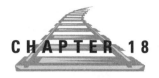

CHAPTER 18

Culturally Specific Strategies for Retention and Adherence to Physical Activity Interventions in Hispanic Women

COLLEEN KELLER
JULIE FLEURY
ADRIANNA PEREZ

BACKGROUND OF THE STUDY

Hispanics continue to be the fastest growing minority group in the United States and are expected to constitute at least 30% of the population by the year 2010 (Centers for Disease Control and Prevention, 2006). Factors linked to low levels of physical activity and associated health disparities in Hispanic women have included socioeconomic, sociocultural, and contextual variables. Equally important, Hispanic women are at increased behavioral risk because of limited access to health education information due to educational, language, literacy, and cultural barriers (Crespo, Smit, Andersen, Carter-Pokras, & Ainsworth, 2000; King et al., 2000). Our work with Hispanic women in community-based physical activity interventions has shown that although recruitment of Hispanic women is successful, we have experienced high levels of dropout and low levels of protocol adherence, particularly in long-term interventions (Gonzales & Keller, 2004; Keller & Gonzales-Cantu, 2008; Keller & Trevino, 2001).

Our work with community-based physical activity interventions has resulted in lessons learned in design, participant retention, and protocol adherence that are specific to Hispanic women. This chapter discusses (1) the challenges of dropout and adherence to physical activity protocols in Hispanic women and (2) resolutions of these challenges through consideration of cultural-contextual strategies and a proactive design strategy that employs Hispanic women as *prosumers* in physical activity interventions.

Few studies have examined the effectiveness of community-based physical activity interventions in older Hispanic women. In one study we examined the effectiveness of two frequencies of walking on cardiovascular risk reduction in sedentary, obese Hispanic women and tested social contextual moderators of treatment effect on physical activity adherence among Hispanic women. This study, *Camina por Salud* (Walking for Health), was a 36-week clinical feasibility study designed to evaluate the effect of two frequencies of walking on serum lipid levels, percentage and location of body fat, blood pressure, and adherence to physical activity. We used a two-group, randomized, repeated measures design with older postmenopausal, obese, (body mass index [BMI] > 30), sedentary, 45- to 70-year-old Hispanic women. A *promotora*, or lay health worker, was employed in this formative study to implement the intervention. The study took place in the Hispanic women's neighborhoods. Group I walked for 30 minutes, 3 days a week; Group II walked 30 minutes, 5 days a week. Our hypothesis was that the length of the treatment at low dose would favorably benefit indices of coronary heart disease (CHD) risk. Data were collected at baseline, 12 weeks, and 36 weeks. Our outcomes included total body fat and BMI, anthropometric measures, blood lipids, and physical activity adherence measured by time walked. We also measured social-contextual factors that might influence response to the intervention in these participants, including the places in which people exercise in neighborhoods and communities with regard to availability, distance, perceived safety, and perceived social support for exercise.

Eighteen women were enrolled, 11 in Group I, the 3-day group (4 remained at study end), and 7 in Group II, the 5-day group (four completing the 36-week study). The mean age of the women in the 3-day group was 56.5 (SD = 6.4), and in the 5-day group, it was 53.5 (SD = 5.8). The number of minutes walked per week for the 3-day group was 63.72 (SD = 44.67), and for the 5-day group, 129.15 (SD = 65.55). The goal was for participants to walk 90 and 150 minutes per week, respectively. At 12 weeks, the dropout rate was 28%; at 36 weeks, it grew to 52%.

THE CHALLENGES

Our work with Hispanic women in several studies across several methods with low-intensity community-based walking programs designed to manage overweight in both young and older Hispanic women showed failure to adhere to walking regimens ranging from 32% to 53% (Gonzales & Keller, 2004; Keller & Gonzales-Cantu, 2008; Keller & Trevino, 2001). Although some women did drop out of the studies, others failed to walk the prescribed amount in the assigned protocol group. Most of the women's attendance at data collection times was adherent, and participation in group activities and walking with study associates or *promotoras* was within the study parameters. The poor adherence to the walking protocol was surprising and led us to ask, "Why do women in general and this subgroup we study fail to adhere to walking regimens when on their own? What can we do about this?"

OVERCOMING THE DIFFICULTIES

Two considerations are needed in a proactive attempt to resolve failure to adhere and dropout issues in hard-to-reach subgroups. Our research and this discussion focuses on addressing these two issues: *Cultural contextual work*—strategies for retention and adherence specific to this subgroup—and the *formation of a women's prosumer group.*

Cultural Contextual Work

In our studies we used several mechanisms to avoid a highdrop out rate. First, we employed culturally relevant mechanisms, such as using *promotoras* and neighborhood walking routes. *Promotoras,* or lay health advisors, are members of the community who are turned to for advice, support, and information (Kim, Flaskerud, Koniak-Griffin, & Dixon, 2005). At the community centers used in the study, the *promotoras* helped participants map out and measure a walking plan in the neighborhood. Together, study participants and *promotoras* assessed the walking route for safety. Before beginning the training and walking, each study participant received athletic walking shoes. Educational sessions were held monthly; the sessions taught heart health information, including nutritional education directed toward low-fat dietary intake and low-fat food preparation methods. Last, we provided positive interpersonal relationships along with social time and snacks. Reinforcement strategies were used, such as having the women walk as partners to encourage and support each other in their walking schedules.

In postintervention debriefings, we conducted focus groups to explore barriers and benefits to the program that might help the participants sustain a community walking program. We collected data by means of semistructured discussions in focus groups, using questions centered on perceived barriers to the initiation of physical exercise and maintenance of physical activity. Participants' answers were audiotaped and transcribed,

and data from the focus groups were analyzed with content analysis procedures and are reported elsewhere (Gonzales & Keller, 2004). This process
yielded significant information about retention and adherence. First, some
of the women who volunteered for *Camina por Salud* regarded caregiving
responsibilities within their families as obligations of greater importance
than their exercise program. Such responsibilities included raising grandchildren or putting the needs of other family members ahead of their own
needs. Consequently, these study participants dropped out and became
inactive once again. Other factors that contributed to participants' inactivity included lack of social support, such as a friend with whom to exercise,
lack of encouragement from a friend, and even the presence of friends who
discredited exercise in favor of other activities, such as going out to eat. The
primary factor that stimulated the Hispanic women to initiate and sustain
their walking was the development of a *gran amiga*, or special friend. Once
special friends were selected, these women became *comadres;* they provided
each other with consistent encouragement to care for themselves and to
promote better health through a planned walking program. Content analysis of the focus group debriefings showed an interesting aspect of *familia
de selección* (selecting the family). The study participants clearly perceived
family obligations to be the primary barrier to the maintenance of regular
physical activity. Yet, paradoxically, these women acknowledged that they
could provide adequate care for their families only if they themselves were
in good health. The women recognized that an increase in regular physical
activity was essential to improved health status.

More cultural-contextual work has been conducted by our research
team. A second study, reported elsewhere (Keller, Fleury, & Perez, 2006),
was conducted to learn more about social-contextual resources and supports for physical activity using photo-elicitation methods. We employed
visual methods, a unique qualitative perspective and approach to data generation to explore the cultural, social, and contextual factors that influence
physical activity (PA) among Hispanic women. The photo-elicitation study
involved a select number of photographs of their physical activity produced
by the participants and used to stimulate interview dialogue. We believe
that the type of physical activity in which Hispanic women engage is both
personally and culturally relevant and is deeply ingrained in life context,
reflecting developmental milestones (marriage and childbirth, divorce), and
embedded in daily activities such as multiple jobs, often with varied shift
work or postretirement volunteer work. We requested the women to record
the ways in which they participated in physical activity, with attention to
factors that made staying active easier or more difficult. Physical activity
was defined by the women themselves, which included moderate-intensity
walking, housekeeping, dancing, playing with the dog, and gardening. Individual qualitative interviews were then conducted and audiotaped, drawing
upon the participant photographs. The photographs were used to elicit the

type, relevance, and meaning of cultural, social, or contextual factors that influenced PA.

We learned more about participant retention and treatment adherence to walking from these study participants. The women talked about the lack of access to health fitness opportunities: "I would like to go to the gym, do a little bit of gym, like that—but since one does not have the possibilities, well, one does not." Instead, the women exercised at shopping malls, walking to and from grocery stores, on children's field trips, and within local casinos (Fleury, Keller, & Perez, in press). We learned that adapting intervention strategies could capitalize on these exercise opportunities. Often, differences in customs surrounding physical activity between the United States and Mexico were mentioned. Older women reported this regarding cultural influences: "When a Hispanic woman gets to be 50 or 55, they just sit and that is it. They sit and watch TV because life is over." And for younger women, walking in public places, particularly to "exercise" was frowned upon: "Well, it's because the husband doesn't want them to [participate in PA]. They don't want them to go out. They are raising children or babies. And so then they give that a priority" (Fleury, Keller, & Perez, in press).

Data indicate that close attention to cultural mores, norms, and values, as well as family inclusion in the intervention design, may enhance protocol adherence and reduce dropout. Attention to what Hispanic women say about aspects of their culture and ethnic affiliation can influence continued participation in our research interventions.

Formation of a Women's Prosumer Group

Overwhelming evidence gained from our research, and from our debriefings and individual and group work with Hispanic women, shows that these women are anxious to take charge of their health, so we formed a prosumer group to advise us on the design of the interventions and to explore intervention adherence strategies. The prosumer concept is credited to Alvin Toffler (1980). Toffler predicted that, in the future, there would be a process whereby the consumer and the producer worked together to create the *prosumer* (Dignam, 2002). Prosumerism works when the consumer "customizes" the product, and this is evident in products offered by Nike, Proctor & Gamble, and even Wikipedia. The consumer of the product or service provides significant input to the product producer to make the product usable, tailored, and relevant to their needs (Tsai, 2002). Hispanic women are the consumers of products, and physical activity is our product. Marketing of the product design (intervention) is best engineered by the consumers, Hispanic women. With this concept in mind, we invited Hispanic women who were interested in PA to join us formally in discussion and strategy development to guide our intervention design.

It must be noted that this effort is distinct from the participatory action research (PAR) method. The PAR method employs communities to define a problem, focusing on the process of community empowerment to resolve community-defined problems. This method is detailed elsewhere and the subject of elegant exemplars in published reports (Minkler & Wallerstein, 2003; Kim et al., 2005). Our efforts in forming a prosumer group were threefold and designed to explore and inform intervention protocols by (1) capturing the experiences of women who engaged in physical activity as useful advice in adherence and motivation strategies, (2) sharing the experiences of Hispanic women who lived in neighborhoods where our walking interventions take place for safety, motivation, and opportunity, and (3) employing these Hispanic women as resources who would serve as leaders in modeling walking and be core personnel in participant-driven sampling. We are currently conducting monthly *prosumer mujeres* (women prosumers) focus group meetings to elicit further information from these women, in their communities and neighborhoods, that will be beneficial to us as we design interventions that include walking for Hispanic women.

LESSONS LEARNED

Poor self-perceptions of health, perceived discrimination in health matters, the stressors linked with migration and acculturation, and the complexity of these links with health behavior are not well understood by minority women, and by Hispanic women in particular. Such stressors include the strain of multiple roles, child or parent care, multiple jobs owing to financial needs, along with low-income earning capacity. Women's health in relation to multiple roles, coupled with workforce obligations, has been well researched. Reports show that for low-income work roles, there is a negative impact on health, and for higher-status employment, work roles influence health positively, which should be the core of designing culturally specific interventions and adherence strategies (Arredondo, Elder, Ayala, & Campbell, 2005; Castro & Alarcón, 2002; Hunt & de Voogd, 2005; Verbrugge, 1983).

Our work with Hispanic women has shown that strong cultural ties greatly influence women's behavior. Both our qualitative work and our postintervention debriefing work showed that the attitudes and ideologies of the culture influence physical activity as part of customs, celebrations, and gathering of friends and families. In our work, we discovered that women's family obligations were a significant barrier to physical activity (Fleury et al., in press; Gonzales & Keller, 2004; Keller, Fleury, & Rivera, 2007). For a few women, multiple jobs and tasks contributed to exhaustion and failure to engage in physical activity. We learned from our cultural-contextual work that adapting intervention strategies could capitalize on exercise opportunities, as well as provide opportunities to relearn exercise habits that would give satisfaction. We learned from our *prosumer mujeres* that specific women, from specific neighborhoods, can address the issues surrounding the structure of an intervention, as well as retention and adherence strategies.

TO READ FURTHER

Keller, C., Gonzales, A., & Fleuriet, J. (2005). Retention of minorities in community based interventions. *Western Journal of Nursing Research, 27,* 292–306.

This report discusses how subject characteristics are assessed to enhance retention of minority participants in research.

Jones, K. M., Gray, A. H., Paleo, J., Bramen, C. J., & Lesser, J. (2008). Community and scholars unifying for recovery. *Issues in Mental Health Nursing, 29,* 495–503.

This article reports the use of a prosumer recovery group interacting with faculty to engage in research collaboration.

REFERENCES

Arredondo, E. M., Elder, J. P., Ayala, G. X., & Campbell, N. R. (2005). Is church attendance associated with Latinas' health practices and self-reported health? *American Journal of Health Behavior, 29,* 502–511.

Castro, F. G., & Alarcón, E. (2002). Integrating cultural variables into drug abuse prevention and treatment with racial/ethnic minorities. *Journal of Drug Issues, 32,* 783–810.

Centers for Disease Control and Prevention. (2006). *Health, United States, 2006 with chartbook on trends in the health of Americans.* Available at *www.cdc.gov/nchs/hus.htm.*

Crespo, C. J., Smit, E., Andersen, R. E., Carter-Pokras, O., & Ainsworth, B. E. (2000). Race/ethnicity, social class and their relation to physical inactivity during leisure time: Results from the third national health and nutrition examination survey, 1988–1994. *American Journal of Preventive Medicine, 18,* 46–53.

Dignam, C. (2002). Prosumer power. *Marketing, 14,* 24–25.

Fleury, J., Keller, C., & Perez, A. (in press). Exploring resources for physical activity in Hispanic women. *Qualitative Health Research.*

Gonzales, A., & Keller, C. (2004). *Mi familia viene primero* (My family comes first): Physical activity issues in older Mexican American women. *Southern Online Journal of Nursing Research, 5,* 21.

Hunt, L. M., & de Voogd, K. B. (2005). Clinical myths of the cultural "other": Implications for Latino patient care. *Academic Medicine, 80,* 918–924.

Keller, C., Fleury, J., & Perez, A. (2006). Diet and physical activity in Hispanic women. *Communicating Nursing Research*. Proceedings of the Western Institute of Nursing Annual Conference, Portland, OR.

Keller, C., Fleury, J., & Rivera, A. (2007). *Dieta en mujeres Americanas Mexicanas* (Diet in Mexican American women). *Western Journal of Nursing Research, 29*, 758–773.

Keller, C., & Gonzales-Cantu, A. (2008). *Camina por salud:* Walking in Mexican American women. *Applied Nursing Research, 21*(2), 110–113.

Keller, C., & Trevino, R. P. (2001). Effects of two frequencies of walking on cardiovascular risk factor reduction in Mexican American women. *Research in Nursing and Health, 24*, 390–401.

Kim, S., Flaskerud, J. H., Koniak-Griffin, D., & Dixon, E. L. (2005). Using community-partnered participatory research to address health disparities in a Latino community. *Journal of Professional Nursing, 21*, 199–209.

King, A. C., Castro, C., Wilcox, S., Eyler, A. A., Sallis, J. F., & Brownson, R. C. (2000). Personal and environmental factors associated with physical inactivity among different racial-ethnic groups of U.S. middle-aged and older-aged women. *Health Psychology, 19*, 354–364.

Minkler M., & Wallerstein, N. (Eds.). (2003). *Community-based participatory research for health*. San Francisco: Jossey-Bass.

Toffler, A. (1980). *The third wave*. New York: William Morrow.

Tsai, A. (2002). The experiences of a "prosumer." *Psychiatric Rehabilitation Journal, 26*, 206–207.

Verbrugge, L. M. (1983). Multiple roles and physical health of women and men. *Journal of Health and Social Behavior, 24*, 16–30.

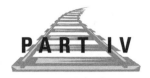

PART IV

STUDY IMPLEMENTATION

Implementing a study is probably its most rewarding, yet most critical, step. The validity of the conclusions, especially in treatment and evaluation studies, depends on delivering the intervention as originally designed, the adherence of the participants—both the providers and the recipients—to the regimen, and preventing contamination and of co-intervention (that is, not having those in the comparison group get the treatment or any "compensatory" treatment). However, the complexity of the real world may limit the investigators' control over the situation and compromise the validity of the study.

Sidani and colleagues (Chapter 19) and van Reekum (Chapter 23) report on challenges encountered when delivering experimental and comparison interventions. In the former, although the intervention was designed on the basis of sound theoretical and empirical evidence, it could not be implemented as planned; it had to be modified to fit the constraints of the practice setting. Van Reekum describes his odyssey in the journey to obtain placebo medications from a drug company. The journey did not have a happy ending and the study did not get off the ground.

Staff involvement at the study site can also present challenges. Many staff members have different experiences and perspectives about the interventions, which affect their willingness to participate, as reported by Cinà and Clase (Chapter 20). In Norman's case (Chapter 21), medical students did not participate in a trial because they viewed the intervention as more cumbersome than the comparison condition. As Filion and Johnston (Chapter 22) found out, the staff's appraisal of the experimental treatment and its benefits influenced their adherence to the protocol to which their patients were randomly assigned, and they worked to provide patients with what they saw as the most beneficial treatment, ignoring the study allocation.

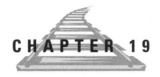

CHAPTER 19

When a Beautiful Intervention Meets Ugly Reality

Implementing an Intervention in the Real World

SOURAYA SIDANI
DAVID L. STREINER
CHANTALE MARIE LECLERC

BACKGROUND OF THE STUDY

Interventions are designed to address the clinical problems of people with various physical and psychosocial conditions. They can be developed from relevant theories underlying our understanding of the condition (e.g., theory of uncertainty in illness), from relevant therapeutic approaches (e.g., cognitive-behavioral), or from a combination of both. New interventions are often carefully planned to ensure optimal implementation of all components, with the most appropriate mode of delivery, and at the right dose or amount required to achieve the intended outcomes. The life cycle of new interventions consists of two main stages, efficacy and effectiveness, before using them in day-to-day practice (Streiner, 2002). In the *efficacy* stage, the intervention is tested under the ideal or best conditions, which include intensive training of staff in implementing the intervention, exactly as planned and in a consistent way, to participants selected on the basis of restrictive eligibility criteria. Interventions that successfully pass this rigorous test then go on to the second stage, which is concerned with examining their *effectiveness*. In this stage, interventions are evaluated in the real-world conditions of day-to-day practice—that is, the actual circumstances under which they will ultimately be delivered (Whitemore & Grey, 2002). Could the interventions be replicated, as originally planned, in effectiveness research? This is what we tried to answer in our trial.

About the Intervention

Dementia is associated with a decrease or loss of abilities needed to carry out daily functions. Persons with dementia living in long-term care institutions require assistance with their personal care, which includes bathing, grooming, dressing, and toileting, usually given in the morning between 7:00 A.M. and 11:00 A.M. During this episode of care, about 86% of persons with dementia exhibit agitation (Sloane et al., 2004). Although the exact reason for agitation is not clear, this disruptive behavior has negative consequences. Agitated persons pose a threat to themselves and to other people living in the institution, are at risk for falls or injury, and often suffer the adverse physical and psychosocial effects of medications used to minimize agitation during personal morning care (Beck et al., 2002).

It has been suggested that the abilities-focused approach to morning care can reduce agitation during morning care in this population. The principle underlying this approach entails respecting persons' abilities and promoting their engagement in activities of daily living, including personal care. It involves using interpersonal interactions to understand the persons' needs and retained abilities, assisting them in performing activities of daily living by using prompts that range in strength from verbal to manual guidance, and creating a pleasant environment, such as by using music (Wells & Dawson, 2000). The selection of appropriate prompts is guided by the individual person's identified needs and abilities.

The effects of specific abilities-focused interventions on relevant outcomes have been looked at in several studies (Lim, 2003; Sloane et al., 2004; Tappen, 1994; Wells, Dawson, Sidani, Craig, & Pringle, 2000). The results of these studies support their efficacy in maintaining the functioning of institutionalized persons with dementia and in reducing agitation during personal morning care. However, the interventions were delivered by highly trained research staff in most studies, or by nursing staff in one study (Wells et al., 2000); that is, they were all efficacy trials. In the Wells et al.'s study, the training consisted of interactive group educational sessions complemented by individual coaching at the bedside. The five sessions involved presenting pertinent content, group discussion, and case study exercises. The bedside coaching entailed discussing problems or concerns the staff encountered when using the interventions in daily practice. This intensive training was consistent with principles of adult learning and was effective in enhancing the staff's knowledge and use of interventions in day-to-day practice, and subsequently in preventing worsening in the functioning and agitation of persons with dementia. The success of this training led us to use it to develop the training program to look at the effectiveness of the abilities-focused approach to morning care.

Study Plan

The study was designed to determine the generalizability and the robustness of the abilities-focused approach in producing the desired outcomes, when delivered by nursing staff to persons with dementia living in several institutions. The plan was to instruct staff members in the use of abilities-focused interventions, to monitor their implementation of interventions in day-to-day practice, and to evaluate the effects of interventions on the functioning and agitation of persons with dementia during personal morning care.

To replicate the training program found effective by Wells et al. (2000), we followed a train-the-trainer model. With this model, we offered a workshop to train advanced practitioners (nurses with a master's degree) who specialized in the care of those with dementia in the abilities-focused interventions. The practitioners were to be responsible for training nursing staff at the various institutions that participated in the study. Staff training included the two components designed by Wells and her colleagues (2000): interactive group educational sessions and individual coaching at the bedside. The educational sessions focused on instructing staff in (1) the effects of dementia on self-care abilities, with an emphasis that some abilities are retained, (2) the specific abilities-focused interventions that could maintain the retained abilities, (3) principles for selecting the appropriate interventions that are consistent with the individual's retained abilities, and (4) the advantages of using the interventions to people with dementia and the nursing staff. The plan was to offer the educational content in five 20-minute sessions, using a number of educational strategies, such as formal discussion, case study exercises, and role play, to actively engage the nurses in learning. In addition, the nurses were informed of the availability of the advanced practitioners for individual consultations related to the application of the abilities-focused interventions in daily practice and, to reinforce learning, were given written material that summarized the steps for implementing these interventions for future reference. Further, we incorporated three strategies that served as incentives for the nurses' attendance at the educational sessions. First, the sessions were offered at various times (e.g., 11:00 A.M. or 2:00 P.M.) that were convenient for staff members working different shifts. Second, refreshments were offered at each session. Third, each staff member who attended the sessions was given a certificate of completion of the abilities-focused training program.

We carefully planned the training program to ensure that it was delivered as originally designed. However, organizational factors prevented the advanced practitioners from offering the educational content as designed.

THE CHALLENGES

As planned, the five 20-minute sessions were to be offered over a 5 week period, one session a week, repeated at various times to reach all unit staff members who consented to participate. Providing the sessions required the endorsement and assistance of the unit managers in relieving nursing staff members from their bedside duties to attend the sessions. That is, the managers had to ensure that a sufficient number of staff members remained to cover the needs of the patients on the unit while other staff members attended each session. During our consultations with the managers, it turned out that the planned schedule was unrealistic, given the financial and human resources constraints. The managers explained that it was neither possible nor efficient to find replacements for several staff members to cover 20-minute absences from the unit on five different occasions. Furthermore, it would be difficult to allow several staff members to attend the sessions at a given time, owing to the limited number of staff members on the unit. In addition, because of scheduling practices and the requirements of shift work, it would have been a scheduling nightmare to ensure that all staff members enrolled in the study participated in all five sessions over the course of several weeks.

OVERCOMING THE DIFFICULTIES

We discussed alternative schedules for giving the educational content with the unit managers. They recommended providing it in one session lasting 1½ hours. In this way, it would be easier and more cost-effective to bring in additional staff to cover for those attending the session. We followed the unit managers' recommendation and the educational intervention was given in one session of 1½ to 2 hours. Although realistic and practical, giving the educational content in one long session may not have facilitated effective learning: Staff members may not have had enough time to absorb all the new information, and to have opportunities to practice their newly acquired knowledge in between weekly sessions as originally planned. Such practical experiences could have both reinforced learning and formed the basis for further discussion about issues related to applying the interventions. Offering the two additional components of training, individual coaching and written material, could have offset to some extent the limitations of having only one educational session. This was suggested by the finding that the average number of abilities-focused interventions that staff members used when providing personal care increased from pre- to posttraining. However, this increase was not maintained at the 3-month follow-up. It appears that the modified implementation of the training program was successful in prompting nurses to use the interventions but did not contribute to the sustainability of the observed effects.

LESSONS LEARNED

Implementing interventions with demonstrated efficacy under the real-world conditions of day-to-day practice is not a simple task. Such interventions are designed for optimal effects and should be carefully delivered to achieve the beneficial outcomes. Although the controlled research environment supports implementing interventions as originally planned, from financial, human resources, and time perspectives, the practice environment does not have this luxury. The transferability and applicability of interventions to practice is at stake.

Two strategies could be useful in this situation. First, researchers conducting clinical effectiveness studies involving staff members could consider earmarking funds to replace members of the staff so that they can be free to participate in training, carry out the intervention, and perform other research activities (e.g., data collection, in some situations). This would also lessen staff members' perception that research studies increase their workload and can minimize their dilemma of balancing the requirements of generating new knowledge with the provision of care. If funding agencies do not approve such requests, researchers may want to try the strategy we used. It involved collaboration with key stakeholder groups in the practice setting, such as unit managers or practitioners, before implementing the intervention. The collaboration aims at finding a compromise that maintains fidelity of delivering the intervention, at the same time ensuring suitability to the setting. Researchers and stakeholder groups should work together to develop a common understanding of the theoretical underpinnings of the intervention, analyze logistical issues that interfere with providing it as planned, explore possible solutions to address these issues, or to suggest modifications in delivery of the intervention. These modifications can be made in the nonspecific, but not in the active, elements of the intervention. The active elements are the essential ingredients of the intervention that are hypothesized to bring about the intended effects. The nonspecific elements are factors that naturally accompany the intervention implementation; they are theoretically inert and not hypothesized to produce the expected outcomes (Bowers & Clum, 1988). Offering interventions that are convenient and fit the constraints of the practice setting may increase the likelihood of their adoption.

TO READ FURTHER

Streiner, D. L. (2002). The 2 "Es" of research: Efficacy and effectiveness trials. *Canadian Journal of Psychiatry, 47,* 552–556.
Whittemore, R., & Grey, M. (2002). The systematic development of nursing interventions. *Journal of Nursing Scholarship, 34,* 115–120.

These two articles clarify the distinction between an efficacy and an effectiveness study, both aimed at delineating an intervention's impact on intended outcomes. Efficacy trials look at whether the intervention *can* work, so everything is done to maximize the effect. Effectiveness studies are done within the real world of day-to-day practice, where the intervention is delivered by various clinicians to persons with diverse backgrounds. These features are associated with limited control (which is a characteristic of efficacy studies), which has implications for the design and conduct of the study in a way that accounts for the naturally occurring variability and possible challenges in study execution.

REFERENCES

Beck, C. K., Vogelpohl, T. S., Rasin, J. H., Uriri, J. T., O'Sullivan, P., Walls, R., et al. (2002). Effects of behavioral interventions on disruptive behavior and affect in demented nursing home residents. *Nursing Research, 51,* 219–228.
Bowers, T. G., & Clum, G. A. (1988). Relative contribution of specific and nonspecific treatment effects: Meta-analysis of placebo controlled behavior therapy research. *Psychological Bulletin, 103,* 315–323.
Lim, Y. M. (2003). Nursing intervention for grooming of elders with mild cognitive impairments in Korea. *Geriatric Nursing, 24,* 11–15.
Sloane, P. D., Hoeffer, B., Mitchell, M., McKenzie, D. A., Barrick, A. L., Rader, J., et al. (2004). Effect of person-centered showering and the towel bath on bathing-associated aggression, agitation, and discomfort in nursing home residents with dementia: A randomized, controlled trial. *Journal of the American Geriatrics Society, 52,* 1795–1804.
Streiner, D. L. (2002). The 2 "Es" of research: Efficacy and effectiveness trials. *Canadian Journal of Psychiatry, 47,* 552–556.
Tappen, R. (1994). The effect of skill training on functional abilities of nursing home residents with dementia. *Research in Nursing and Health, 17,* 159–165.
Wells, D. L., & Dawson, P. (2000). Description of retained abilities in older persons with dementia. *Research in Nursing and Health, 23,* 158–166.
Wells, D. L., Dawson, P., Sidani, S., Craig, D., & Pringle, D. (2000). Effects of an abilities-focused program of morning care on residents who have dementia and on caregivers. *Journal of the American Geriatrics Society, 48,* 442–449.
Whittemore, R., & Grey, M. (2002). The systematic development of nursing interventions. *Journal of Nursing Scholarship, 34,* 115–120.

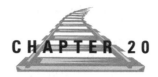

CHAPTER 20

When Saving Blood Goes Wrong

CLAUDIO S. CINÀ
CATHERINE M. CLASE

BACKGROUND OF THE STUDY

Surgery requiring replacement of the thoracic and abdominal aorta (the major artery coming from the heart) is a highly invasive procedure associated with major blood loss, often exceeding the patient's total blood volume. Further, there are often complicated bleeding problems during and after surgery (Fernandez, MacSween, You, & Gorelick, 1992; Oba et al., 1995; Aramoto, Shigematsu, & Muto, 1994), necessitating large volume transfusion of blood products (a median 50–60 units, in which a unit is the amount donated by a volunteer at a single session, which varies from 150 to 300 mL; Cinà & Bruin, 1999; Svensson, Crawford, Hess, Coselli, & Safi, 1993). Massive blood loss and the transfusion of large amounts of stored blood products can lead to bacterial and viral infections, as well as the inability of blood to clot (called coagulopathy) and hemorrhage. Of patients who die following this procedure, bleeding is responsible in 12 to 38% of the cases (Janusz, 1994; Gilling-Smith & Mansfield, 1995; Gilling-Smith, Worswick, Knight, Wolfe, & Mansfield, 1995) and frequently is the consequence of severe coagulopathy, rather than technical problems.

There is a debate in the literature regarding the effect of diluting the blood by infusing nonblood solutions but maintaining the same total blood volume (acute normovolemic hemodilution [ANH]) as an intervention to reduce blood losses and improve coagulation. ANH is a technique used by anesthesiologists. Immediately before or soon after induction of anesthesia, blood is removed from the patient's vein, stored in bags during surgery, and retransfused as indicated during or soon after the surgical procedure. During the blood collection process, crystalloids or colloids (acellular fluids) are infused in order to maintain the blood volume. This leads to dilution of the blood circulating in the patient (Stehling & Zauder, 1991).

Two systematic reviews (Bryson, Laupacis, & Wells, 1998; Loubser & Dejuan, 1998) suggested that ANH has the potential to reduce transfusion of red blood cells, but they did not address the impact on coagulation parameters and the use of blood products other than red blood cells. In addition, the conclusions from these studies were limited because of issues with inclusion and exclusion criteria of the studies that were evaluated, heterogeneity of the findings, the quality of studies, and a lack of an established protocol to define when to administer blood transfusion.

We hypothesized that the benefits of this technique might be greatest when large volumes of blood were obtained with ANH, and that the reinfusion of the patient's own whole blood would have a beneficial effect on the capability of the blood to clot beyond what could be achieved with blood product transfusion and the use of drugs (Cinà, Clase, & Bruin, 2000). This beneficial effect would be due to preservation of intact coagulation factors and inhibitors of thrombolysis, which may directly promote or inhibit coagulation.

THE CHALLENGES

One of the anesthetists in our group was particularly interested not only in the type of surgery but also in the possibility of reducing blood transfusions and improving hemostasis (the physiological processes that stop bleeding). To test the feasibility of our hypothesis with this anesthetist, we began a prospective, nonrandomized, historically controlled study of the effect of ANH in patients undergoing replacement of the thoracic and abdominal aorta (Cinà et al., 2000). We saw a clinically and statistically significant reduction in the total number of units of blood products transfused in the ANH-treated group as compared with controls (30 vs. 68 units). The ANH group received fewer transfusions of platelets (8 vs. 22 units) and of blood components aiming at improving the patient's capability to clot during surgery. Drugs that promote clotting were also used in a smaller proportion of patients (0 of 7 vs. 4 of 15 patients). Postoperatively, APTT (activated partial thromboplastin time, a measure of how quickly blood clots) values were less prolonged (26 vs. 34 seconds) and the number of platelets (cellular fragments that promote clotting) in patients' blood was higher in the ANH group than in controls.

Armed with the theoretical construct of the possible benefits of ANH and the results of the feasibility study, we proposed a randomized controlled trial (RCT) comparing ANH with standard transfusion management in 110 patients undergoing repair of thoracic or thoracoabdominal aortic aneurysms (bulges on the aorta that can break, with possibly fatal consequences). The two of us (with specialties in internal medicine, vascular surgery, and methodology) were the principal investigators, and we recruited the help of a hematologist with a particular interest in coagulation disorders as a co-investigator. We aimed to compare total intra- and postoperative blood product use in the two groups.

This study had the potential to reduce blood product use in a population whose current transfusion requirements are extraordinarily high. If our hypothesis was correct, and we were able to show a reduction of 25% in the use of blood products as suggested by our pilot study, this would have been immediately generalizable to other centers that perform this surgery. The intervention was simple, requiring only the inexpensive bags used to collect blood as additional equipment. Considering that approximately 100 to 150 such operations are carried out annually in Canada, the potential reduction in blood products transfused annually in Canada was 1700 – 2550 units, translating into savings of $272,000 to $408,000.

(NOT) OVERCOMING THE DIFFICULTIES

We know that surgical trials are often difficult. We solicited the opinion of leaders in vascular surgery and in transfusion medicine, which showed that the project was regarded as clinically important by both groups. We also discussed and circulated our proposal with other surgeons with interest in this surgery and enrolled two other centers. We designed a study with control and intervention arms in which transfusion strategies were carefully carried out using a written protocol, derived from all available evidence and consensus statements available at the time. The protocol included transfusion during surgery, at the end of surgery, and in the postoperative period in the intensive care unit. We soon became aware that in the management of these patients, although the number of surgeons could be limited (likely a maximum of three, who in addition could work together during the surgery to standardize other interventions that may be required), a very large number of other individuals were involved, providing anesthesia and intensive care. All of them had different traditions, experience, interpretation of the available evidence, and ideas about transfusion in these settings.

In addition, our pilot study was conducted in the late 1990s and published in 2001, whereas the randomized controlled study was supposed to start in 2005. During that time, another intervention aimed at improving coagulation during surgery became available (Factor VII concentrates; DiDomenico, Massad, Kpodonu, Navarro, & Geha, 2005; Boffard et al., 2005). This was another variable that needed to be accounted for in our study—should its use follow a strict protocol, be excluded, or given at the discretion of the anesthetists? This further multiplied the number of reasonable differing opinions.

Now having our available evidence and a detailed draft operational manual, we began meeting with the several anesthetists and specialists in intensive care who would have been involved in the study. In spite of the evidence that we presented, the providers of the intervention to be studied (anesthetists) and the individuals involved in following the transfusion protocols (during surgery and in intensive care) did not feel that they could follow the study design because of concerns with the transfusion strategies and the protocols we suggested. The RCT did not get off the ground.

LESSONS LEARNED

In theory there is no difference between theory and practice. In practice, there is.
—Yogi Berra

1. Research on topics involving collaboration among different disciplines (e.g., surgeons, anesthetists, intensivists) requires careful planning to obtain buy-in of all involved. Early involvement of other disciplines before developing the protocol may facilitate this.

2. For technical or complex interventions, each participating center needs at least one credible opinion leader who is committed to both following the protocol (once agreed on) and the idea of a trial.

3. It is probably a good idea to have direct input from at least one person from each discipline, with these contributors as investigators (rather than collaborators) in the grant proposal.

4. Testing any innovative strategy, such as surgery, may be subject to changes in the strategy itself (as evolution of knowledge occurs) or in the equipoise (the state of uncertainty regarding the risks and benefit of an intervention) of providers and subjects involved in the research project.

5. Even a good idea tested in a pilot study may not succeed when applied to an RCT.

6. The pilot study and the RCT need to be temporally close to avoid changes based on new research or nonevidence-based shifts in practice.

TO READ FURTHER

McCulloch, P., Taylor, I., Sasako, M., Lovett, B., & Griffin, D. (2002). Randomised trials in surgery: Problems and possible solutions. *British Medical Journal, 324*, 1448–1451.

In RCTs, committed buy-in from all clinicians is essential. Although most may seem willing to participate, in practice individuals may be unwilling to comply with the protocol or to enroll participants in the study. In addition, rare conditions cause difficulties with recruitment, consent, and randomization. This article gives some suggestions about overcoming these problems.

Weinberger, M., Murray, M. D., Marrero, D. G., Brewer, N., Lykens, M., Harris, L. E., et al. (2002). Issues in conducting randomized controlled trials of health services research interventions in nonacademic practice settings: The case of retail pharmacies. *Health Services Research, 37*, 1067–1077.

This article addresses the issues faced in conducting RCTs in nonacademic settings and possible solutions.

REFERENCES

Aramoto, H., Shigematsu, H., & Muto, T. (1995). Perioperative changes in coagulative and fibrinolytic function during surgical treatment of abdominal aortic aneurysm and arteriosclerosis obliterans. *International Journal of Cardiology, 47*(Suppl. 1), S55–S63.

Boffard, K. D., Riou, B., Warren, B., Choong, P. I., Rizoli, S., Rossaint, R., et al. (2005). Recombinant factor VIIa as adjunctive therapy for bleeding control in severely injured trauma patients: Two parallel randomized, placebo-controlled, double-blind clinical trials. *Journal of Trauma, 59*, 8–15.

Bryson, G. L., Laupacis, A., & Wells, G. A. (1998). Does acute normovolemic hemodilution reduce perioperative allogenic transfusions: A meta-analysis. *Anesthesia and Analgesia, 86*, 9–15.

Cinà, C. S., & Bruin, G. (1999). Acute normovolemic hemodilution (ANH) in surgery of the thoracoabdominal aorta: A cohort study to evaluate coagulation parameters and blood product utilization. *Journal of Cardiovascular Surgery, 40*, 37–43.

Cinà, C. S., Clase, C. M., & Bruin, G. (2000). Effects of acute normovolaemic haemodilution and partial exchange transfusion on blood product utilization, haemostasis and haemodynamics in surgery of the thoracoabdominal aorta. A cohort study in consecutive patients. *Panminerva Medica, 42*, 211–215.

DiDomenico, R. J., Massad, M. G., Kpodonu, J., Navarro, R. A., & Geha, A. S. (2005). Use of recombinant activated factor VII for bleeding following operations requiring cardiopulmonary bypass. *Chest, 127*, 1828–1835.

Fernandez, L. A., MacSween, J. M., You, C. K., & Gorelick, M. (1992). Immunologic changes after blood transfusion in patients undergoing vascular surgery. *American Journal of Surgery, 163*, 263–269.

Gilling-Smith, G. L., & Mansfield, A. O. (1995). Thoracoabdominal aortic aneurysm. *British Journal of Surgery, 82*, 148–149.

Gilling-Smith, G. L., Worswick, L., Knight, P. F., Wolfe, J. H., & Mansfield, A. O. (1995). Surgical repair of thoracoabdominal aortic aneurysm: 10 years' experience. *British Journal of Surgery, 82*, 624–629.

Janusz, M. T. (1994). Experience with thoracoabdominal aortic aneurysm resection. *American Journal of Surgery, 167,* 501–504.

Loubser, P. G., & Dejuan, I. A. (1998). Effect of acute normovolemic hemodilution on allogeneic blood tranfusion during cardiac surgery: A meta-analysis. *Anesthesia and Analgesia 86*(4S), SCA21.

Oba, J., Shiiya, N., Matsui, Y., Goda, T., Sakuma, M., & Yasuda, K. (1995). Alterations in coagulation and fibrinolysis after surgery for aortic aneurysm. *Surgery Today, 25,* 532–535.

Stehling, L., & Zauder, H. L. (1991). Acute normovolemic hemodilution. *Transfusion, 31,* 857–868.

Svensson, L. G., Crawford, E. S., Hess, K. R., Coselli, J. S., & Safi, H. J. (1993). Experience with 1509 patients undergoing thoracoabdominal aortic operations. *Journal of Vascular Surgery, 17,* 357–368.

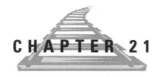

CHAPTER 21

PDA = Pretty Darned Awful
The Trials and Tribulations of Running Trials of PDAs

GEOFFREY R. NORMAN

BACKGROUND OF THE STUDY

Although the BlackBerry has pretty well monopolized the market for portable vest pocket digital thingies, there was a time not many years ago when PalmPilots were all the rage. Moreover, they appeared to have some particular advantages in educational settings. Students and teachers spend a lot of time filling out forms with ratings on 7-point scales—of teachers, of students, of other students, of learning resources, of libraries, of cafeterias, and on and on. Someone then has to enter these numbers into a spreadsheet so the multiple evaluations can be summarized and feedback provided. All too often, this never happens and the bits of paper languish in bottom drawers until the statute of limitations expires and they find their way into blue boxes or shredders. Imagine the appeal, then, of turning the primary data entry into digital form. Instead of dealing with all those bits of paper that then have to be copied, mailed, digitized, and analyzed, all one need do is plug the personal digital assistant (PDA) into a computer somewhere and send the file downstream by e-mail, and a spreadsheet program can then read the data, calculate means and medians or whatever, and send the results on to whoever needs them.

This technological revelation coincided with some developments in clinical education. Traditionally, medical students in clinical placements were assessed by a supervisor at the end of each placement (typically 4–8 weeks) with some kind of global rating; a piece of paper with anywhere from 5 to 25 categories such as "History-taking skills," "Communication skills,"

"Clinical reasoning," "Use of tests," "Responsibility," and 5- or 7-point scales with descriptors like "Poor" through "Excellent" or "Much below average" to "Much above average." These forms are ubiquitous; I have never met a medical school that did not use them. And they are commonplace in work settings everywhere. All this is despite the fact that evidence more than 20 years old showed repeatedly that (1) the interrater reliability of these ratings was awful, typically lower that .3, and (2) internal consistency was, conversely, far too high, typically .90 or more, showing that the raters were unable to distinguish between the categories (Streiner, 1985).

There were several reasons for this situation. Frequently, raters had minimal contact with the trainee, far too little to base an assessment on. In fact, in one unpublished study conducted in South Africa, the investigator mailed out rating forms, for assessing fictitious residents, to various clinical settings. Twenty percent of these were returned completed, and on these, 80% of residents were rated "above average." This highlights two other problems. First, even if the supervisor remembers a trainee, he or she may well not remember much in the way of specifics, except for particular incidents that were memorably good or awful, which is not a good basis for an overall assessment. Second, all of these factors conspire to ensure that raters will take the path of least resistance and simply rate everyone "above average." Indeed, our residency program had a policy for some time requiring that if a resident was rated "average" in anything, that person was called on the carpet, because he or she must be awful.

One solution to this problem was to do a series of small performance "biopsies," whereby the supervisor, after having an exchange with the trainee over some matter of patient care, would complete a brief form with only one to four scales. Over a period of time, these assessments would accumulate, and eventually the trainee would have 10 to 15 assessments. Studies showed that the average over these assessments was actually quite reliable (Turnbull, MacFayden, van Barneveld, & Norman, 2000).

These results were sufficiently encouraging that an approach called "Clinical Work Sampling" (CWS), was adopted in several clinical programs at McMaster University. In particular, the undergraduate medical program required each student to have 10 of these assessments completed for each rotation (pediatrics, obstetrics, medicine, surgery, etc.). In order to track all the assessments, the form was made into a multipart form, and every student carried one of them around with him or her. It was also adopted by the anesthesiology program, and the chair of anesthesiology, a techic (it goes with the territory) put the whole thing on a PalmPilot and gave one to each resident. In turn, the residents were required to complete a minimum number of assessments each year. He also hired a technician to do all the programming to summarize the scores and create a feedback form for each resident.

That approach seemed so promising that we decided to turn it into research. We put a proposal together that involved four residency programs—radiology and anesthesiology at McMaster and at another Ontario university. We were going to look at reliability and validity in each program. Dead simple—we already had 2 years' worth of data from anesthesiology, and the principal investigator at McMaster was the residency program director in radiology. And the program director was good friends with the program directors at the other university.

Well, the best laid plans of mice and men.... We got the funding, just about the same week that the anesthesia program chair decided precipitously to leave the academic game and go into private practice. Yet that was not a big issue, as we had 2 years' worth of archival data, or so we thought. However, the program chair put the data on his secretary's computer, and some time between the decision to write the grant and getting the money, her hard drive died, with no backup. And since the chair's departure, the department was no longer using PDAs. We still had the programs at University X, we thought. But they were just too gosh darn busy, so they too packed it in. Eventually, we managed to pull off a small study in the radiology residency program, and actually published it (Finlay, Norman, Stolberg, Weaver, & Keane, 2006). Nevertheless the grand thoughts of a multicenter trial were dashed on the rocky shores of reality.

However, that's not what this story is about. Like the losing gambler who just can't walk away from the slot machine, because he has put so much into it that it has to pay off soon, we went back and tried again—and failed again. But we're getting ahead of ourselves.

Remember all those multipart forms that were implemented in all the clinical rotations? Well, not surprisingly, they all got collected religiously in every rotation and put into files. And someone looked at them at some point. But no one ever set up the mechanism to have them entered into a spreadsheet so that means and standard deviations could be reported. It seemed an ideal opportunity to implement a PDA approach and give students really useful feedback. Further, we had colleagues in pediatrics and obstetrics/gynecology who were keen to pursue some educational research.

At about this time, a federal granting agency, the Medical Council of Canada, announced a special competition for research on the use of PDAs in clinical evaluation. It was a large sum of money, but there was one catch—it had to be a multicenter competition. However, even that was not an issue, as I had supervised a faculty member in obstetrics/gynecology at the University of Ottawa who had done a study of CWS, using phone-recorded assessments. Things were beginning to fall into place. We could do the study in pediatrics and obstetrics—both 6-week rotations and natural partners. We had a co-investigator in three of the four rotations, and we soon recruited a pediatrician at Ottawa to help out.

Things got better and better. It turned out that each rotation actually involved two hospitals, so we had the makings of a really neat randomized trial, with students at one hospital using paper and at the other using the PDA. We wrote the proposal and, soon after, received funding for a 3-year study. To ensure that we would not have any loose ends at the partner institution, the funding covered several trips to Ottawa to meet with the faculty and staff there. We even did surveys at both institutions to estimate how many students carried PalmPilots and how many we would have to have on hand to lend out; this too was built into the budget.

Once we received the funding, we were off and running. We received full ethics approval (after all, what harm can befall someone from carrying a PDA?). Of course, because this was a research project, students had to actively consent to be randomized into the paper or PDA arm. We foresaw that we might have trouble getting students to go along with the paper, particularly when we were offering them the loan of a brand new state-of-the-art PalmPilot, but this bridge would be crossed when we came to it.

Programming the Palms went smoothly. It was very clever; we even had the assessor sign his name onto the PDA and digitized the signature. Mind you, it was a bit awkward by the time we had screens to enter the ID of the student, the ID of the faculty members, the date, their PIN numbers, and so forth. But it was easy enough to understand, just took a bit more time.

We put together a PowerPoint show that would be used to introduce the study to students at the beginning of each rotation. We met with the program directors and made sure they were on board. We met with the administrators' secretaries to make sure they could put all the data into their computers. We devised websites to show students how to download the special software onto their PDAs.

THE CHALLENGES

And then we began. For the first rotation we presented the study during the orientation on the first day. All the students were present—attendance was required. The talk was well received, we think. We explained that this was a randomized trial of PDA versus paper for CWS assessments. All the students had to do was go to our website and download the special software into their PDAs and complete a consent form. If anyone didn't own a PalmPilot, we would lend one to him or her for the duration of the study. When the students were observed by a staff person or resident, they would get the observer to record his or her observations and comments on the PDA. Then when they had completed the prerequisite 10 forms, they would hot-synch the PDA to a computer and upload the data to our website. In return, they would receive quantitative feedback about their performances relative to their peers'.

At the first rotation, only a couple of students signed up to be in the study, so we improved the presentation, made sure that faculty talked up the study, and so on. At about this time, we began recruiting students from Ottawa; here the presentation was done by an administrative person who was in daily contact with students. But again, very few students stepped up to the plate. We kept up the charade for a few more rotations, but things never got much better. The horrible truth is shown in Table 21.1. Fewer than one-third of students agreed to participate, 6% went so far as to complete any evaluations, and 4% completed the full complement.

(NOT) OVERCOMING THE CHALLENGES

After considerable soul-searching, we pulled the plug on the study after 1 year, and sent the last 2 years of funding back to the agency. But to salvage something from the disaster, over the last few months of the study we systematically surveyed students; this time at least, the response was a bit better, at about 25%. Three-quarters of them owned a PDA, mostly a PalmPilot, although informally, we discovered that only about one in three owners had actually hot-synched it to a computer.

It was clear from the comments that the students recognized what we had missed. Despite the gloss of the new technology, it had more disadvantages than strengths. It took time to download the software and master the specifics of the program. It took time to go through all the identification pages for both student and supervisor (it was really like trying to do telephone banking, only worse), and it took time to explain the specifics to the supervisor. In contrast, an evaluation card could be whipped out and completed in seconds, or left with the supervisor for later completion. Further, students had lots of experience with other e-based systems and all the

TABLE 21.1. Number and Percent of Clerks Who Were Invited to Participate, Agreed to Participate, Uploaded Any CWS Records, and Completed the Study

	Invited	Agreed		Uploaded		Completed	
	N	N	%	N	%	N	%
School A	122	20	16	9	7	7	5
School B	54	32	59	2	4	0	0
Overall	176	52	29	11	6	7	4

Note. From Norman, Keane, and Oppenheimer (2008). Reproduced by permission of Taylor and Francis.

glitches that are routinely encountered along the way. Finally, about half the students were concerned that, given the less than optimal performance of such systems, there was a good chance that their data might be lost somewhere in cyberspace between the PDA and our computer; and this was a risk they were not prepared to take.

But all was not completely lost. The description of the failed study was published (Norman, Keane, & Oppenheimer, 2008).

LESSONS LEARNED

There are three lessons to be learned from the study. First is the technological lesson. All of us have experienced the frustrations that accompany attempts to master new digital technology. Perhaps we thought that students in this wired generation were more adept and more enamored of the technology than we were, and hence more likely to assume the small risk involved. If anything, the reverse is likely true. Students viewed the PDA, correctly, as a somewhat cumbersome and primitive technology whose small size had advantages in basic record keeping, such as for appointments, addresses, and activities. But even though two-thirds of them owned a PDA, most restricted the use to just these basic functions, recognizing that more advanced and special-purpose functions would require a much greater investment of time and effort, an investment that they were not prepared to make. And the liability of the technology in terms of questionable reliability was not something they were prepared to take on. So, as we should have known from the outset, there are times when technology does save labor and does justify an investment, but there are many other times, as we have all experienced, when technology simply creates obstacles. As the sage said, "Computers are labor-saving devices that increase work."

The second lesson is more universal. It is often far too easy to go from an idea to a grant proposal to a study without adequate time spent in actually understanding the context. If we had really reflected on the impact of dropping PDAs into the clerkship, or, better still, if we had spent some time talking to clerks about the idea, we would have easily seen that this was an idea whose time would never come. Over my research career, the studies that turned into horrors were those in which too little time was spent in really understanding the context.

The final lesson is still more universal. Even if the study had succeeded, it amounted to little more than a demonstration and could hardly qualify as good science. It had no theoretical underpinning and led nowhere. It was hardly the making of anything resembling a program of research. It might, perhaps, have shown that PDAs could replace paper, but within a year or two, as the technology went from Palm to BlackBerry, the study would have been quickly forgotten.

ACKNOWLEDGMENTS

I wish to thank the Medical Council of Canada for funding the original study; Drs. Lawrence Oppenheimer and David Keane for co-investigating the study; faculty and students from McMaster and Ottawa who participated in the study; and *Teaching and Learning in Medicine* for permission to reuse some of the materials from the journal article.

TO READ FURTHER

There are many articles about ethical research, informed consent, and the like. There are even some that talk about educational research specifically, and how sometimes research can be viewed as quality control and consent is not necessary, although generally they come down on the "better safe than sorry" side. But there are few or no resources we know of that state what you can do when informed consent scuppers the whole enterprise.

Callahan, C. A., Hojat, M., & Gonnella, J. S. (2007). Volunteer bias in medical education research: An empirical study of over three decades of longitudinal data. *Medical Education, 41,* 746–753.

A longitudinal follow-up study of graduates from Jefferson Medical School from 1970 to 2004. The 5,500 who granted permission and participated performed better in medical school and beyond than the 500 who did not.

Dauphinee, W. D., & Frecker, R. C. (2007). Routinely collected educational data: Challenges to ethics and to privacy. *Medical Education, 39,* 877–879.

This article deals with routinely collected educational performance data, such as exam scores. It argues that such data may be used for research without signed consent, as long as ethical standards are adhered to. It also raises the issue of privacy and confidentiality in educational data. But the purview is routinely collected data.

Eva, K. W. (2007). The yin and yang of education research. *Medical Education, 41,* 724–725.

Eva argues that all educational research should go through formal ethical review.

REFERENCES

Finlay, K., Norman, G., Stolberg, H., Weaver, B., & Keane, D. (2006). In-training evaluation using hand-held computerized clinical work sampling strategies in radiology residency. *Canadian Association of Radiology Journal, 57,* 232–237.

Norman, G. R., Keane, D. R., & Oppenheimer, L. (2008). An attempt to persuade medical clerks to use personal digital assistants to record in-training assessments. *Teaching and Learning in Medicine, 20,* 295–301.

Streiner, D. L. (1985). Global rating scales. In V. R. Neufeld & G. R. Norman (Eds.), *Assessing clinical competence* (pp. 119–141). New York: Springer.

Turnbull, J., MacFadyen, J., van Barneveld, C., & Norman, G. (2000). Clinical work sampling: A new approach to the problem of in-training evaluation. *Journal of General Internal Medicine, 15,* 556–561.

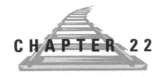

CHAPTER 22

When Sugar Is Not So Sweet
Camera Shyness and Intentional Cointervention Almost Derail a Study

FRANÇOISE FILION
C. CÉLESTE JOHNSTON

BACKGROUND OF THE STUDY

Pain in preterm neonates has been the focus of many studies in the past decade. It is still studied today as we know that pain management for this vulnerable group of infants continues to be problematic (Johnston, Collinge, Henderson, & Anand, 1997; Simons, van Dijk, Anand, Roofhooft, van Lingen, & Tibboel, 2003; Stevens et al., 2003; Johnston et al., 2008). Our main interest has been in nonpharmacological interventions for pain caused by various procedures during the preterm infant's stay in the neonatal intensive care unit (NICU). Most studies focus on the most common procedure, which is a heel lance to draw blood, looking at an older preterm population, and always as a *single* procedure. A number of studies have consistently shown the analgesic effect of 0.05 to 2 ml of orally administered sucrose (sugar water) for a single painful event (Stevens et al., 2003; Stevens, Yamada, & Ohlsson, 2004). We were interested to relieve *repeated* procedural pain with very low birth weight infants (those born at less than 1,500 grams) in the NICU. For a very premature infant, the number of painful events is more important during his or her first week of life. When the research protocol was written in 1995–1996, no other study had used sucrose repeatedly to decrease procedural pain in preterm infants. Therefore, we decided to use sucrose for every painful procedural event during the first week of life of preterm infants born at less than 32 weeks gestational age, looking at developmental, physiological, behavioral, and hormonal outcomes. The data from this research project were collected from 1997 to 2000, and the results were published in 2002 (Johnston et al., 2002).

To measure the effectiveness of a sucrose intervention, it is imperative to quantify pain in neonates. The measure that we and many others have used is the Premature Infant Pain Profile (PIPP; Stevens, Johnston, Petryshen, & Taddio, 1996), which includes both physiological indicators of pain—heart rate, oxygen saturation (the amount of oxygen in the blood)—and three facial actions. For research purposes, the physiological data are taken with a pulse oximeter that downloads the data to a computer for later analysis. A camera is used for coding of the three facial actions.

The primary outcome of this study was the evaluation of the development of the infant, which was measured with two subscales of the Neurobehavioral Assessment of the Preterm Infant (NAPI; Korner & Thom, 1990) at 32, 36, and 40 weeks of gestation. This measuring tool proposed seven subscales but we used only two, which were theoretically more relevant to the intervention: Motor Development and Vigor, and Alertness and Orientation.

The primary hypothesis of the study was that an infant's receiving sucrose for every painful procedure in the first week of life would improve developmental outcomes. Secondarily, we were interested in seeing if the sucrose remained analgesic over time, inasmuch as that had never been tested. The study design was a randomized, double-blind clinical trial (RCT). Only the research nurse knew the assignment of the infant as she prepared the syringes with the 0.1 ml of liquid (sterile water or 24% sucrose solution) with the label including the neonate's identification and date of preparation. No one caring for the infant or coding or analyzing the data knew the group assignment.

In order to verify that the infant received a syringe for every painful procedure, we wished to record all events that happened to the infant. We also proposed to videotape and record, second-by-second, the physiological data of heart rate and oxygen saturation each time the infant had a painful procedure carried out. The recording equipment we used combined a small camera placed on top of the infant's incubator and a pulse oximeter attached to the foot or hand of the infant, which tape-recorded in synchrony during the painful procedure. All the invasive events were included for the entire week of data collection, which included tissue-damaging procedures (e.g., heel lance, venipuncture, lumbar puncture) and non-tissue-damaging events, such as suctioning or chest physiotherapy.

In order to trigger the tape-recording in synchrony with the visual and physiological data, a device was installed, imbedded in a rubber carpet on the floor in front of the incubator. The carpet was 2 × 3 feet and as such was large enough that anyone interacting with the neonate, mostly parents or healthcare professionals, would be stepping on it.

A large lettered sign on the incubator provided instructions to anyone approaching the infant. The instructions were simple and straightforward: People had to identify themselves as soon as they stepped on the carpet and state why they were approaching the infant. Examples included mother, visiting baby; nurse, doing routine care; doctor, examining infant; physiotherapist, doing chest physiotherapy. We needed this information in order to verify how many procedures the infant had, who approached the infant, and whether the infant received the syringe of study solution by mouth. The camera focused only on the infant, and the sound was recorded for the identification of the person and the care given to the infant. The tape-recording lasted as long as the person was on the carpet and for 5 minutes more after he or she stepped away from the carpet. In this way, not only could we ensure the integrity of the study intervention for painful procedures, we could also score the infant's pain responses using the PIPP.

THE CHALLENGES

Camera Shy

Upon reviewing the videotapes, we realized that almost none of the healthcare professionals or parents identified themselves while approaching the infant. Furthermore, as the study progressed and the staff members became accustomed to the presence of the research nurse in the unit, many of them avoided the carpet by kicking it out of the way, under the incubator. When the carpet was subsequently secured on the floor in front of the incubator, we also witnessed many nurses avoiding stepping on the carpet by using the nonergonomic position of putting a foot on each side of it. We inquired why they did not like to step on the carpet; the answers were that they did not want to be tape-recorded during their care of the infant.

Overcoming the Difficulties

This problem was related to our data collection; without this tape-recorded visual and marking of the physiological data, we were missing vital information for the painful outcomes using the PIPP as our measuring tool, as well as being unable to verify if the infants were receiving the study protocol. As mentioned before, the PIPP is a multidimensional pain assessment tool whereby we need the visual aspect to measure three facial actions (brow bulge, cheek wrinkle caused by crying, and eye squeeze) and the state of the infant (quiet sleep, agitated sleep, quiet awake, crying). The PIPP also requires the physiological aspect of the data with heart rate and oxygen saturation in 30-second sequences.

The research nurse made a quick survey of the bedside nurses working during the day shift to discover more about their reluctance to use the carpet to trigger the data collection. The problems included the following: They did not want to be filmed themselves, they did not want anyone to watch them while they were giving care to the infant, they were concerned that the head nurse or the chief neonatologist would find mistakes or errors in their care, they did not want the researchers to know about their conversations unrelated to their infant care, or simply that they were not interested in this research project.

Following this anecdotal survey, the research nurse organized a meeting with the chief neonatologist, the head nurse, and the clinical nurse specialist of the unit to discuss different strategies to improve compliance in data collection for the research project. It was decided that the bedside nurses needed more information and education about the importance of following the research protocol, and about the methodology of randomized clinical trials, the consequences of a breach in protocol during data analysis, and the interpretation of results. Finally, it was important to emphasize the magnitude of their involvement in the research in order to improve the future care of very premature infants.

Various strategies were discussed; the main objective was to reach as many nurses as possible with the education/information sessions. The research nurse prepared three different sessions, none lasting more than 10 minutes. The research nurse met with only two or three nurses at a time and at the bedside of the infants for the three shifts (night, day, evening). The clinical nurse specialist provided appropriate time during each shift to talk to the nurses. In the first session, anecdotal comments were reviewed and validated with the nurses; the research nurse let the nurses express themselves and corrected their misconceptions. For the second session, the research nurse explained the design of the study in lay terms and how the design was linked to data collection, analysis, and interpretation. She gave many examples to facilitate an understanding of how researchers would not be able to generate appropriate conclusions if a research protocol was not followed. Finally, the last session gave positive feedback to the nurses and emphasized the importance of their participation to improve very premature infants' care.

These three sessions were not necessarily sequential; they were repeated as needed and to new staff. The head nurse and clinical nurse specialist also supported the action of the research nurse. There was some improvement: The research nurse did not see the carpet pushed under the infant's incubator; however, she still saw nurses straddling the carpet. It does not appear that the information/education and positive reinforcement strategy was effective enough to completely correct the data collection challenge.

Intentional Cointervention

As mentioned earlier, the design of the study was a randomized controlled trial; the intervention consisted of orally giving the preterm infant a solution of 24% sucrose, 0.1 ml placed in a small syringe (1 ml capacity). The control solution, in a similar syringe and with the same volume, consisted of sterile water. Several syringes were placed in a basket for each participating infant, identified by name, in the NICU's medication refrigerator.

The bedside nurses needed to retrieve the research solution from the refrigerator before performing any painful procedure on the infant under their care. This was not unusual for them, because all of their infants' medications were kept in the same refrigerator. The bedside nurses were also instructed to retrieve the research solution before any painful procedure performed by another health professional.

The active solution did not differ in color or volume from the control solution; however, the nurses intuitively knew how to distinguish between them by observing an infant's reaction: the sucrose solution relaxed the infant, or, when they were cleaning the infant's mouth, they saw that the sucrose solution was more viscous. To confirm their intuition, some nurses tasted the solution; this was reported to the research nurse by other bedside nurses.

The research nurse also found the wrong research solution, labeled for another included infant, on top of a participating infant's incubator. The mistaken solution found was the active solution, even though the infant had been randomized to the control solution. In this particular NICU, the research nurse observed low compliance when an infant had been randomized to the control solution.

Overcoming the Difficulties

The research nurse discussed this problem with the head nurse and clinical nurse specialist in an informal meeting. A short information and education session was coconducted with two or three bedside nurses at their incubators. The sessions lasted 10 to 15 minutes, explaining the RCT design and the rationale of the nurses keeping themselves and the research participant blinded to the active solution.

A second session stressed the difficulty in interpreting the results when the RCT was not blinded. The last session again promoted the positive aspects of data collection and gave constructive and encouraging feedback to the bedside nurses.

Another solution to the problem was suggested to the research nurse during her meetings with the bedside nurses: Better identify the solution for each participating baby. Each solution had a white label including the name and unit number of the infant and the date of preparation. It was decided to improve the labeling of each participant infant's solution by using the same information but with a label of a different color for each included infant; we ended up using very bright colored labels. Each basket for each infant was also identified with the same information and colored label. For a bedside nurse in a hurry, this eased the task of getting the infant's solution from the refrigerator.

The sucrose solution was not prepared under sterile conditions; this was the main reason that the syringes were kept in the refrigerator. However, the hospital's infection control person told us that the solution could be kept at room temperature for 4 hours. The research nurse suggested to the bedside nurses that they take four to six syringes at the beginning of their shifts, keep them at their incubators until lunchtime, and discard the solutions that were not used. They could repeat the same procedure after their lunch break. The proximity of the research solution was intended to ease compliance.

Better identifying a participant's research solution was a good decision; the research nurse did not see another case of mixed up solutions. However, the idea to increase access to the research solution by bringing the syringes to the incubator did not increase compliance more than 60%, compared with another research site in the same study which had a 100% compliance rate. Even with the education/information sessions tailored to this particular unit, compliance stayed below our expectations.

LESSONS LEARNED

This particular unit had a very high rate of nurse turnover; using bedside nurse champions could have disseminated the information regarding the protocol and data collection procedures in a more efficient way. The champions could have worked closely with the research nurse during the information/education sessions and given positive reinforcement targeted to specific bedside nurses.

Moreover, involving the chief neonatologist, the head nurse, and the clinical nurse specialist more closely with the research, in concert with the bedside nurses, would have reinforced the importance of this research in this particular unit. We realized that a research unit with a high rate of staff turnover requires special care in order to follow a research protocol. Perhaps involving a more clearly defined and stable authority figure, such as the chief neonatologist, during the daily medical rounds to explain our research study and the importance of the research protocol could have improved implementation on this particular neonatal intensive care unit. Furthermore, the medical rounds could have provided opportunities for the research nurse to inquire about the progress of the research participants over the course of the study.

TO READ FURTHER

Elwood, J. M. (2007). *Critical appraisal of epidemiological studies and clinical trials* (3rd ed.). New York: Oxford University Press.

Chapter 5, on error and bias in observation, gives useful information to avoid errors and bias during data collection in experimental studies.

Weiss, R. B. (1998). Systems of protocol review, quality assurance and data audit. *Cancer Chemotherapy and Pharmacology, 42*(Suppl.), S88–S92.

This article is a bit older but gives a good example of the way the U.S. National Cancer Institute implemented a protocol to ensure reliability of data. This can give readers some good clues on how to ensure data quality.

Plost, G., & Nelson, D. P. (2007). Empowering critical care nurses to improve compliance with protocols in the intensive care unit. *American Journal of Critical Care, 16*, 153–157.

This article gives a good example of how medical personnel can be empowered to follow protocols; it gives readers ideas about how to improve protocol compliance.

REFERENCES

Johnston, C. C., Barrington, K., Taddio, A., Carbajal, R., Brintnell, J., Byron, J., et al. (2008, May). *Comfort measures for procedural pain in Canadian NICU's: Have we improved over the past decade?* EPIPPAIN Canada. Abstract for Pediatric Academic Society Meeting, Honolulu, HI.

Johnston, C. C., Collinge, J. M., Henderson, S., & Anand, K. J. S. (1997). A cross sectional survey of pain and analgesia in Canadian neonatal intensive care units. *Clinical Journal of Pain, 13*, 1–5.

Johnston, C. C., Filion, F., Snider, L., Majnemer, A., Limperopoulos, C., Walker, C. D., et al. (2002). Routine sucrose analgesia during the first week of life in neonates younger than 31 weeks' postconceptional age. *Pediatrics, 110*, 523–528.

Korner, A. F., & Thom, V. A. (1990). *Neurobehavioral assessment of the preterm infant: Manual.* New York: The Psychological Corporation.

Simons, S. H., van Dijk, M., Anand, K. J. S., Roofhooft, D., van Lingen, R. A., & Tibboel, D. (2003). Do we still hurt newborn babies?: A prospective study of procedural pain and analgesia in neonates. *Archives of Pediatrics and Adolescent Medicine, 157,* 1058–1064.

Stevens, B., McGrath, P., Gibbins, S., Beyene, J., Breau, L., Camfield, C., et al. (2003). Procedural pain in newborns at risk for neurologic impairment. *Pain, 105,* 27–35.

Stevens, B., Johnston, C., Petryshen, P., & Taddio, A. (1996). Premature Infant Pain Profile: Development and initial validation. *Clinical Journal of Pain, 12,* 13–22.

Stevens, B., Yamada, J., & Ohlsson, A. (2004). Sucrose for analgesia in newborn infants undergoing painful procedures. *Cochrane Database of Systematic Reviews, 3,* CD001069.

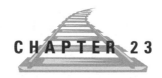

CHAPTER 23

Placebo Problems
Power and Persecution, or Paranoia?

ROBERT VAN REEKUM

BACKGROUND OF THE STUDY

In the late 1990s, cholinesterase inhibitors (CIs), which are a type of medication that increases memory function, became available for treatment of cognitive impairment in Alzheimer's disease. The study team wondered whether CIs might also be efficacious in the treatment of cognitive impairment in individuals who have developed these impairments following a traumatic brain injury (TBI). TBI is common in the United States and Canada and frequently causes cognitive impairments that affect functioning and quality of life and lead to significant societal impact.

To allow us to address this question, we entered into preliminary discussion with the distributors of the then-available CIs in Canada to see if they would be interested in funding a randomized controlled trial (RCT) in the TBI population. When we learned that no funding would be available to us through the pharmaceutical companies, we continued with our grant application to the Canadian Institutes for Health Research (CIHR). This process also proved to be time-consuming and difficult (and is nearly a chapter in and of itself), as some of the reviewers for CIHR had concerns related to public funding for research involving a medication which, pending results of the study, might lead to profit for the private sector (a pharmaceutical company). Ultimately, and with considerable delays and effort, we were able to argue that it was in the best interest of the Canadian public to fund this research at arms length from the pharmaceutical company that stood to profit from use of the medication (to avoid a potential conflict of interest and biases that might flow from this). With funding finally approved, we needed to purchase active medication (which was not a problem, as we could do so through our hospital pharmacy), and an identical placebo. We had no idea that purchasing a placebo would become as difficult a process as it eventually became, nor that this issue would have the dramatic impact on our study, and its implementation and execution, that it proved to have. Was the pharmaceutical company simply vulnerable to bureaucratic bumbling, or was it exerting its power over us (e.g., perhaps in an attempt to maintain control over the data)? Or, as it sometimes seemed on our "bad days" (see below), was it deliberately persecuting us (or, at least, contributing to delays in order to achieve some gain, such as perhaps providing us with motivation to agree to their contractual demands)? Alternatively, were we simply becoming paranoid (in addition to being frustrated, depressed, anxious, agitated, and perhaps ultimately at homicidal risk)?

THE CHALLENGES

The following is excerpted from a letter I wrote to CIHR on March 29, 2004, in which I had to explain the reason for the delay in initiating our study (i.e., the placebo issue), and to advise the organization that the delay had led to cost overruns. I also felt that CIHR needed to be made aware of what had occurred, particularly given the relatively recent (at that time) initiatives for joint CIHR/industry funding of research studies in Canada. I have made only minor changes to the text of the letter, such as masking the name of the medication (in order to avoid identifying the pharmaceutical company and its representatives) and adding some commentary (in *italics*).

After an introductory paragraph, the letter read:

The chronology of events is as follows (note that the quotes are taken from documentation that we can make available to you should you require it):

July 11, 2002—Notification of receipt of grant.

October 21, 2002—Preliminary ethics approval from Baycrest Centre for Geriatric Care (the primary investigative site).

October 28, 2002—Request for purchase (*i.e., we made it clear we were no longer requesting a grant or funding*) of active medication and placebo. The request included a copy of the research protocol, which stipulated that this was to be a Randomized Clinical Trial comparing outcomes in active, and identical placebo, groups.

November 8, 2002—Follow-up e-mail to the Clinical Scientist (whom we were advised would assist us with the process) at the Canadian branch of the pharmaceutical company (as we had not heard back from her).

December 5, 2002—The Clinical Scientist apologized for "not getting back to you sooner" and advised that the company's "review committee" had decided not to fund or provide medications to us.

December 9, 2002—I left a voice mail for the Clinical Scientist advising that we had not requested funding from them, but rather that we were specifically requesting <u>purchase</u> of the medication and placebo. Later in the day the Clinical Scientist e-mailed back her apology "for the misunderstanding" and promised to "look into" our request to purchase active medication and placebo. The Clinical Scientist also queried the quantities required, and I provided her with this information by reply e-mail later that day.

December 11, 2002—The Clinical Scientist suggested we "check the possibilities via your hospital pharmacy" as regards to purchase of active medication, and advised that the pharmaceutical company's "global review committee" had received our request for purchase of placebo. The committee was to meet "at the end of January."

December 12, 2002—The Clinical Scientist confirmed that we should "proceed via your hospital pharmacy" as regards purchase of the active medication. I replied on December 13, 2002, to thank her, and to advise that it had been the pharmaceutical company's own Sales Department that had initially advised me to contact her as regards purchasing the active medication and the placebo (*bit of chasing the tail here!*).

March 14, 2003—I e-mailed the Clinical Scientist reminding her that when I called in early February she had advised that the committee would make its decision on February 28th, 2003, and requesting the results of the committee's deliberations.

March 17, 2003—The Clinical Scientist replied that she understood we were eager to get an answer, assured me that she was regularly following up with the committee, and expressed her hope that "we will be able to resolve this shortly."

April 10, 2003—The Clinical Scientist advised that our request for purchase of placebo had been "granted," and requested a formal letter from us (the letter was sent on April 14, 2003). The Clinical Scientist advised that it would be "approximately 3 months from the time of order to delivery of supplies."

May 6, 2003—We received a letter from the U.S.-based head office of the pharmaceutical company, advising that our "request for clinical supplies" had been forwarded to them, and had been further "forwarded to the (*name of medication deleted here*) Medical Grants Committee" for "scientific review and funding consideration." I phoned the identified contact person at the head office, and advised that we were <u>not</u> requesting funding, that we had already been reviewed by the firm's Canadian office, and requested delivery of the placebo. I asked our research assistant to call the Canadian Clinical Scientist to advise her as to the receipt of this letter, and to request her help in obtaining the placebo ASAP.

July 16, 2003—We sent another letter (this time to our identified contact in the U.S. head office) formally requesting purchase of the balance of placebo that we would need to complete the study (the initial request had only been enough for a "start-up" period). We also met with Baycrest's Pharmacy Department, and ordered the full allotment of active medication.

September 11, 2003—The Canadian Clinical Scientist advised that "a first shipment was made" of placebo tablets related to our initial letter. She further advised that the placebo tablets related to our second letter of request were "being prepared." (Please note that we had yet to receive <u>any</u> placebo tablets, despite a number of calls and e-mails requesting they be forwarded to us). The Clinical Scientist then advised that as they had been "reviewing your file, it came to our attention that **the placebo tablets and the commercial tablets won't match, and that you will not be able to blind your study adequately.**" To address "this inconvenient situation," the Clinical Scientist advised that the pharmaceutical company had "agreed to provide you with the active medication." The Clinical Scientist requested copies of our governmental approval for the study (required as we were studying a medication outside of its accepted clinical indication), and the quantity of active medication required. She advised that we would need to sign a contract.

September 17, 2003—I wrote to the Clinical Scientist advising that we had already purchased active medication through our Pharmacy (per her previous directions!), that the pharmaceutical company had refused to accept return of these tablets, and that our grant did not allow for the purchase of two full allotments of active medication. I also advised that we had removed the active tablets (that we had already purchased) from the blister packs that they were packaged in (making it even less likely that a commercial provider would be willing to have the tablets returned to them). I requested urgent assistance to address our dilemma, and advised that the study was ready to start upon receipt of the active and placebo medications (and indeed had been for several months).

September 24, 2003—The Clinical Scientist requested a formal letter of intent related to the "medication request."

September 26, 2003—I wrote another formal letter to the Clinical Scientist requesting unmarked active medication (the "unmarked" tablets were apparently going to match the placebo).

October 21, 2003—Our research assistant e-mailed the pharmaceutical company advising that we had received the contract they wished us to sign. Our research assistant requested the promised attachment to the contract (*which they had neglected to attach*), and this was sent later in the day (at which time our contact at the pharmaceutical company asked her shipping department to advise us as to when we could expect receipt of the placebos, and noted that she had seen a "ship notification dated September 8th").

October 29, 2003—Our research assistant requested an electronic copy of the contract/letter of agreement, and this was sent later in the day.

November 11, 2003—We involved legal counsel for Baycrest Centre, and upon legal review of the contract, it was sent back, with revisions, to our contact at the pharmaceutical company. Our legal counsel wrote, "Baycrest believes CIHR would be concerned if they thought (*name of pharmaceutical company deleted*) was providing a grant or sponsorship for this research." Our legal counsel further advised the pharmaceutical company that the proposed changes to the contract were intended to "dispel any such misconceptions and to clarify that this is really a commercial transaction to correct a purchase error."

November 12, 2003—I e-mailed our contact at the pharmaceutical company following up on an e-mail that our research assistant had sent a week earlier requesting that the placebo be sent to us from Quebec (*where it apparently had been shipped to; note that Baycrest is in Toronto, Ontario*). The contact at the pharmaceutical company replied later in the day, advising that they could not proceed "with active medication" until the agreement is signed (and noting that Baycrest's "extensive changes to the contract" would require further review by the pharmaceutical company's attorneys).

November 17, 2003—I e-mailed our contact at the pharmaceutical company, arranging to have the placebo forwarded to us, and noted that in our view this was independent of the contract related to the active medication as "we have purchased it" (the placebo). The pharmaceutical company's contact person replied that the placebo had not, in her view, been purchased (contrary to our request to purchase it, and our belief that we were in fact purchasing it). She forwarded our request for shipment on to another individual in the company, who advised that the shipment would be delayed until the end of January due to the holidays (*this was in mid-November!*). I then e-mailed her back, to advise her that we had repeatedly and expressly requested "purchase" of the placebo, and that we thought it was vital to all concerned (the study itself, CIHR, readers of publications related to the study, and perhaps to the pharmaceutical company itself) that the study remain at arm's length from the pharmaceutical company. I requested an invoice for the purchase of the placebo. The contact person replied that it was illegal for the company to sell us placebo. She advised that the placebo was "a grant, or gift." I replied that this was the first we had heard that the placebo was a gift. I thanked her for the "gift," and noted that since we had not received a request to sign a contract for this gift whether we might also consider the active unmarked medication (that they had promised to provide us with) to not require a contract. The contact person replied that a contract would be required for "release of active substance" due to "regulatory and safety reporting requirements." Please note that the contract stipulated that we would provide to the pharmaceutical company a copy of any manuscripts arising from the study (and also the results and findings of the study).

December 8, 2003—The Clinical Scientist wrote to advise that the active unmarked medication "should be ready to ship out in January."

January 13, 2004—Baycrest legal counsel advised that the Executive Director for Medical Affairs of the pharmaceutical company (at U.S. head office) needed information from me, and asked that I call him. I did so shortly thereafter, and provided the information required (basically a summary of the events to date, as I saw them).

February 4, 2004—Legal counsel for the U.S. head office of the pharmaceutical company e-mailed Baycrest's legal counsel with some further revisions to the contract (relating to liability issues, and concern with my individually indemnifying the pharmaceutical company as I would lack adequate insurance to cover any potential claims that may arise out of the study). I subsequently contacted the Canadian Medical Protective Association, which is the group that insures physicians.

February 10, 2004—Baycrest legal counsel advised me that in order to move the matter forward, Baycrest was prepared under the contract to agree alone to indemnify the pharmaceutical company in order to avoid potential problems with my insurance coverage. She was prepared to send her revisions back to legal counsel for the pharmaceutical company, but raised with me an issue related to the CIHR "guidelines on other funding sources" (which stipulate that CIHR must be made aware of any potential "overlaps" between a CIHR grant and grants from other sources). Because I had never considered the pharmaceutical company's offer to reimburse us for what I thought was an error on their part, and because I had insisted that the placebo be purchased, I had not thought to advise CIHR of this so-called "grant" (although I had certainly planned to advise CIHR of the reasons for the delay of this study). For me this became yet another hurdle posed by the arrangement with the pharmaceutical company, and given the history to date, and the likelihood of even more delays in future, we decided to discontinue our discussions with the pharmaceutical company, and to proceed with repackaging the commercial active medication we had purchased the previous July (along with preparing our own identical placebo).

OVERCOMING THE DIFFICULTIES

Ultimately, we were forced to place the active medication tablet into a larger capsule, which was then filled with a biologically inactive substance (masking the presence of the active tablet). We prepared placebo capsules by using the same outer capsule and filling it with the same biologically inactive substance. Clearly, this was less than ideal, as blindness was at risk (by breaking open the capsule) and as both the capsule and the biologically inactive filler might theoretically have affected the bioabsorption of the study medication.

LESSONS LEARNED

1. Attempting to work with industry, from within the public sector, will pose significant potential barriers. Considerable assistance (e.g., legal, administrative, etc.) will be required.

2. Our experience raised issues that are likely best met at senior (e.g., institutional, national) levels, as individual research teams are unlikely to have the resources, or clout, to effect significant change over matters that are as "simple" (yet seemingly incredibly complex, given the multitude of issues we were confronted with) as the purchase of an identical placebo!

3. We spent roughly 2 years seeking industry funding for the study, and more than 2 years obtaining CIHR funding. After that, it took us almost 2 more years before we realized that we would not be able to purchase an identical placebo. Needless to say, patience is required when conducting clinical research! Note that, in Chapter 16 of this book, we present some further challenges (this time related to participant recruitment) that we experienced when trying to implement this study. These challenges led to even greater demands on our reserve of patience.

TO READ FURTHER

Boffey, P. M. (1987, April 12). Experts find lag on testing drugs in AIDS patients. *New York Times.*

This investigative report documents many cases of drug companies failing to cooperate with universities, drug regulators, and others.

PART V

DATA COLLECTION

Researchers are familiar with the advice to develop a protocol that guides data collection. It should delineate the *what* (the nature of measure), *how* (the specific procedures), *when* (time point, sequence), and *where* (the context or setting) for gathering data. No matter how well planned, implementing this protocol is subject to Murphy's law. Data collection is the research step where the law strikes most frequently, as judged by the number of stories describing such occurrences. Of the 42 stories included in this book, 9 report events or things that "went wrong" while gathering data.

The nature of the events and their consequences varied within and between the studies discussed in the next nine chapters. In Chapter 24, Spencer and Patrick's experience was that two interrelated factors contributed to a low response rate to a mail survey of a marginalized (i.e., gay and lesbian) population: the sensitive nature of the topic, and the potential for incomplete anonymity; that is, the names of participants and their responses, although coded, could potentially be linked. Changing the method for administering the survey, from mail to online, reassured concerned participants and increased the number of respondents.

Advances in technology have led to increased efficiency in data collection. Computer-based administration of surveys has the advantages of promoting enrollment, speeding administration, and ensuring completeness of data. This may be true if the sites have enough computers that can handle the survey software. But when the computers are slow, the time needed to administer the survey may jeopardize completing the study, as Roberts found out (Chapter 25) to her dismay.

Collecting data at a prespecified times is critical when the data are time-sensitive. Reminding participants to complete the measures is important in this situation. However, to be effective, the reminders should get to participants on time. Streiner (Chapter 26) reminds us of unforeseen delays in postal services and reports that calling participants is more efficient (albeit more time-consuming) in reminding them to complete their diaries.

In Chapter 27, Cairney and colleagues remind us that events, while seemingly minor, can work together to jeopardize the integrity of a study. The events span different stages of data collection: gaining entry into schools, obtaining consent, traveling to the various sites, and finding appropriate room and equipment to gather the data. Similarly, Carpenter and Balsis (Chapter 28) report on their experience with an observational study that involved inviting family members to a meeting held in the participants' home. The issues encountered relate to the participants' refusal to have the researchers and/or other family members visit them at home, difficulty in scheduling the meeting at a time that was convenient to all those invited, difficulty in setting up the equipment needed to videotape the meeting (e.g., finding a plug, temperature and light in the room), gaining access to buildings, equipment failure, and interruptions by visitors.

Bryant (Chapter 29) and Watson (Chapter 30) touch on an equally important issue, that of having an adequate number of research staff members to collect the data from different sites and at the appropriate time. Bryant also highlights the need for enough funds to cover the staff's expenses. In Chapter 31, Shannon describes a challenge frequently encountered in historical research: incomplete records. McKnight and McKnight (Chapter 32) focus on the negative consequences of using inadequate measures for gathering data. They discuss three consequences: error of measurement, bias, and changing the nature of what is being measured by the very act of measuring it. They illustrate their points with examples taken from various studies.

In addition to describing what happened, the authors also present strategies they improvised on the spot to address a challenge. They also mention strategies they later incorporated in the data collection protocol to overcome the barriers encountered. Although these strategies are unique to the particular studies, they provide other researchers with food for thought, pointing to aspects of the protocol that require careful consideration to prevent what may have been "unexpected."

CHAPTER 24

Revisiting Traditional Survey Methodology to Recruit and Survey Lesbian, Gay, and Bisexual Older Adults

S. MELINDA SPENCER
JULIE HICKS PATRICK

BACKGROUND OF THE STUDY

Population aging in the United States has led to increased diversity and service needs among older adults. Consequently, gerontologists are faced with providing information about a rapidly growing heterogeneous group. One contributor to this increasing heterogeneity is sexual orientation. In the United States alone, the number of lesbian women and gay men over age 65 has been estimated to range between 1.75 and 3.5 million (Claes & Moore, 2000). This number is expected to increase dramatically as the Baby Boom generation ages. Similar to same-aged heterosexuals, older lesbians and gay men are a diverse group whose lives have been shaped by the sociohistorical period in which they have developed, lived, and worked (Reid, 1995). Lesbian, gay, and bisexual (LGB) adults also share a unique history of negative stereotyping, discrimination, and marginalization (Kimmel, 1978). However, few studies of older adults have examined the influence of sexual orientation on adaptation to aging (see, e.g., Berger, 1982, 1984; Dorfman et al., 1995; Friend, 1987; Kehoe, 1986; Kimmel, 1978; Quam, 1982).

As with other age groups, social support is a significant correlate of physical health, psychological well-being, and mortality (Krause, 2001). Differences in the nature of social interactions within one's social network can contribute to differences in well-being. Research with relatively small samples has shown that the family support systems of lesbian and gay adults are reinforced by support from friends (Berger, 1982, 1984; Friend, 1987). Cultural ethnographers refer to these strong friendship networks as fictive families or fictive kin (Berger & Kelly, 1996). Differences across sexual orientation in the structure of social networks have also been noted in previous literature. In one study, lesbian and gay adults reported having significantly more friends and fewer family members from whom they received support than same-age heterosexuals. Moreover, there were no overall between-group differences in either social support or depression (Dorfman et al., 1995). Variations in the structure or composition of social networks do not guarantee that the quality of these networks will differ by sexual orientation, but information on both the structure and function of social networks is necessary to fully understand social support among LGB older adults.

Although lesbian and gay adults are generally well integrated in their social networks (Berger & Kelly, 1996), it remains unclear whether and to what extent these associations are observed among middle-aged and older adults. The purpose of our study was to examine (1) the influence of gender and sexual orientation on perceived social support among middle-aged and older adults and (2) contributions of gender, sexual orientation, and social support to psychological well-being. In this chapter, we describe the traditional survey methodology we used to recruit and collect data on 105 study participants, the challenges we encountered during this process, and the strategies we used to modify our study protocol to address these challenges. Sample recruitment and procedures are presented in two phases: Phase I describes recruitment and procedures consistent with the initial study protocol, and Phase II reflects adjustments that we made to improve LGB participation.

THE CHALLENGES

Sexual orientation is a sensitive subject for individuals of any age, and older adults might be a particularly vulnerable population for this kind of social-scientific research. We designed the study with a number of traditional safeguards in place to protect our research participants. First, we recognized that the stigma attached to same-sex orientation might place LGB participants at a heightened risk for negative consequences if their personal information were to become known to others (Herek, Kimmel, Amaro, & Melton, 1991). The original plan was to use a self-administered, mail-back survey format to increase anonymity and decrease social desirability responses (Dillman, 2000). Because we did not plan on follow-up, the participants did not need to provide any identifying personal information.

Another way to protect the privacy of LGB participants is to ensure that recruitment procedures are nonintrusive (Herek et al., 1991). Therefore, we took a very "hands-off" approach to recruitment; although we made study announcements at specific interest groups and organizations, we did not solicit potential participants on an individual basis.

Phase I: Traditional Methodology

Initial recruitment efforts focused on adults 60 years of age and older in the tristate area surrounding our university. A number of recruitment strategies aimed at diverse and otherwise invisible sections of the community were used (Herek et al., 1991), all of which are standard approaches to survey research. In the first step of a three-tiered approach to recruitment, we distributed research announcements to agencies and organizations that specifically served older LGB adults (i.e., support groups, social clubs and restaurants, and political and religious organizations). We also asked study participants to forward these announcements to friends and/or family who might be interested in the study. This strategy has been described in the literature as particularly useful for recruiting participants who do not frequent LGB groups or organizations (Berger, 1984). Finally, ads were placed in area LGB and feminist newspapers, bookstores, coffeehouses, and newsletters. A heterosexual group was also a convenience sample recruited with strategies that paralleled this three-tiered approach.

Individuals who were interested in participating in the study contacted us by e-mail, standard mail, or by calling a toll-free number. We explained the purpose of the study at that time and answered any questions. We then mailed interested participants a packet that contained a detailed cover letter, two copies of the information and consent form, a questionnaire, a self-addressed stamped envelope, and a token prepaid $5 financial incentive. Research has shown that including a prepaid incentive improves response rates significantly, whereas promised incentives do not have as great a response or have been found to have no effect at all (Dillman, 2000). Approximately 2 to 4 weeks after the packet was mailed, we sent either a personalized thank-you card to individuals who completed and returned the survey or a reminder to nonrespondents. All surveys were returned, and the $5 token prepaid incentive was returned in 15 of the 105 cases (all LGB participants).

Our traditional Phase I recruitment strategies worked for the heterosexual sample but were relatively unsuccessful for recruiting LGB participants. After approximately 2 months, we received surveys from a total of 56 heterosexuals and only 8 LGB adults. We found that advertising was difficult because LGB social and political organizations were not very active in our area. More important, many of the LGB adults who were interested in the study were reluctant to provide mailing addresses. There seemed to be a level of participant distrust in psychological research on sexual orientation. This was understandable, given that heterosexism and negative stereotyping have characterized much of the social science research. We felt that the only way to complete our study in a timely manner would be to modify the protocol. We used the following Phase II recruitment and data collection strategies to encourage the participation of LGB older adults and improve the overall success of our study.

OVERCOMING THE DIFFICULTIES

Phase II: Modifying the Protocol

We modified the study protocol to allow greater flexibility and anonymity for LGB participants. Our first step in the modified design was to lower the age criterion to include middle-aged adults at least 45 years old. Although this is no longer considered "older" as traditionally defined, we felt that middle-aged LGB adults had experienced the effects of the pivotal 1969 Stonewall Riots (Blumenfeld & Raymond, 1993). Thus, lowering the age of the study participants still provided meaningful information about a group of individuals who share a common sociocultural history.

The most important modification we made to the research protocol was to use the Internet as a way to add legitimacy to the study and provide an easy, viable option for participants to take the survey online. We circulated new recruitment advertisements to online LGB newspapers, to Listservs, and to the contacts listed on LGB social group websites. The new research announcement offered two options; participants could either contact us for a mail-back survey or complete the anonymous survey in an identical, online format. Respondents who were interested in completing the online survey went directly to the website and could access the survey without providing any personally identifying information. Additional heterosexuals were also recruited through online methods to reduce potential sample bias resulting from the Phase II recruitment efforts.

The domain name for this study was purchased on a 6-month contract. The survey website was designed using Javascript code and Microsoft FrontPage and maintained by a professional web developer for the duration of data collection. The heterosexual and LGB welcome pages used the same code and linked to the same survey, but with semantic differences to tailor the welcome pages to each particular group (i.e., affirmative pride symbols/colors for the LGB welcome page). A nontraditional consent and information form allowed the participant to click a button to indicate consent, and no IP addresses or other traceable data were recorded. When a participant chose to take the online survey, he or she was prompted to the subsequent pages by selecting a "submit and continue survey" button.

Form data were posted via Simple Mail Transfer Protocol (SMTP) transfer protocol to a password-protected e-mail address. Each page of the survey was then e-mailed to the researcher as the participant was entering data through a redirect, which allowed for total user anonymity and enabled us to calculate how many surveys were not completed (3 of 62, or 4.8%).

Modifying the initial study protocol to include an online survey option catalyzed a shift in the success of the project. Not only were LGB participants completing the online version, but a number of e-mails were received from individuals who had visited the professionally designed site and wanted one of two things. First, many stakeholders in various LGB social organizations wanted to be included on the list for study updates. Second, participants sent e-mails requesting the survey packet. Study participants claimed that visiting the site offered legitimacy to the research announcements. From this website, potential participants could both read more about the importance of the project and view the .pdf version of the survey. We continued to receive online and mail-back surveys and met our target sample of 105 approximately 3 months later.

LESSONS LEARNED

An unexpected result of this research was the ability to incorporate online technology and mixed-mode data collection in our modified study. Internet research has gained considerable momentum in recent years, in part because it has improved access to research participants through targeted advertising and because it is so cost-effective (Nosek, Banaji, & Greenwald, 2002). Results from a study that compared a large sample of Internet questionnaires with an archival set of 510 articles indicated that the Internet-based findings were consistent with those achieved by traditional methods. In addition, anonymity online did not necessarily threaten data integrity (Gosling, Vazire, Srivastava, & John, 2004). We believe that including an online format for data collection may be especially attractive for researchers interested in collecting data on "sensitive" topics.

To our knowledge, our study was the first to integrate the Internet with traditional survey methodology to examine social support among middle-aged and older LGB adults. If we had not made an effort to gain support for this research from the LGB community and modified the protocol to meet the participants' needs, the end result would have been unlikely. As a result of this project, we developed a conceptual approach to negotiating some of the challenges associated with conducting research with older LGB adults. The "CRAFT" model outlines five strategies for working with understudied, difficult-to-reach populations and is based on the success of various approaches we used over the course of this research project.

The CRAFT Model

The first strategy of the CRAFT model is Communication with the LGB community to determine which research issues are the most socially-relevant. This also meant communicating with more senior researchers in the field of LGB aging for advice and guidance when we encountered difficulties in recruitment. The second strategy is a focus on Responsibility in the ethical treatment and protection of participants, which includes acknowledgement of culture, use of appropriate measures, and timely dissemination of results to the LGB community. Related to responsibility is the issue of Access, or gaining entrée to the LGB community. Our recruitment efforts would have failed had we not directly involved key gatekeepers from the various social organizations and showed a clear respect for organizational boundaries. Sufficient research funding is another important component of access. Although all research is more likely to be successful when adequately funded, we could not have recruited participants without a research budget. In the LGB community, many of the organizations and publications are not-for-profit entitles and require compensation for advertising.

The last two strategies outlined in this model are directly related to research methodology. Flexibility, or an investigator's willingness to employ a multimethod approach to recruitment, helped to maximize the quality and scope of our research project. Our flexibility was best illustrated by the decision to place the survey in an anonymous, online format in response to the participants' needs. Ideally, the online version of the survey should have been extensively piloted and compared with the traditional mail-back versions before data collection began (Kraut et al., 2004). Future research should take more preventative measures so that its protocol does not require modification in the middle of data collection. Related to flexibility is the final aspect of this model, Technology. For participants, the Internet has enabled older LGB adults to maintain privacy, meet new people, and become connected to targeted support services. For researchers, online resources are more helpful than ever, offering greater access to, and protection for, participants.

Conclusions

Internet methodology has the potential to make a sizable contribution to the field of LGB psychology. Limitations and sample bias are introduced by using this method, but participants are truly anonymous and therefore more protected. Generally, what we know about social support comes from one mode of data collection, which makes it necessary for future studies to consider multiple methods of data collection to better reflect the complexity of the LGB social support network. Although we are taught and continue to teach our students that quality empirical work adheres to strict a priori protocols, the reality of the research process may be much different. For example, in the study discussed here, difficulties in recruitment necessitated modifications to the protocol. Investigators need to be sensitive to the needs of participants and adjust research plans accordingly. When such changes are necessary, we have the analytic tools to assess their effects. Thus, these modifications may increase our knowledge in the content domain, as well as our understanding of effective and appropriate research designs.

TO READ FURTHER

Nosek, B. A., & Greenwald, A. G. (2002). E-research: Ethics, security, design, and control in psychological research on the Internet. *Journal of Social Issues, 58,* 161–176.

Discusses a number of the ethical issues related to online research and presents several strategies to reduce threats to validity.

Dillman, D. A. (2007). *Mail and internet surveys: The tailored design method* (2nd ed.). New York: Wiley.

An updated version of the classic Dillman text, this is a crucial resource for understanding everything about surveys, from design to administration. Includes a new Internet, visual, and mixed-mode guide.

Gosling, S. D., Vazire, S., Srivastava, S., & John, O. P. (2004). Should we trust web-based studies? A comparative analysis of six preconceptions about Internet questionnaires. *American Psychologist, 59,* 93–104.

Clear and accessible article that outlines six of the common preconceptions about Internet research. The authors address each preconception by systematically comparing a large Internet sample with 510 more traditional published samples.

REFERENCES

Berger, R. M. (1982). The unseen minority: Older gays and lesbians. *Social Work,* 27, 236–242.

Berger, R. M. (1984). Realities of gay and lesbian aging. *Social Work, 29,* 57–62.

Berger, R. M., & Kelly, J. J. (1996). Gay men and lesbians grown older. In R. P. Cabaj & T. S. Stein (Eds.), *Textbook of homosexuality and mental health* (pp. 305–316). Washington, DC: American Psychiatric Press.

Blumenfeld, W. J., & Raymond, D. (1993). *Looking at gay and lesbian life.* Boston: Beacon Press.

Claes, J. A., & Moore, W. (2000). Issues confronting lesbian and gay elders: The challenge for health and human services providers. *Journal of Health and Human Services Administration, (Fall),* 181–202.

Dillman, D. A. (2000). *Mail and Internet surveys: The tailored design method.* New York: Wiley.

Dorfman, R., Walters, K., Burke, P., Hardin, L., Karanik, T., Raphael, J., et al. (1995). Old, sad, and alone: The myth of the aging homosexual. *Journal of Gerontological Social Work, 24,* 29–44.

Friend, R. A. (1987). The individual and social psychology of aging: Clinical implications for lesbians and gay men. *Journal of Homosexuality, 14,* 307–331.

Gosling, S. D., Vazire, S., Srivastava, S., & John, O. P. (2004). Should we trust web-based studies?: A comparative analysis of six preconceptions about Internet questionnaires. *American Psychologist, 59,* 93–104.

Herek, G. M., Kimmel, D. C., Amaro, H., & Melton, G. B. (1991). Avoiding heterosexist bias in psychological research. *American Psychologist, 46,* 957–963.

Kehoe, M. (1986). Lesbians over 65: A triply invisible minority. *Journal of Homosexuality, 12,* 139–152.

Kimmel, D. C. (1978). Adult development and aging: A gay perspective. *Journal of Social Issues, 34,* 113–130.

Krause, N. (2001). Social support. In R. H. Binstock & L. K. George (Eds.), *Handbook of aging and the social sciences* (5th ed., pp. 272–294). San Diego: Academic Press.

Kraut, R., Olson, J., Banaji, M., Bruckman, A., Cohen, J., & Couper, M. (2004). Psychological research online: Report of Board of Scientific Affairs' Advisory Group on the conduct of research on the Internet. *American Psychologist, 59,* 105–117.

Nosek, B. A., Banaji, M. R., & Greenwald, A. G. (2002). E-research: Ethics, security, design, and control in psychological research on the Internet. *Journal of Social Issues, 58,* 161–176.

Quam, J. K. (1982). Adaptation and age-related experiences of older gay and lesbian adults. *The Gerontologist, 32,* 367–374.

Reid, J. D. (1995). Development in late life: Older lesbian and gay lives. In A. R. D'Augelli, & C. J. Patterson (Eds.), *Lesbian, gay, and bisexual identities over the lifespan: Psychological perspectives* (pp. 215–240). New York: Oxford University Press.

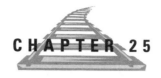

CHAPTER 25

Technology
Help or Hindrance?

NASREEN ROBERTS

BACKGROUND OF THE STUDY

The detailed background of this study is presented in Chapter 40, *What Happened to Cooperation and Collaboration?* (pp. 337–343). To avoid repetition I present only a brief summary of the project here.

Studying the prevalence of mental health problems in adolescents is important for prevention and program planning. Epidemiological studies have the potential to elucidate the need and provide the necessary support for program development to meet this need. At present there are no epidemiological studies of adolescents between 16 and 18 years of age in Canada. Data from Statistics Canada in 1997 showed that among 15- to 18-year-olds there were 529 deaths from unintentional injuries and 261 deaths from suicide. There were 3,674 hospital admissions due to suicidal attempts in this age group, a rate of 18.3 per 100,000 (Health Canada, 1997). This is second only to deaths due to motor vehicle accidents in this age group. The overall prevalence of diagnoses in children and adolescents based on the text revision of the fourth edition of the *Diagnostic and Statistical Manual of Mental Disorders* (DSM-IV-TR), which is the current classification system for mental disorders in North America, is generally about 8–22% for studies conducted in the United States (Gould, Greenberg, Velting, & Shaffer, 2003).

This study was undertaken by me, the author, as a preliminary step in response to a request from a local school board for an expedited psychiatric assessment program for its students. We (my supervisor and I) felt that it was essential in responding to this request that we establish the extent of the need, to enable us to weigh the costs and benefits of implementing this additional program. We are aware that prevalence of mental health problems may vary in the population as a function of factors such as sociodemographic characteristics, catchment area, or type of school.

A two-stage cross-sectional design for this study of high school students in a midsize city in Ontario was chosen. The primary goal was to estimate the number of students potentially in need of further psychiatric diagnostic assessment on the basis of the 12-month-period prevalence of child and adolescent psychiatric disorders. A secondary goal was to evaluate the construct validity of a mental health screen against the gold standard National Institute of Mental Health–Diagnostic Interview Schedule for Children (NIMH-DISC; Schaffer, Fisher, Lucas, Dulcan, & Schwab-Stone, 2000) for any child or adolescent psychiatric diagnosis.

THE CHALLENGES

The first hint of all not being well on the western front arose when we were cross-examined about our motivations and the secondary gains for us, for about 2 hours, by not only the district school board members, but also the school's parent council separately. Both groups repeatedly and in different words wondered if we had thought about the damage it could do to the students by stigmatizing them with psychiatric labels. This was, however, nothing compared to being confronted with a much larger challenge at the school computer room when we arrived to start testing.

I had been assigned the school's computer room and test-ran the study instruments on a couple of the computers to ensure all worked smoothly. Alas, we did not test each of the computers, which, with hindsight being 20/20, we know should have. Not only did we discover that the computers were very slow, but 3 days later, perhaps as a consequence of the time that was needed to complete each questionnaire, we were evicted from this room and asked to use library computers. We rejoiced and thought these would certainly be up to snuff—wrong again! Not only were there fewer computers, they followed the same pattern of technological distribution as those in the computer room; that is, only a couple of the five computers were able to handle the study software adequately.

I won't talk about our frustration or sense of disappointment as I do not want to portray us as theatrical, but let me say there was much clutching at hearts and rending of hair. But deterred we were NOT. So onward we marched intrepidly.

OVERCOMING THE DIFFICULTIES

The first step happened to be an exercise in being totally disillusioned about the "collaboration" chant, which is addressed in another chapter. Suffice it to say it took a couple of months of meetings with various committees and then waiting for their deliberations before we could go ahead.

The next monumental challenge was the horrendous realization that we did not have enough fast computers to get the study completed in the time we had stipulated (2 weeks), and that we could not take the kids to the university computer labs. So off we went to our department and brought in all the latest laptops we could beg, borrow, or steal (not really) from our colleagues and got the kids plugged in and roaring along. However, this meant that every night we had to download all the information from each of these computers into the one we had designated our study computer; the hourglass was turned hundreds of times.

Despite all our efforts to get the testing done within the time we had predicted in our proposal, we knew we weren't going to be able to get all of the kids to complete the questionnaire in the 2 weeks. We requested another 10 days to complete the study, but were asked to discontinue within that week. This, of course, reduced an already small sample size even further. We made as dignified and professional an exit as we could muster (I will tell you that all those annoying times past my 10th birthday, when my mother kept reminding me to say "Please" and "Thank You," really worked).

LESSONS LEARNED

Keep your cool; do not blow a gasket at the participants, colleagues, or computers. Expect things to not go smoothly; if they do, hey! it's a megabonus. If you are someone who is easily frustrated by bank lineups, I suggest practicing breathing, relaxation, and finding your inner Zen place before undertaking research.

Being annoyingly obsessive beforehand (for instance, personally checking each and every computer the school had offered) would have really helped avoid this challenge.

We could have used paper copies of the screening questionnaire rather than the computer version for the students. Although it would have meant a lot more data entry time for us, it would have been less time-consuming or disruptive for the school. As I state in Chapter 40, I learned many a good lesson for future projects—and, of course, got to write this chapter.

TO READ FURTHER

Trivedi, M. H., Kern, J. K., Marcee, A., Grannemann, B., Kleiber, B., Bettinger, T., et al. (2002). Development and implementation of computerized clinical guidelines: Barriers and solutions. *Methods of Information in Medicine, 41,* 435–442.

This article discusses a number of issues pertaining to the use of technology, including the barriers of implementation, the importance of the user's role in development, implementation, and adherence, and some methods that can improve acceptance and use of technology.

Holroyd, B. R., Bullard, M. J., Graham, T. A., & Rowe, B. H. (2007). Decision support technology in knowledge translation. *Academic Emergency Medicine, 14*, 942–948.

This article highlights the importance careful consideration of the workflow and culture of the environment where a system is to be used for its successful implementation.

REFERENCES

Gould, M. S., Greenberg, T., Velting, D. M., & Shaffer, D. (2003). Youth suicide risk and preventive interventions: A review of the past 10 years. *Journal of the American Academy of Child and Adolescent Psychiatry, 42*, 386–405.

Health Canada. (1997). Leading causes of hospitalization and death in Canada. Available at *www.hcsc.gc.ca/hpb/lcdc/publicat/pcd97/mrt_mf_e.html.*

Shaffer, D., Fisher, P., Lucas, C., Dulcan, M., & Schwab-Stone, M. (2000). NIMH Diagnostic Interview Schedule for Children version IV (NIMH DISC-IV): Description, differences from previous versions, and reliability of some common diagnoses. *Journal of the American Academy of Child and Adolescent Psychiatry 39*, 28–38.

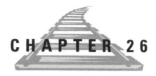

CHAPTER 26

Hoist on Our Own Postcard

DAVID L. STREINER

BACKGROUND OF THE STUDY

For many years there has been a debate in the literature regarding the relationships among stress, social support, and people's susceptibility to illness. The homeostasis hypothesis states that anything that disrupts our lives, either positively or negatively, results in some degree of stress; and with too much stress, we become more susceptible to falling sick (Holmes & Masuda, 1973). It is obvious, though, that people differ greatly in this regard; given the same degree of stress, one person may become ill and another may not. So, researchers have looked for other factors that can account for individual differences. One possible suspect is social support—the degree to which we feel we can rely on others for emotional, financial, or instrumental help in times of need. However, the mechanism by which social support exerts its influence is open to question.

The buffering hypothesis holds that social support is a moderator between stress and illness, in that those with a high degree of stress and low social support are more prone to fall ill, whereas those with an equivalent level of stress who have high levels of social support are less likely to do so (Cohen & Wills, 1985; Power, 1988). However, the direct, or main effect, hypothesis states that social support has a direct influence on health; socially rewarding roles provide positive experiences, and integration in a social network helps people avoid negative experiences (e.g., financial problems) that could have negative consequences (e.g., Levinger & Huesmann, 1980).

The difficulty with many previous studies was that they were cross-sectional, so that it was impossible to establish causation. Whether the stress came before the illness, or vice versa, depended on the participants' recall, and we know that the recall of events is notoriously poor (e.g., Cohen & Java, 1995; Glickman, Hubbard, Liveright, & Valciukas, 1990; Monroe, 1982). Moreover, stress itself interferes with the recall of stressful events (Steele, Henderson, & Duncan-Jones, 1980). The only way around this problem was to do a longitudinal study, in which participants could be followed over time, and this is what we did.

Our study (McFarlane, Norman, Streiner, Roy, & Scott, 1980) involved 500 healthy people, recruited from the practices of family physicians. At baseline, and then every 6 months over 2 years, there was a home interview, during which these people completed a standardized measure of stressors they had experienced during the previous 6 months (Rahe, 1974), which we modified for this study (Streiner, Norman, McFarlane, & Roy, 1981), a scale of social support (McFarlane, Neale, Norman, Roy, & Streiner, 1981), plus some other measures, such as health locus of control (Wallston, Wallston, & DeVellis, 1978) and a modification of Rokeach's Value Survey (1973). The main outcomes were various aspects of illness. Strain was captured with Langner's (1962) measure of impairment, and a patient encounter form recorded all visits to the family physician. Finally, the participants also recorded any symptoms and their severity, and actions taken (e.g., use of prescription or nonprescription medication, time taken off from work); these were captured in a diary that the participants completed on 3 consecutive days every 2 weeks in order to reduce the demand on their time (Norman, McFarlane, Streiner, & Neale, 1982).

So as to eliminate any possible bias caused by day of the week, such as a person's not working on weekends, we very carefully worked out a schedule so that one-seventh of the people filled out the diaries on Monday through Wednesday, one-seventh on Tuesday through Thursday, and so forth. Moreover, we tried to reduce any other bias by changing the start day for each round of diaries; those who completed them on Monday, Tuesday, and Wednesday in one week filled them out Tuesday, Wednesday, and Thursday 2 weeks later. Our plan was to give the people a package of diaries and a note indicating on which days they were to complete them and mail them back to us.

THE CHALLENGES

In our first pilot study to look at the feasibility of this scheme, the four of us on the research team each took 2 weeks' worth of diaries that we were to fill out on designated days and then bring in to our next planning session. At that meeting, after some beating around the bush, we all had to 'fess up—each of us had completed the whole package the night before the meeting; our compliance rate in regard to doing them on time was zero. Needless to say, this was a major problem. If the members of the team, who were presumably the most motivated in regard to doing the study right, weren't able to adhere to the task, then it was highly doubtful that the participants would be any better at completing the diaries on the specified days. So, we had to come up with an alternative plan, one that would increase the likelihood that the diaries would be filled in when they should be.

Plan B consisted of mailing the forms ahead of time to the participants, and then sending a postcard reminder to tell the people when to start completing the diaries. This led to our second pilot study, to determine how long it would take for postal reminders to reach different parts of the city. We got a pile of postcards, and, over a period of a few weeks, mailed them to ourselves, dutifully noting the date of mailing and when we received them. With the exception of a few outliers, among which it took 30 days for one card to arrive (we say here that postal rates are so high because Canada Post charges for storage), we figured we should mail the cards 3 days before the people were to start their diaries.

With this in mind, we geared up to begin the study. Just as we were to mail the first batch of reminders, an annual Canadian tradition kicked in—a postal strike!

OVERCOMING THE DIFFICULTIES

Given the uncertainties of when the diaries and the reminders would reach the people, we modified the procedure yet again. Once the strike was over, we mailed batches of diaries to the participants. But as we were never sure if another strike would occur, we resorted to having the research assistant call the people the day before they were to begin filling out the diaries. As it turned out, this wasn't any more expensive than using the mails. The time spent calling people, and the cost of the calls, was roughly equivalent to the time it would have taken to address the cards (this was before the days when computerized mailing lists could have sped up the task) and the cost of the cards themselves.

The final result turned out well; the combination of telephone reminders, plus a lottery ticket that was given to the participants with every third mailing of diaries, proved to be extremely successful. Over the 2-year span of the study, we mailed a total of 18,708 diaries, of which 15,923 were returned, for an overall compliance rate of 85.1%.

From a statistical perspective, we should note that over the course of the 2 years, we mailed out approximately 2,000 lottery tickets. One person won $10. That is why we call lotteries a tax on the statistically challenged.

LESSONS LEARNED

Be flexible! Methods that seem eminently feasible on paper rarely are in real life. People are not as compliant as we would like, and procedures that sound good must be pretested to see if they work. Even when they do, circumstances change, and you must be prepared to change your methods to accommodate them.

TO READ FURTHER

Dillman, D. A. (2006). *Mail and internet surveys: The tailored design method.* New York: Wiley.

Don't think of this as a book; it is a bible. Ever since the first edition appeared in 1978, it has been *the* guide to designing questionnaires and maximizing the return rate. It has now been updated to cover surveys done on the Internet.

Streiner, D. L., & Norman, G. R. (2008). *Health measurement scales: A practical guide to their development and use* (4th ed.). Oxford, UK: Oxford University Press.

Only modesty prevents me from also calling this book a bible. However, it is a step-by-step guide to designing scales, with a chapter about increasing adherence rates.

REFERENCES

Cohen, G., & Java, R. (1995). Memory for medical history: Accuracy of recall. *Applied Cognitive Psychology, 9,* 273–288.

Cohen, S., & Wills, T. A. (1985). Stress, social support, and the buffering hypothesis. *Psychological Bulletin, 98,* 310–357.

Glickman, L., Hubbard, M., Liveright, T., & Valciukas, J. A. (1990). Fall-off in reporting life events: Effects of life change, desirability, and anticipation. *Behavioral Medicine, 16,* 31–38.

Holmes, T. H., & Masuda, M. (1973). Life change and illness susceptibility. In J. P. Scott & E. C. Senay (Eds.), *Separation and depression* (pp. 161–186). Washington, DC: American Association for the Advancement of Science.

Langner, T. S. (1962). A twenty-two item screening score of psychiatric symptoms indicating impairment. *Journal of Health and Human Behavior, 3,* 269–276.

Levinger, G., & Huesmann, L. R. (1980). An "incremental exchange" perspective on the pair relationship. In K. J. Jurgen, M. S. Greenberg, & R. H. Willis (Eds.), *Social exchange: Advances in theory and research* (pp. 165–188). New York: Plenum Press.

McFarlane, A. H., Neale, K., Norman, G. R., Roy, R. G., & Streiner, D. L. (1981). Methodological issues in developing a scale to measure social support. *Schizophrenia Bulletin, 7,* 90–100.

McFarlane, A. H., Norman, G. R., Streiner, D. L., Roy, R., & Scott, D. J. (1980). A longitudinal study of the influence of the psychosocial environment on health status: A preliminary report. *Journal of Health and Social Behavior, 21,* 124–133.

Monroe, S. M. (1982). Assessment of life events: Retrospective vs concurrent strategies. *Archives of General Psychiatry, 39,* 606–610.

Norman, G. R., McFarlane, A. H., Streiner, D. L., & Neale, K. (1982). Health diaries: Strategies for compliance and relation to other measures. *Medical Care, 20,* 623–629.

Power, M. J. (1988). Stress-buffering effects of social support: A longitudinal study. *Motivation and Emotion, 12,* 197–204.

Rahe, R. H. (1974). The pathways between subjects' recent life changes and their near-future illness reports. In B. S. Dohrenwend & B. P. Dohrenwend (Eds.), *Stressful life events: Their nature and effects* (pp. 73–86). New York: Wiley.

Rokeach, M. (1973). *The nature of human values.* New York: Free Press.

Steele, G. P., Henderson, S., & Duncan-Jones, P. (1980). The reliability of reporting adverse experiences. *Psychological Medicine, 10,* 301–306.

Streiner, D. L., Norman, G. R., McFarlane, A. H., & Roy, R. G. (1981). Quality of life events and their relationship to strain. *Schizophrenia Bulletin, 7,* 34–42.

Wallston, K. A., Wallston, B. S., & DeVellis, R. (1978). Development of the Multidimensional Health Locus of Control (MHLC) scales. *Health Education Monographs, 6,* 160–170.

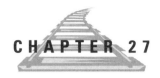

CHAPTER 27

On the Finer Points
of Handling Googlies

*Reflections on Hits, Near Misses, and Full-Blown
Swings at the Air in Large, Population-Based Studies
Involving School, Parents, and Children*

JOHN CAIRNEY

JOHN A. HAY

BRENT E. FAUGHT

BACKGROUND OF THE STUDY

The term "googly" is one that the first author (J. C.) has been trying for some time to incorporate into his academic writing.[1] Although foreign to most North Americans, the googly is familiar to those with some knowledge of the sport of cricket. It refers to a type of bowling delivery in which the ball takes an unexpected and often dramatic twist before reaching the batsman. If the googly is successful, the batsman is left chopping foolishly at empty air.[2] The nearest equivalent in North American parlance is the "knuckleball"[3] in baseball, and there, as in cricket, it involves the fine art of making the strong and skilled look weak and helpless.[4]

So what do googlies and knuckleballs have to do with research? Quite a lot when the research in question is played out "in the field" or "on the ground." Training, practice, and hard-won experience are all very well, but the art of doing this type of science is, above all, the art of spotting and responding to googlies. The very reason we pose many of the questions we attempt to answer is that individual humans do not act in a predictable and stable manner. Our hope is that by studying populations of reasonably similar persons, we may come to a general understanding of the likely tendencies of most. Unfortunately, gaining a true understanding of individuals means observing and measuring them in their natural habitat, and it is in that habitat, far from the carefully controlled setting of the lab, that googlies consistently appear. Although we take every reasonable precaution to avoid problems before they arise, we can never fully anticipate all the challenges research, especially the kind with real, live human beings living in their natural environment, will throw our way. Perhaps the best preparation is to accept that googlies will appear, that some will evade you, and that some will make you look (and feel) utterly foolish. Ultimately, it is how we respond to these events that counts, and that probably determines whether we continue to attempt doing field research at all.

In this chapter we consider a few lessons learned while conducting a large school-based prospective study of children. We have tried to focus on a few points that might be helpful to other researchers contemplating similar work. We are not claiming that these lessons are unique to us or to our specific area of research. In fact, it is likely that other researchers have had similar experiences and crafted similar or identical responses to the problems. Were a soundtrack to accompany this discussion—and if the technology were cheaper—it would include repeated "whoosh" noises, muffled cursing, and perhaps the odd cry or two.

Context and Study Design

In 2004, we began a large prospective school-based study that we dubbed PHAST (Physical Health and Activity Study Team). We collected a wide variety of data, hoping to explore a range of issues related to health and physical activity in children. One of our particular interests centered on children who seemed to be behind their peers in the development of motor skills and coordination. These children, about 6% of the total pediatric population, are thought to have a condition known as developmental coordination disorder, or DCD (American Psychiatric Association, 2000; Gibbs, Appleton, & Appleton, 2007; Hay & Missiuna, 1998). Our own work has shown that these children tend to be less physically active than their nonaffected peers (Cairney, Hay, Faught, Mandigo, & Flouris, 2005) and that this in turn is associated with poorer physical fitness (Faught, Hay, Cairney, Flouris & Klentrou, 2005; Cairney, Hay, Faught, & Flouris, 2007) and obesity (Cairney, Hay, Faught, & Hawes, 2005).

To further explore the relationship between physical health and motor coordination, we proposed to follow an entire cohort of children from grade 4 through to grade 6 in a public school board in southern Ontario, Canada. Twice yearly, once in the fall and again each spring, we sent trained research assistants (RAs) into the schools to administer surveys, conduct anthropometric assessments, and perform fitness testing on all consenting children.

In order to combat concerns about the representativeness of our sample, we succumbed to the seductive logic of one of us (J. H.) and decided to propose "testing them all". This logic was sufficiently compelling to garner funding from the Canadian Institutes for Health Research, and in September of 2004 we began, full of enthusiasm and, as it turns out, an utter lack of appreciation of the enormity of the undertaking.

A brief précis: We gained ethics approval from the school board and Brock University, permission from 75 of 92 possible school principals (82%), and informed consent from the parents of 2,262 of 3,030 children (75%). We established testing and training protocols and completed baseline testing. Ninety-seven percent of our target sample (2,164 children) have been evaluated for physical activity, height, weight, body mass index, hip and waist girth, aerobic capacity, and self-efficacy in physical activity twice annually for 3 years, and motor coordination assessments have been carried out. We have published a number of journal articles on our findings. Our funding has been renewed for a further 3.5 years. Looks impressive on paper, but the reality on the ground, however, is less pretty. What follows are accounts of what really happened in the course of producing those dry but, we hope, coherent additions to the scientific literature.

THE CHALLENGES

The Consent Process

School Bureaucracy[5]

The first googly offered by studies of this kind typically involves some aspect of the consent process. This process is, in a word, multilayered (or, in two words, multilayered and hideous). First, there is consent at the board level. Representatives of the school board, either a research board and/or an ethics board, are required to approve all studies involving the children in their jurisdiction. In our case, this was relatively painless, and our access was greatly facilitated by having had an insider (a school board consultant for health and physical education) as part of the research team. We also found it invaluable that one of us (J. H.) among the principal investigators was experienced with research in school settings, but insufficiently wise to desist.

It must be understood, however, that we mean "relatively painless" not as "almost painless," but rather, "much less painful than things that were to follow." At one point the entire project was almost derailed when the school board became concerned about the implications of diagnosing well over 100 children with a disorder like DCD. Those children would require special support or therapy—a situation with which the board was poorly equipped to deal. It was suggested to the special needs coordinator of the board that we would not provide a diagnosis, but rather simply report the results of an assessment to the parent. A keen awareness of semantics—along with politeness, thorough planning, and pure, mindless obstinacy, one of the most important weapons in the field researcher's arsenal—was crucial at this stage. The word "identification" was the issue. Removing any implication that we would be providing diagnoses—which we were not staffed or equipped to do anyway—exorcised the specter of another group of special needs children requiring treatment and support, and the board relented. This solution, however, provided a potential flash point for the university's ethics review board. Again, however, the distinction between an assessment and a diagnostic evaluation proved our salvation. We provided parents with results, material on DCD, and a special notice if their child appeared to meet the criteria for motor coordination problems. We advised these parents to approach their physician to pursue a formal assessment if their child's results were of concern. To be frank, this was a hollow solution for the investigators. Many of those children who most needed assistance were likely to come from families lacking either the insight or wherewithal to pursue the matter. To our knowledge, only one family pursued the issue with its family physician. To mix sporting metaphors, we dealt with this googly by hitting a foul ball. We weren't out, but we also weren't satisfied.

Oh Yes, Principals and Teachers

The next layer of the consent process involves school principals. Even if a board enthusiastically and wholeheartedly endorses your proposed work, it cannot—it turns out—force schools to cooperate. The final decision to let researchers in lies with the principals and, in some cases, the parent–teacher councils (apparently, schools are run somewhat more democratically than we would have thought). Most principals were enthusiastic, or at least willing, but 21 initially rejected our study. Their reasons for declining to participate included "we don't do research," "the grade 4 teacher is new and I don't want to overburden her," and "I'm a new principal and don't want to impose this on my staff." The most common, however, and also our favorite, was "I don't think this is important research for a child's education and so we don't wish to be involved." Attempts to establish our bona fides, including a presentation at a principals' meeting, led to acceptances from four more schools. We ended with acceptance by 75 of 92 schools in the region.

Googlies are hard to anticipate—that's the whole point of them. One practical problem that regularly astonishes people studying change over time is that *things change over time*. In our case, we were surprised by the migratory behavior of principals within school boards. It is, we discovered, entirely possible for a principal who had turned down the study in the first year to be transferred to a school where his or her predecessor had been only too happy to grant us permission. And principals, it turns out, are not obliged to honor the commitments of their predecessors. Here, the best defense proved to be the relationships already established with teachers and parents. Both parties came to our aid on at least one occasion, and we lost no schools as a result of principal transfer. We now track principal changes when they occur and are proactive in ensuring that there is not the faintest hint of any possibility of withdrawing from the study.

Finally, we had the dubious fortune to discover a new, heretofore unsuspected consent barrier between layer 2 (principals) and layer 3 (parents). Teachers, though not formally part of the decision-making process, could refuse to participate and not allow access to their classrooms. To sidestep this potential, "layer 2.5," we made use of another important tool of the field researcher: judicious use of threats. We arranged a preemptive strike in the form of a letter from the school board clearly stating that failure to collaborate with a board-approved project would be noted on a teacher's performance appraisal. We lost no classes.

The Positive Power of Pizza

Assuming you have not thrown in the towel during the first two stages, the next challenge in a school-based study is to secure the consent of parents. In this step, we anticipated the googly and took it out of the hands of the gremlins.[6, 7] We borrowed a page from McDonald's marketing strategy—a willingness to emulate evil examples being yet another essential item in the field researcher's toolbox—and used the children to sell the consent to their parents. Our first concern was the reliability of mail delivery via grade 4 students. Our second was our suspicion that parents were likely to have limited interest—given the large number of "things to be signed" that come to every parent—in signing, let alone reading, an informed consent form. We solved these problems with an adroit application of pizza. All classes who returned 100% of the consent forms, signed (whether providing or withholding consent) within 1 week "won" a pizza party. For those wondering about the ethics of this practice, we emphasized again and again to teachers and children that agreement to participate was not a prerequisite for the magical pie. Simply returning the sheet (signed "yes" or "no") was all that was required. To enlist the aid and goodwill of the teachers, they were given full control over the timing of the event, including the authority to cancel it for poor behavior. Reports from the field indicated that the children stormed home demanding that their parents sign and return the forms—some classes achieving full consent in 24 hours. Children who forgot were badgered by their classmates and reminded by their teachers. For an investment of roughly $500 (less than 15% of the cost of mailing self-addressed, stamped envelopes to parents), we received back almost 95% of the consent forms, with nearly 100% approval. For the few classes that did not quite achieve 100%, we demonstrated our good nature and provided pizza in any case—a small investment in the future goodwill of students and teachers alike. In fact, it was never our intent to deny anyone pizza—how could we?

Testing in the Field

Securing consent, while trying at times, was to be the easy part.[8] The real challenges arose from trying to test more than 2,000 children from more than 100 classrooms in 75 schools scattered across more than 3,000 square kilometres (approximately 1,200 square miles). The simple solution to these challenges is not to do studies like this one in the first place. But, assuming you are compelled,[9] here is what we learned about the process of testing.

Getting There and Getting Started

Googlies frequently come flying out of matters that seem so simple that there is no need to plan for them. One issue we honestly did not think would be a problem was getting to the schools on testing day. Useful preparations—appropriate for any trip, we have since learned—include ensuring (1) that there is gas in the car and (2) that the map you have is the map you need. We had at least one recorded instance of a team running out of gas. Unfortunately, the culprits were two of us, the principal investigators (PIs), one of whom (B. F.) apparently had a history of this sort of thing, much to the chagrin of another PI (J. C.), who was in the car, and the delight of the third (J. H.), who wasn't. In another instance, a phone call received at the office of PHAST from a cell phone on a Tuesday afternoon brought to light another potential problem in getting to schools. As scientists, we initially felt compelled to present a complete transcript of the call, thereby, as qualitative researchers would say, allowing the "voice" of the participant (J. C.) to be heard. But, in the interests of good taste, and to ensure that this book does not need a parental warning label for explicit material, we will summarize the event instead. Having downloaded a map to his destination, the PI was surprised to discover that the road (a rural route deep in heart of God's country) simply ended—with no warning—in the middle of what appeared to be an abandoned farm field. Getting out and scanning the horizon, he found that the road did indeed continue, about 800 meters (half a mile) farther on, past a patch of uneven (read: swampy, hilly, and possibly sinkhole-filled) terrain. Not having had the foresight to drive his amphibious vehicle that day, the PI had no choice but to turn his car around and try to find an alternate route. Ultimately, the whole trip had to be abandoned when it became clear that the testing would be over before the trip could be completed. Solutions? In the first case, look at the gas gauge prior to leaving; and, in the second, recognize that local knowledge always supersedes any map available on the Web. Although uncomfortable for many male investigators, asking the school secretary for the best way to arrive and park at the school is an investment in humility that will pay handsome dividends.[10] In any case, we note that our belief that the RAs, at least, would have the sense to put gas in their cars and obtain reliable maps was vindicated.

Other frustrations upon arrival included showing up and not being expected by the school principal, in spite of a confirmatory call the day before and a clear record of that phone call in the principal's Day-Timer (clearly marked when she looked it up to demonstrate that we had not called; one of us [J. H.] was there for that one), which led us to adopt the practice of confirming our test date and time with the school secretary, the principal, and the teacher. Twice each.

Given the nature of the testing we conducted, the use of a gym was essential. However, even today, not all schools have gyms, some gyms are small, and some architects who design gyms do so under the influence of daring but fundamentally unsound artistic theories and/or mind-bending drugs. All gyms, if present, are precious commodities, jealously guarded by zealous physical education teachers, coaches, and the occasional custodian ("you can't go in there with those shoes!"). We recorded at least one instance of a teacher demanding use of the gym, despite our having booked it much earlier, to conduct a badminton practice with four children. An on-site solution was eventually identified—we simply split the gym in two, and our research team aided in the setup of the badminton nets as a show of good faith.

Gyms that existed in the schools, but were less than 20 meters (66 feet) long, posed a particular challenge for us, as one of our key measures, the 20-meter shuttle run, requires ... well, enough said. Although we knew before going in that some schools were not equipped with a gym, we were surprised at the number of interesting rooms (in regard to shape and size) that principals, with an awareness of the power of semantics reminiscent of a successful field researcher's, call gymnasia. In the cases where a gym, by any definition, was not present, we surveyed the field outside the school, considered the weather conditions, and made provisions to perform the shuttle run outside. In the case of schools with gyms less than 20 meters in length, more creative adjustments were made. If we could offer one piece of advice, it is that it is important to remember that the hypotenuse is longer than the adjacent and opposite sides of a triangle, so that a few children may be able to run 20 meters safely on the diagonal—in theory, if not in practice.

Surprises on Beginning to Test

Although there were numerous challenges during testing, one of the most interesting phenomena we observed involved our testers and a sudden, inexplicable change in their behavior that Zimbardo (1972) would have appreciated. Although we admire and envy their ability to check gas gauges and find accurate maps, we found, much to our alarm, that university students such as our RAs, on returning to an elementary school setting to carry out research, can regress to a stage of development more consistent with that of their subjects. Upon completion of the aerobic testing, our assistants often found themselves in the gymnasium with a large group of children and no teacher supervision. Gyms are for games, and games are fun. In one case, the group decided to play dodgeball. Unfortunately, the competitive natures of some male assistants were aroused, and balls were soon flying at alarming speeds. Several children suffered minor bruising, and many more suffered, quite understandably, psychological trauma. We learned of these events when an enraged parent called one of us (J. H.) the next day. This was followed, in short order, by calls from the school principal, the dean of the faculty, and the school board offices. Our response was to immediately apologize to the parents and the school, interview the assistants to determine what had taken place, remove the offenders from our team, and then communicate our response to the parents, school, and board. We then arranged with the school principal for all the RAs to come to the school to apologize to the children and to serve them lunch—again making use of the soothing powers of pizza. The end result of our taking immediate responsibility and acting to make amends was that we did not lose the school, or a single subject, and that our reputation with the board actually improved. As a result of this learning experience, we instituted a policy of forbidding researchers to play with the children and requested that a teacher be present at all times during testing. We had made this request before, but with limited success. Some teachers who dealt with unruly classes on a daily basis were more than pleased to see our research team arrive—seeing an opportunity for a mental health break. This left two RAs to control an undisciplined class, with no authority, while also providing assistance to children with learning challenges. Because pepper spray would never have made it past an ethics review board, we began sending larger teams to those schools identified as problematic and, more important, reminded teachers that the board required their presence in class. It took the dodgeball incident, however, for the school board to throw its weight behind this policy, recognizing that, in some instances, the teachers had abdicated their responsibility as much as our assistants had abused theirs.[11]

And then there are the host of little annoyances and minor shocks that make the ability to problem solve on the fly a vital characteristic for a team leader in the field. These included the absence of electrical outlets in the gym (or outside) for test equipment (*policy solution: always bring an extra-long extension cord*), children with no running shoes or gym clothes (*policy solution: test in bare feet if possible, bring extra T-shirts*), and children physically unable to complete the testing. We soon appreciated the need to ask all children before we started our assessments if they had any significant impairments that might interfere with their ability to complete the necessary tasks. This allowed us to identify children recovering from long illness, with severe asthma, and at least one with the telltale symptoms of gastrointestinal upset very near full expression. The word "significant" in the question was vital, as that did not include lack of motivation or interest—a fairly common affliction prior to aerobic testing.

LESSONS LEARNED

Throughout this chapter we have described specific examples of how we addressed some of the unexpected challenges we faced over the past 3 years in this particular study. These can be summarized into more general observations. A successful school-based researcher's tool kit needs to include an awareness of the power of semantics, politeness, mastery of logistics, obstinacy, a willingness to employ a steel fist in a velvet glove (*read judicious use of threats*), and the emulation of highly successful (*or exploitative*) fast-food marketing practices. And of course, pizza. Ashamedly, we must include paying attention to fuel gauges and obtaining directions from knowledgeable sources, and with no shame whatsoever, recognize the importance of both humility and improvisation. The ability to set up badminton equipment competently and cheerfully is not a core part of the field researcher's tool kit, but some sort of training in the research area never hurts either.

A reasonable question to ask at this juncture is, would we do such a study again, given what we now know about the challenges of doing large-scale school-based research projects? The answer is, unequivocally, yes, but with some equivocation. From a methods perspective, there is a certain appeal in doing school-based research. In Canada, more than 90% of all children are enrolled in the public school system, which is very convenient for drawing representative samples. Moreover, subjects are captive for long periods during the day, and in most cases, teachers and parents seem to be interested in lending their children out as research subjects, especially when the topic is related to health and well-being. At the same time, these benefits must be weighed against the other challenges of doing school-based research, some of which have been discussed here. Although some problems have a nasty habit of staying hidden until you are already knee-deep in data collection, we hope some of our stories may be useful as inducements to think beyond design and measurement and to consider the googlies that may pop up. There is an old expression that goes, "Hope for the best, plan for the worst." Sage advice for all researchers undertaking school-based research.

NOTES

1. This has proven supremely difficult, despite the fact that most of his writing is in the field of psychiatric epidemiology.
2. And, ideally, spins around and falls over.
3. Actually, there are probably several options here—screwball, changeup—that would also work. The important point is that they're all deliveries that are intended to surprise the batter and that are difficult to hit.
4. We believe it was Bob Uecker who said, "The best way to catch a knuckleball is to wait until the ball stops rolling and then pick it up."
5. University bureaucracies, or hospital bureaucracies in the case of one of us (J. C.), we felt, would be a given to most readers and not really worth covering. Suffice it to say, we had challenges at all levels of research administration—but none that would surpass the expectations of anyone who as worked in these environments long enough to administer a grant.
6. In the metaphor we have been pursuing, the opposition is a team of gremlins.
7. Also, we know that taking the ball out of the bowler's hand is not a legal tactic in cricket. We apologize if this metaphor is becoming difficult to follow, but we can't abandon it now.
8. Again, we mean "easy" relative to some other things that were really remarkably annoying, not in the customary sense of "simple" or "not intensely aggravating."
9. Contractually obligated, threatened at gunpoint, driven by an overwhelming conviction that it is your destiny, and so forth.
10. Including, to choose an example at random, not finding yourself parked at the edge of a desolate field in rural Ontario in the early morning, cursing into a cell phone and wondering whether your Saturn could navigate a sinkhole if it really had to.
11. Well, maybe not that much, but you see what we mean.

TO READ FURTHER

There is a rich literature on conducting research in schools, including negotiating research interests with key stakeholder partners (teachers, parents, and principals) and ethical consideration about issues such as consent. A example of a recent, introductory textbook is:

Wilson, E. (2009). *School-based research: A guide for education students*. Thousand Oaks, CA: Sage.

There is an equally rich (and large) literature on assessing physical activity, health, and physical fitness in children. We suggest the following references, which include discussions on field-testing with children:

Armstrong, N., & Welsman, J. (1997). *Young people and physical activity.* Oxford, UK: University Press.

Rowlands, T. W. (2005). *Children's exercise physiology* (2nd ed.). Champaign, Ill: Human Kinetics.

REFERENCES

American Psychiatric Association. (2000). *Diagnostic and statistical manual of mental disorders* (4th ed., text rev.). Washington, DC: Author.

Cairney, J., Hay, J. A., Faught, B. E., Flouris, A., & Klentrou, P. (2007). Developmental coordination disorder and cardiorespiratory fitness in children. *Pediatric Exercise Science, 19,* 20–28.

Cairney, J., Hay, J. A., Faught, B. E., & Hawes, R. (2005). Developmental coordination disorder and overweight and obesity in children aged 9–14y. *International Journal of Obesity, 29,* 369–372.

Cairney J., Hay, J. A., Faught, B. E., Mandigo, J., & Flouris, A. (2005). Developmental coordination disorder, self-efficacy toward physical activity and participation in free play and organized activities: Does gender matter? *Adapted Physical Activity Quarterly, 22,* 67–82.

Faught, B. E., Hay, J. A., Cairney, J., Flouris, A., & Klentrou, N. (2005). Increased risk for coronary vascular disease in children with developmental coordination disorder. *Journal of Adolescent Health, 37,* 376–380.

Gibbs, J., Appleton, J., & Appleton, R. (2007). Dyspraxia or developmental coordination disorder? Unravelling the enigma. *Archives of Disease in Childhood, 92,* 534–539.

Hay, J., & Missiuna, C. (1998). Motor proficiency in children reporting low levels of participation in physical activity. *Canadian Journal of Occupational Therapy, 65,* 64–71.

Zimbardo, P. (1972). Pathology of imprisonment. *Trans-Action, 9* (Apr.), 4–8.

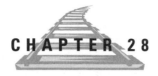

CHAPTER 28

Pets, Pies, and Videotape
Conducting In-Home Observational Research with Late-Life Intergenerational Families

BRIAN D. CARPENTER
STEVE BALSIS

It is impossible to create in the laboratory the frequency, duration, scope, complexity, and magnitude of some important human conditions. In this, psychology has something in common with meteorology. Some of the principles of the whirlwind and the thunderbolt can be studied in the laboratory, but to extend the curves into the high values, and to include all complicating factors, it is necessary to go to the plains and to observe these events as they occur under natural conditions
—BARKER (1968, p. 3)

BACKGROUND OF THE STUDY

Barker (1968) draws a vivid analogy between the science of meteorology and the science of human behavior, encouraging researchers to take their questions into the field where the action is. Observational research in naturalistic settings gives researchers access to behaviors that are elusive in laboratory settings. In the case of our interests (late-life families), this methodology also opens doors to otherwise inaccessible populations, such as frail elders who live at home. But conducting research outside the lab brings its own challenges. In this chapter we describe our efforts to conduct a research project that involved videotaping late-life families as they interacted in their own homes. As it turns out, Barker was on the mark when he chose whirlwinds and thunderbolts as metaphors.

Adult children often collaborate with their older parents on a wide range of decisions in areas such as healthcare, housing, and finances. How late-life families work together to make these decisions is still something of a mystery. But with upcoming demographic changes—in particular, the aging of the baby boomers—more and more families will need to work in partnership to make sure older adults get the care and support they need.

The goals of our study were (1) to examine the ability of adult children to predict the care preferences of their older parents and (2) to clarify the factors that differentiate children who are more knowledgeable about their parents from children who are less knowledgeable (see Carpenter, Lee, Ruckdeschel, Van Haitsma, & Feldman, 2006, for partial results). We used a set of self-report questionnaires to assess parents' preferences and children's predictions of parent preferences, along with perceptions of family dynamics. Of course, asking people to describe their family relationships invites potential bias—underreporting, overreporting, minimization, exaggeration—all damaging to the validity of the research. So, we also decided to bring the family together to participate in structured problem-solving tasks and conversations, which we videotaped and analyzed to see if there were process features of how the family members behaved with one another that might be predictive of children's knowledge about their parents.

In an earlier study we conducted these "family meetings" in our lab. In that setting we were able to enhance reliability through standardization. We arranged the physical space the same way for every family. We controlled the task lighting (an important feature when working with older adults). We minimized the potential for unexpected interruptions or distractions. And we were able to observe the families behind a two-way mirror, minimizing the obtrusiveness of our microphones, our audio and video recorders, and ourselves.

Gains in the lab in terms of predictability and control can be offset, however, by compromised ecological validity (Rosenthal & Rosnow, 1991). Put simply, families may behave differently in the lab than they would at home. What we observe in the lab may not be an accurate representation of how families really communicate, make decisions, and express affection (or don't). No matter how researchers try to create a home-like environment in the lab, with plants and decorative lamps and sofas and carefully chosen watercolor paintings, it is still not a home, and, more important, still not *that family's* home. More natural behaviors are likely to occur when the family members are in their own space, surrounded by the objects they know, in a place where countless previous interactions have taken place.

Another advantage of taking the research to families is that we may enhance the sample we can recruit and thereby the generalizability and validity of the research (Cavanaugh & Whitbourne, 1999). Older adults who have stopped driving or modified their driving habits (e.g., driving shorter distances, not driving at night), or older adults with mobility restrictions caused by arthritis or stroke, may refuse a trip to the lab. Participants should be representative of the people who are actually involved in the real-world analogue of the research task (Czaja & Sharit, 2003). In the case of our research, we are interested in family decision making regarding housing, healthcare, and finances, topics that are particularly relevant to more frail older adults. Therefore, meeting families at home increased the likelihood that we studied families actively facing the issues of interest to us. Nonetheless, it turned out that we weren't quite prepared for all the decisions and challenges we would face in making home visits.

THE CHALLENGES AND OVERCOMING THEM

Even as we were designing the study, we realized that conducting in-home observations would make it difficult to get the entire family to participate. Our research is guided by family systems theories, so we want as many family members to participate as possible. But geographical dispersion of adult children was an immediate obstacle, as many families had children spread over many states. To deal with this, we scheduled family meetings when out-of-town children were visiting, often around holidays or birthdays. We soon found that this was not possible for every family. Consequently, we ended up studying some incomplete families, which we knew was not ideal. For instance, a child in one of these families commented, "You know, the conversation wouldn't be going this way if my bossy brother were here." So much for ecological validity.

Our next decision point was whose home to visit. During recruitment, some older adults gave vague refusals, which we later learned were due to discomfort with inviting a stranger into their homes. In this era of senior-targeted scams, older adults may be (justifiably) reluctant to have visitors to their homes. Sending a preliminary letter before we called (on university letterhead) seemed to help. Even when a family agreed to participate, however, we discovered that the location could influence what we observed. The hosts, whether parents or children, were on their home turf, whereas the others were guests. And place, we learned, is power. For example, we witnessed a lengthy and heated conversation about the expected use of coasters on a parent's coffee table. Although it sounds minor, it set a confrontational tone for at least the first task in our protocol.

Including multiple people in the family meeting led to another challenge in scheduling the home visit. Middle-aged adult children had many competing demands and time commitments associated with their own families and jobs; this "sandwich generation" is pulled in many directions. We should say, though, that despite stereotypes, many older adults were tough to schedule too. They had active lives of their own, with commitments to social clubs, volunteer organizations, and travel. Even older adults in poor health had limited availability because of the amount of time they spent preparing for, going to, and recuperating from lab tests, rehabilitation appointments, or other outpatient visits. Flexibility in scheduling was key. We found it most efficient to ask one family member to coordinate scheduling with the rest of the family and then relay the date and time to us. With two mobile research assistant teams, we were able to tell families, "You tell us when, and we'll be there." Naturally, this meant being available evenings and weekends. We also tried to keep the in-home protocol brief, relying on preliminary phone and mail contacts to gather some data, thereby reducing the time of the in-home session. It helped during recruitment to be able to tell families that we would be there for only an hour.

Earlier we mentioned the advantage of capturing a more frail sample by traveling to participants' homes, but we also discovered that there were complications when our recruitment was based on telephone contact alone. On a few occasions we arrived to discover that the older parent would not be able to complete tasks because of a cognitive or physical impairment. At the start of the project we screened for cognitive impairment but discovered that some older adults were able to pass the screen yet were unable to participate in problem-solving tasks with their children. Adjusting the screening cut point was necessary.

Upon arrival, an unexpected complication was figuring out how to get into the homes, literally. At some apartment buildings we could not get in without knowing the code to use on an external call box. And our frequent visits to retirement communities and congregate housing facilities taught us to ask beforehand whether we would need permission from a gate guard or doorman to enter. We also found it necessary to ask the family if we should know an apartment or unit number. On occasion we arrived at a street address only to be faced with a building directory arranged by apartment numbers, with no names listed.

Once inside, our next challenges were in setting up our equipment. We encountered a number of issues associated with the space itself. Some older adults lived in very small apartments, which required creative positioning of the equipment, research assistants, and family members. We also discovered that we had in mind an ideal seating arrangement—all family members seated around something like a dining room table with a smooth, open work surface—that was impossible, given the actual layout of most homes. Some families made it clear they wanted to sit in a room without a table nearby, in other families the members sat at a distance from one another, and in still other families the members positioned themselves so that participation by everyone was discouraged.

Two other important aspects of the physical environment were the lighting and the temperature. The lighting needs to be sufficient so that the family members can see what they are doing, particularly older parents who may have some visual impairment, but not so bright that it causes glare or washout in the camera image. Some homes we visited were cave-like, with drapes drawn and dim 20-watt lightbulbs flickering here and there; others had bright halogen spotlights, large wall mirrors that multiplied the family infinitely, and direct sunlight streaming into the room, which made for a confusing or bleached video. Creative positioning of family members and the camera helped overcome some of these obstacles. We had one research assistant (RA) lead the family through the informed consent process, while the other RA took on the task of setting up a room for taping, assuring the family that we would return all the furniture to its original place. Regarding room temperature, our advice is to dress in layers. We mention this because some older adults, owing to normal physiological changes with age, keep their homes warmer than you might expect, and even though we needed the wool sweater on the way to the home, we didn't like being trapped in it for 60 minutes in the equivalent of a sauna.

Despite our best attempts to have adequate recording resources, we learned a few technical tips to share. One is to be prepared for equipment failure. We began taking two complete sets of equipment after one camera failed. Although some of our equipment could run on batteries, we discovered we needed access to an electrical source (we use a microphone preamplifier that requires an electrical supply), which meant we needed to be near an electrical outlet. We learned to travel with a 12 foot industrial extension cord, grounded three-prong adapter, and power strip that could accommodate all our equipment. Here again we sometimes needed to move furniture, or at least be ready to crawl around on the floor to find an outlet. Once the equipment was set up, we conducted a brief audio and video test to make sure our connections were working properly. This, too, we learned by experience. After our first family observation, we returned to the office, pleased with the excellent picture quality but humbled by the lack of sound.

Space and equipment issues aside, other practical considerations included the presence of unexpected participants, interruptions, and offers. In rare circumstances a family member we expected to be present was not there or someone we didn't expect was there. Our protocol was of the sort that we could include extra people if they wished. That may not always be true, and you may have to contend with people being upset at their exclusion or at least influencing the interaction by their presence, even if they are not participating. We hadn't anticipated the participation of in-laws, but at one visit a son appeared with his wife, and it became clear she was important to the conversation (our solution: have extra materials on hand). At another family visit, a friend of the parent had come over out of interest to watch, and we had to ask that person to sit in another room, out of view and earshot, so she wouldn't influence the interaction (our explanation: "We will be asking the family some personal questions").

Interruptions occurred when visitors dropped by unexpectedly in the middle of taping (neighbors, the mail person, solicitors) or the phone rang in the middle of a task or sensitive conversation. A "Do Not Disturb" sign on the front door can help, and we started to ask families not to answer the phone during a meeting. Even less predictable was the behavior of pets. We had little trouble from fish and cats, but dogs could be distracting during the conversation, and some birds were quite loud, disrupting clear audio. It's also wise when making assignments to ask participants about pets and research assistants about allergies. Finally, we often dealt with offers of food or drink. As a rule, we declined politely. Yet we were guests in their homes, and the social norms of older adults are different from those of younger generations, so we tried to consider what would most facilitate our relationship with the participants.

Earlier we mentioned that one advantage of lab observations is that the recording equipment and the researchers can be less obtrusive. In the home, that's not the case, which can mean significant reactivity effects (Lyman, 1994). Indeed, participants made more glances and comments toward us at home in comparison to the lab-based version of the study. Nonetheless, we're hesitant to conclude that our visibility was damaging. Comments directed to the researchers in the midst of the protocol can clarify what is happening at the moment. For example, during a discussion of one older mother's desires regarding aggressive medical intervention, her daughter commented to us, "It's important for you to know this conversation would be entirely different if we hadn't been through the kind of death my dad had." Her offhand comment helped us put the conversation in context and identify a variable we had not considered before. Although the literature seems to suggest that reactivity effects are minor (e.g., Christensen & Hazzard, 1983; Jacob, Tennenbaum, Seilhammer, Bargiel, & Sharon, 1994; Johnson & Bolstad, 1975), we should point out that these studies have not examined late-life families, in which cohort differences in familiarity with technology and norms of privacy may accentuate reactivity.

A final issue concerns confidentiality. It is essential to make sure everyone in the family is aware beforehand of what will take place at the home visit and what information will be shared with other family members. We spoke with some family members who were willing to do most of the tasks we described but were unwilling, for example, to talk explicitly about family relationships (perhaps interesting in itself). Family members should also be clear about who will see their videotape, what it will be used for, and how long it will be retained. In one case family members requested at the conclusion of the meeting that we not use their tape (also perhaps interesting, given that this family had heated disagreements during tasks). For the most part, though, aside from quips about ill-prepared wardrobe and hair, families tended to be receptive to the taping.

LESSONS LEARNED

By the end of the study we felt as though we were finally ready to begin the study, given what we had learned, which we summarize here. First, during recruitment, determine whether your research question influences whether you should contact adult children or older parents first. Next, when multiple family members are eligible and interested, but not all are needed, decide who will actually participate. When screening, consider cognitive, sensory, and functional impairments that could interfere with participation, and set adequate screening cut points. Gather contact information for *all* family members. And be flexible when scheduling appointments; evenings and weekends may be necessary.

Before leaving for an in-home visit, make sure research assistants are trained to respond to medical emergencies. It may seem morbid to mention, but working with more frail research participants increases the likelihood that researchers will encounter circumstances that call for intervention (e.g., falls or other adverse events). We had a mobile phone with us at all times, and our research assistants had basic training in CPR just in case. More ambiguous are situations in which the researcher encounters an unsafe living situation (e.g., a home without heat or air conditioning, an environment of squalor, an older adult whose nutritional status may seem tenuous, or comments and interactions with adult children that suggest elder abuse or neglect). Researchers should be aware of the ethical and legal requirements for mandatory reporting. It may be worthwhile to consult with an Institutional Review Board when drafting consent forms, in case a provision about reporting should be added. Send appointment confirmation letters to all family members, and call them all the day before as a reminder. Get good directions to the home, including specifics about parking and entry. Develop a checklist to make sure you have all your equipment and supplies before leaving the office.

Upon arrival, be prepared for more or fewer family members to be present than you expected, and give some forethought to what family relatives are eligible (in-laws? extended family?). As you begin with the family, discuss how you would like to handle potential interruptions. Be ready to move furniture (and move it back). And don't forget to double-check the operation of your equipment for video and sound quality.

In-home observations with late-life families have the potential to expand our knowledge of family dynamics beyond information obtained by self-report questionnaires. Observations in the home enhance the ecological validity of research findings by placing the family in a setting that maximizes their comfort and willingness to act naturally. Despite this benefit, home observations come with costs, including demands on investigators for flexibility in scheduling, a willingness to travel, and challenges associated with unpredictable assessment conditions. When studying late-life inter-generational families in particular, the complications extend to complex recruitment decisions and the unique features of some older adults' situations and homes. In this chapter we highlighted some of the pragmatic issues we faced when going into the homes of late-life families. Our intent is not to discourage observational research. On the contrary, our experience has sharpened our belief that in-home observations with intergenerational late-life families provide a window into family dynamics unavailable with other methods.

ACKNOWLEDGMENTS

The research described in this chapter was supported by grants from the Brookdale Foundation, the Harvey A. and Dorismae Friedman Research Fund at Washington University in St. Louis, and the Administration on Aging (90AM2612) and the State of Missouri in grants to the Jewish Federation of St. Louis.

TO READ FURTHER

Dallos, R. (2006). Observational methods. In G. M. Breakwell, S. Hammond, C. Fife-Schaw, & J. A. Smith (Eds.), *Research methods in psychology* (3rd ed., pp. 124–145). Thousand Oaks, CA: Sage.

A good overview of observational methods, describing their central features and related theoretical frameworks. The chapter also includes examples of different types of observations and ways of coding subsequent data.

Friedman, S. L., & Wachs, T. D. (Eds.). (1999). *Measuring environment across the life span: Emerging methods and concepts.* Washington, DC: American Psychological Association.

This text can help researchers start to think about the important influence the environment has on behavior (including environments in which researchers may choose to do observational research). Its chapters explore ways of conceptualizing and measuring the environment across the life span.

Montgomery, B. M., & Duck, S. (Eds.). (1993). *Studying interpersonal interaction.* New York: Guilford Press.

A great introductory resource for people just getting into the study of inter-personal interactions. Its chapters lay out important theoretical considerations, discuss what kind of data can be collected, and how those data can be analyzed. It also contains a chapter by Sillars on observational methods, including a discussion of sampling and reactivity.

REFERENCES

Barker, R. G. (1968). *Ecological validity: Concepts and methods for studying the environment of human behavior.* Stanford, CA: Stanford University Press.

Carpenter, B. D., Lee, M., Ruckdeschel, K., Van Haitsma, K. S., & Feldman, P. H. (2006). Adult children as informants about parent's psychosocial preferences. *Family Relations, 55,* 552–563.

Cavanaugh, J. C., & Whitbourne, S. K. (1999). Research methods. In J. C. Cavanaugh & S. K. Whitbourne (Eds.), *Gerontology: An interdisciplinary perspective* (pp. 33–64). New York: Oxford University Press.

Christensen, A., & Hazzard, A. (1983). Reactive effects during naturalistic observation of families. *Behavioral Assessment, 5,* 349–362.

Czaja, S. J., & Sharit, J. (2003). Practically relevant research: Capturing real world tasks, environments, and outcomes. *The Gerontologist, 43,* 9–18.

Jacob, T., Tennenbaum, D., Seilhamer, R. A., Bargiel, K., & Sharon, T. (1994). Reactivity effects during naturalistic observation of distressed and nondistressed families. *Journal of Family Psychology, 8,* 354–363.

Johnson, S. M., & Bolstad, O. D. (1975). Reactivity to home observation: A comparison of audio recorded behavior with observers present or absent. *Journal of Applied Behavioral Analysis, 8,* 181–185.

Lyman, K. A. (1994). Fieldwork in groups and institutions. In J. F. Gubrium & A. Sankar (Eds.), *Qualitative methods in aging research* (pp. 155–170). Thousand Oaks, CA: Sage.

Rosenthal, R., & Rosnow, R. L. (1991). *Essentials of behavioral research: Methods and data analysis* (2nd ed.). New York: McGraw-Hill.

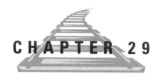

CHAPTER 29

Underfunded but Not Undone

DIANNE BRYANT

BACKGROUND OF THE STUDY

When reporting the results of clinical trials comparing two interventions, investigators often include a description of patients' pretreatment (baseline) health status to illustrate similarity between groups before the intervention is applied. In addition, baseline data often provide a covariate for statistical between-groups comparisons to adjust for any differences that were present before treatment began, increasing the power to demonstrate the effect of the intervention.

Often, clinicians involved with trials evaluating surgical interventions are unable to fully assess a patient's eligibility before surgical evaluation. In fact, depending on the specificity of preoperative evaluations to diagnose the disease of interest and to identify concomitant pathology, the number of patients who are found to be ineligible following surgical examination can be high, introducing huge inefficiencies in the process of data collection, inasmuch as the research assistant collects baseline data for patients before surgical evaluation.

A recent example of this inefficiency occurred as part of a randomized trial to compare the effectiveness of inside-out suturing (i.e., sewing the torn pieces of meniscal cartilage together using a needle and thread introduced through an incision) to bioabsorbable Arrows (i.e., holding the torn pieces of meniscal cartilage together using "darts" introduced through arthroscopic instruments) for reparable meniscal lesions[1] (Bryant et al., 2007). During the course of the trial, 700 patients undergoing anterior cruciate ligament reconstruction[2] or isolated knee arthroscopy[3] who were suspected of having a meniscal tear gave their consent to participate and completed baseline assessments before surgery (each requiring approximately 40 minutes to complete). Following arthroscopic evaluation, however, only 100 of these patients remained eligible for the study, which meant that 85.7% of patients who had completed baseline measurements were excluded from further participation.

Because patient-reported outcomes are often the primary outcome of interest to measure treatment effects in orthopedic populations, we began to wonder whether researchers could collect baseline data retrospectively, following surgical determination of the patients' eligibility, and whether these data would accurately represent data that would have otherwise been collected preoperatively.

To address this question, my colleagues and I designed a randomized clinical trial (RCT) to investigate patients' ability to recall their presurgical quality of life, function, and general health at their first postoperative clinical follow-up (approximately 2 weeks after surgery) (Bryant et al., 2006). Eligible patients who gave consent were randomly allocated to one of two groups. Group I underwent assessment at 4 weeks preoperatively, on the day of surgery, and at 2 weeks and 12 months postoperatively. Group II underwent assessment at 2 weeks and 12 months postoperatively.[4] At the 2-week visit patients were asked to complete two sets of questionnaires; the first set asked them to think back to before their surgery and to complete the questionnaires according to their status before surgery. The second set of questionnaires asked patients to respond according to their current status.

THE CHALLENGES

Experience has taught us that patients are more likely to agree to participate in a study if the assessments correspond with regular clinic checkups with their surgeons. For our study, this meant that the data assessor needed to be available during clinic hours. Because one of our assessments was in addition to regular clinic visits (4-week preoperative assessment for Group I), patients were unlikely to participate if it meant taking time from work, which meant that this assessment may have to take place outside regular business hours. Further, if the patient was scheduled for the first surgery of the day (8:00 A.M.), assessments that needed to take place on the day of surgery (Group I patients) could start as early as 6:30 A.M. Given that there were four surgeons at one center and two surgeons at another, with at least one surgery day and up to two clinic days per week per surgeon, it seemed we would need at least a full-time research assistant at each center.

In addition, because of the multicentered nature of the study, the complexity of the design, and the volume of data being collected (five patient-reported questionnaires per assessment, surgical details, demographic information, and adverse events), we needed a fairly elaborate plan for data management. Ideally, we would need a study coordinator to monitor data for completeness—both that the assessment took place according to protocol and that the case report forms for each assessment were complete and made sense. Further, we needed a data entry clerk and/or a fairly intricate database.

At first pass, the budget to run this study totalled just over $225,000 over 3 years—relatively inexpensive for an RCT, because we did not have to consider any of the usual costs associated with taking expensive images of the knee, special tests, or the intervention itself. Because this project's sole purpose was to address a methodological question, however, we were limited by the number of agencies willing to consider funding questions of this type. Furthermore, the dollar amounts available from these agencies were usually much less than our current budget required. In the end, we managed to secure Can$45,000; $30,000 from an industrial partner and $15,000 from an internal hospital competition—more than a bit shy of where we needed to be.

OVERCOMING THE DIFFICULTIES

Given our own interests in pursuing this project, we decided to reassess the budget—were there means to address our research objectives within our fixed budget? As usual, the greatest proportion of the budget was allocated to supporting research staff. One option to reduce this spending was to pay assistants for data collected and not for the time actually spent collecting the data, which was something we had seen more and more as a center contributing to other multicenter trials. For example, the budget would allocate $500 per eligible patient, so that if there were five visits, each time data for a visit was submitted and the study coordinator deemed the data complete and query-free, the center would receive $100 until the patient had completed all five visits. In general, this method can reduce a study's budget because it does not reimburse for the time spent screening, recruiting, and gaining consent from potential participants who are not eligible or those who are eligible but who refuse to give consent. Furthermore, if eligibility cannot be fully determined until during surgery (just before the surgical intervention), then it also ignores the cost of conducting the presurgical baseline visit of patients who are deemed ineligible following surgical evaluation.

In my experience, this option works well if two things are true: (1) that centers can agree on a reasonable amount of reimbursement per patient (by reasonable I mean an amount that would allow the budget to be substantially reduced) and (2) that there is a full-time research assistant already at each center who has time available to allocate to your project. Usually this is someone who is paid for full-time work at that center but who divides his or her time between projects.

In our case, because nearly every patient was eligible for study participation, this method reduced the overall budget by only 5%, or $15,000, which was not going to reduce costs sufficiently within our funding means. Second, one of the centers did not have a research assistant in place and was not participating in any other research. We needed another plan.

Fortunately at that time, I was teaching a third-year undergraduate course in research design and critical appraisal. Many of the students in this course were interested in pursuing a career in research and/or some health-related field. Quite often I had students approach me to inquire about opportunities to volunteer their time (which is part of the application package for many graduate or medical schools) or to participate in an independent study or a fourth-year thesis under my supervision, which was a requirement for their undergraduate degrees. After speaking with the associate dean of their program about the opportunity for students to gain practical experience in a clinical research setting, I posted a brief summary of the project.

Within the week, I had more than 90 applications from interested students. From this pool, I selected 20 students whose varying availabilities meant that we would have access to a research assistant beginning from 6:30 A.M. to 6:00 P.M. each weekday and a few hours on weekends to meet with patients, who would agree to participate only if study assessments did not interfere with their time at work.

The students were responsible for designating the position as either volunteer work or as an independent study for credit, whichever they felt was in their best interest. For students who chose to complete an independent study, we defined their objectives and responsibilities together—some worked to create teaching materials (e.g., models, poster boards, videos, websites) for patients undergoing knee surgery, and others conducted a search and critical appraisal of the existing literature concerning some of the orthopedic surgeries that patients were having done. The majority of projects were designed to meet mutual objectives so that students could maximize their experience while I minimized my participation in tasks that would not advance my own research agenda.

One of the most important aspects that contributed to the success of this approach was the effort put forth in training, organization, and management. In terms of training, students attended two sessions that were organized by me and an experienced study coordinator, in which they learned how to screen and recruit patients, how to randomize patients, and how to conduct assessments so as not to bias patients' responses on self-reported outcomes. We discussed ethics in terms of obtaining informed consent, privacy, and safety issues. Arrangements were made for the students to attend hospital safety and privacy seminars.

In terms of organization, we used an online limited access calendar through LearnLink that allowed students to add patient appointments to the schedule, identify the student responsible for conducting assessments during a particular time slot, and send an e-mail to that student to make him or her aware of the upcoming appointment. I met with students as a group on a biweekly basis for the first few months, and then monthly thereafter, so that they could share their experiences and problem solve together. These meetings quickly advanced their skills as data collectors and allowed me to closely monitor the progress of the project and the integrity with which data were being collected.

Although we were able to reduce our budget quite considerably by the methods described here, we did support a quarter-time experienced study coordinator/data manager ($32,000) and built and maintained a database to house the data ($6,000). The data manager was absolutely key to monitoring the quality of incoming data, generating queries, communicating with students and investigators, and resolving issues.

The database was generated using the DataFax platform. We shared the licensing and maintenance fees between numerous projects led by us or colleagues. Using the DataFax platform meant that case report forms could be faxed in from any fax machine and data entry was automatic and direct. In addition, this platform allowed us to build in logic and edit checks so that the system would automatically alert us to missing or late data, or data that were nonsensical. Although there was an upfront expense to create the database and a yearly cost to maintain it, there were minimal costs associated with data entry, and minimal translation errors.

At the end of the project, in just over a year, we had screened more than 1,000 consecutive patients and randomized 398. Patient follow-up lasted for 1 year postsurgery. Overall, only 15 patients were lost to follow-up (4%), which is quite remarkable.

LESSONS LEARNED

Maximize the efficiency of funding dollars by hiring qualified personnel and limiting their tasks to higher-level operations—overall study coordination and data management. By sharing the costs of licensing and maintenance, you can take advantage of "smart" databases that will assist with data management and further reduce the number of person-hours spent managing data. There are ways to assemble qualified personnel willing to give their time if they are getting something in return—monetary compensation is not always the currency.

NOTES

1. Menisci are disks of cartilage that sit between the surfaces of the bones that make up the knee joint and are responsible for distributing weight through the knee and improving the stability of the knee joint.
2. The anterior cruciate ligament (ACL) is one of the most important of four strong ligaments connecting the bones of the knee joint. Its function is to provide stability to the knee and minimize stress across the knee joint.
3. In an arthroscopic examination, small incisions are made to allow the insertion of pencil-sized instruments that contain a small lens and lighting system to magnify and illuminate the structures inside the joint. By attaching the arthroscope to a miniature television camera, the surgeon is able to see the interior of the joint and determine the amount or type of injury and then repair or correct the problem, if it is necessary.
4. The purpose of including Group II was to determine whether there was evidence that Group I patients' prior exposure to the instruments (4 weeks preoperative and day of surgery) influenced their recalled ratings. We assumed that by virtue of randomization, Group I and Group II would have similar characteristics and so should have similar recalled and current ratings at 2 weeks postoperatively.

TO READ FURTHER

Sackett, D. L. (2001). On the determinants of academic success as a clinician-scientist. *Clinical and Investigative Medicine, 24*, 94–100.

This remains the best article I've come across to describe the roles and responsibilities of the mentor and mentee to each other and to self.

Bhandari, M., & Joensson, A. (2008). *Clinical research for surgeons*. Stuttgart: Thieme.

Chapter 31 of this book, "How to Budget for a Research Study," provides detailed guidance for budget planning for multicenter and single-center studies.

REFERENCES

Bryant, D., Dill, J., Litchfield, R., Amendola, A., Giffin, R., Fowler, P., et al. (2007). Effectiveness of bioabsorbable arrows compared with inside-out suturing for vertical, reparable meniscal lesions: A randomized clinical trial. *American Journal of Sports Medicine, 35*, 889–896.

Bryant, D., Norman, G., Stratford, P., Marx, R. G., Walter, S. D., & Guyatt, G. H. (2006). Patients undergoing knee surgery provided accurate ratings of preoperative quality of life and function 2 weeks after surgery. *Journal of Clinical Epidemiology, 59*, 984–993.

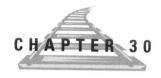

CHAPTER 30

Community-Based Participatory Research
A Lesson in Humility

DENNIS WATSON

BACKGROUND OF THE STUDY

Community-based participatory research, a form of applied research, is an effective tool for achieving positive change in communities because it helps to form working relationships between community organizations and researchers through organizations' participation in research activities. Participatory research itself requires the involvement of individuals who make up organizations or communities in the research process. This form of research takes into account the idea that every member of a community or organization has something to provide, and tapping into the abilities of individuals, as resources within the community, is the best way to engage in community-based research. Three elements common to most participatory research projects that distinguish them from traditional academic methods are that they (1) are useful (i.e., able to be applied to solve a problem in some manner), (2) use mixed methods, and (3) focus on the collaborative process (Stoecker, 2005, p. 30).

The project I outline here is a participatory evaluation that was carried out for a graduate-level sociology course in engaged methodologies. Our class was required, as a team or as individuals, to find a community partner with which to conduct an applied research project in order to gain firsthand experience in participatory research methods. The project was designed to last for 1½ semesters.

Northtown, a neighborhood with a very rich history, is located in a large Midwestern urban center. Having once been a site of mansions and vacation homes for the wealthy, Northtown has transformed over the last 80 or so years into having a large concentration of social service organizations, homeless individuals, single-room-occupancy hotels, and low-income housing units that disguise its history of affluence. In addition to having this economic mix, Northtown is one of the most racially and ethnically diverse communities in the city, with large numbers of African, Latino, and Asian Americans, as well as a large immigrant population composed mainly of Asian and African immigrants.

At the time of this writing, Northtown is currently in a period of rapid gentrification, which has become a polarizing force within the community. Divisions within gentrifying communities are nothing new and reflect the diversity found within them. Past research on similar gentrification issues has shown that polarization happens when higher-income residents see neighborhood diversity as a sign of neighborhood decline and lower-income residents see it as a sign of displacement (see Maly, 2005; Maly & Leachman, 1998; Patillo, 2007). But, although many of the traditional residents of Northtown may not trust their new neighbors, the gentrification of Northtown can be seen as a mixed blessing for low-income residents because, even while it is causing them to be blamed for problems in the community and resulting in a loss of affordable housing, new money coming into the area is also bringing a number of services and businesses that never previously existed. This is a benefit because it means people of low income can now obtain much needed goods and services without spending the money or time required to get them from other areas. It also means that there are more available job opportunities in the area for individuals to pursue.

As mentioned, gentrification is both a blessing and a burden to the people of low income in Northtown. This is also true for the small businesses of Northtown, many of which are run and owned by people from ethnic and racial minorities, and these ethnic minority business owners were of particular concern to our community partner for this project.

Our Partner's Focus and Problem in the Community

Our partner in this project was a community development corporation (CDC) that is partnered with the local chamber of commerce. The broad mission of the organization is to promote community development through supporting businesses in Northtown. The first reason that the organization is concerned with ethnic minority businesses is that many of them are not faring well in the community. According to staff at the CDC, the owners are just barely getting by on what they make, and there are many cultural barriers that stand in the way of their being competitive in the American business world. This leads to the second issue with these businesses, which is that these cultural barriers also make it difficult for our partner and the local chamber of commerce to gain participation and membership from these ethnic minority businesses—two things that would allow them to help these at-risk establishments survive. These cultural barriers, from our partner's perspective, include language difficulties, trust issues, basic ideas of business practice, and concepts of hygiene and cleanliness, to name a few.

Our partner had made a number of attempts to get the ethnic minority business members to become more involved in the community, but this job has been difficult. The research team I was part of sought to specifically address this issue through a participatory evaluation. The research itself underwent a number of methodological adjustments in response to time and resource restraints, as well as cultural barriers, which left me as the sole researcher on the project.

Overview of the Original Study

The original evaluation team consisted of me and two other students in my sociology course. Our professor arranged a meeting for the team with the CDC that we partnered with. This and a subsequent meeting were used to discuss the various projects and issues the CDC was facing in the community in order to brainstorm ideas for ways in which we could help the organization through a research partnership.

Our team listed and discussed the various issues that were brought to light at the two meetings. We decided early on that the ethnic minorities' lack of involvement and trust in the CDC, as well as in each other, was a major issue that the organization was facing. We proposed an evaluation of the outreach efforts directed toward these businesses, which would look at the attitudes and needs of the business owners and managers as well as the effectiveness of the communication between the CDC and these businesses.

We had our work cut out for us because there was little previous research on this topic to guide our efforts. Whereas a portion of the literature looking at minority businesses focuses on how to help them through outreach, most of this research, although paying significant attention to racial differences, fails to look at or discuss in detail the ethnicity of business owners. Another factor not adequately addressed by research to date is the immigration status of business owners. For example, most research considers only four or five generic racial categories that lump ethnically diverse groups together when considering this issue: Black/African American, Latino, Asian, Asian Pacific Americans, and American Indian. In fact the term "ethnic" is rarely used to describe minority businesses in the

United States unless it is used to describe a firm that specializes in providing ethnic products (Logan & Alba, 1994).

Our initial proposal was for an outcome evaluation using a 32-question survey to determine how aware the various businesses in the area were of the CDC and the chamber of commerce's activities, as well as the benefits of participation and/or membership. In addition, we also wanted to assess possible problems that might be interfering with communication issues (e.g., language barriers, lack of Internet access to obtain e-mails, lack of trust in outsiders). We believed that a survey would be a good tool to evaluate the minority business outreach because it would allow us to reach a large number of individuals and lend itself to both quantitative and qualitative analysis (with our professor's advice, we decided to give the survey to all businesses, not just those owned or operated by ethnic minorities).

The program manager of the CDC voiced various misgivings about the proposed method because she believed the business owners, not trusting the evaluators for cultural reasons, would refuse to participate in a survey, but we decided to proceed with the survey regardless. The reason we made this decision was due to constraints related to the length of time available to complete the project and our individual group members' other priorities (i.e., we had no extra time because we were in graduate school). Another issue affecting the team's decision was the researchers' conceptions about what constituted appropriate and objective research methods, which were derived from previous education and training in fields other than sociology (business and psychology).

THE CHALLENGES

The evaluation faced various time and resource constraints. Early in the data collection phase, one of my team members left the project for personal reasons. To address new constraints related to loss of this team member, my remaining partner and I amended the original method from a survey to be conducted in person to one that would be conducted over the phone. Because of the lack of time before the end of the semester, the university's urban research center, of which our professor was the director, allowed us to engage two undergraduate students to help conduct the survey (only one of the students eventually completed any work allocated to them).

In addition to these constraints, a poor response rate of 3%, of which none of the respondents was a member of an ethnic minority, led us to further reevaluate our methods. Reasons for poor response included, among others, not being able to reach a person authorized to speak as the owner/manager, having a wrong number, or the business being closed. The main reason, though, was the outright refusal by businesses to participate (see

TABLE 30.1. Results of Initial Survey Attempts

Reason	Number
Refused	33
No answer	15
Not attempted[a]	14
Told to call back	13
Left message	9
N/A	6
Disconnected phone line	5
Survey completed	3
Hung up on	2
Total = 100	

[a]These were assigned to an undergraduate assistant who we later learned did not finish the work.

Table 30.1). The CDC staff reminded us of their previous caution that we would have a hard time collecting survey data because of mistrust in the community. Although we were unable to verify the reasons behind the refusals—the businesses contacted over the phone did not explicitly state that they mistrusted us when refusing—we were quite convinced that cultural barriers, and possibly lack of trust, had something to do with our poor response rate.

OVERCOMING THE DIFFICULTIES

On the basis of a literature review of various methodological approaches' strengths and weaknesses, it was decided that "snowball sampling," a method more appropriate for working with hard-to-reach or mistrustful populations, and qualitative interviewing would lead to a better result (see Bamberger, Rugh, & Mabry, 2006, pp. 105–109). We also decided that, if possible, it would be a good idea to accompany the CDC staff members into the community and collect field notes while they were attempting to conduct outreach to businesses in the community. The reason we decided to collect field notes was lack of time and the apparent possibility that we would be unable to conduct enough interviews before the final project was due. Because of this change in data collection methodology, we understood that our evaluation would have to shift from an outcomes focus to a process-based study, looking at the CDC's outreach efforts in order to better help it understand what techniques it was using and how they were working in its immediate practice in the community.

It was at this time that my other team member left the project, leaving me to finish the evaluation myself. Although the loss of the majority of the evaluation team may have seemed daunting, in actuality, it allowed me to form closer ties to the CDC, which served me well.

Unable to conduct the interviews of business owners, owing to time constraints (the class would be over) and because the CDC had requested that I not bother the business owners with interviews (because of another project it was starting, which it was afraid I would interfere with), I had to rely solely on field observation.

I was able to collect a variety of field notes from my trips into the community with the CDC program coordinator and by engaging in and listening to discussions at the CDC office. These field notes reflected interactions with immigrant business owners of different ethnicities—nine Asian, five African, two Middle Eastern, and two European. Moreover, because I kept detailed notes on all meetings and conversations I had with the CDC staff, I was able to use them, along with my e-mail correspondence, as additional data. These observations led to a detailed analysis of the communication patterns between the CDC and ethnic minority business owners, as well as how the outreach process itself worked—that is, how it worked in different contexts (with different types of people)—the views of CDC staff in regard to business owners, and business owners' (both minority and majority) views of the community and each other.

In the end, I was able to provide the CDC with a report and program theory model (a model that showed the underlying logic of their efforts), detailing its outreach process and the issues affecting it (see Table 30.2). I was informed by the project manager that I had helped her to better understand her own behaviors/process in engaging with businesses in the community.

In addition to these results, during the course of the evaluation I learned that the project manager position had been implemented only shortly before our research project began. The most important aspect of the position for its current holder was the need to conduct in-person outreach to businesses, which had never been done at such a level in the organization's history. The effect of this was that the program manager was making personal connections with individual business owners in the community, which caused them to see her more as a friend and less as a representative of a neighborhood organization. This phenomenon was in fact leading to progress in the community, but this progress was so new and on such a low level that the CDC could not see it. In addition, it was something that our proposed survey would never have been able to pick up by asking questions specifically about the CDC because, even if certain business owners were working with the program manager, most of them knew her only by her first name and did not associate her with the larger organization. This was largely due to the need for the program manager to keep as informal a relationship as

TABLE 30.2. Summary of the Three Major Themes Found in the Field Observation Data

What is going on in the businesses	• Business owners want success, but do not know how to attain aid. • Ethnic minorities are the majority of patrons in minority businesses, but business owners want to attract other types of patrons.
Issues with trust	• Afraid of being charged for free services by the CDC • Mistrust of strangers stemming from treatment in home country • Problems with local government affects trust of outside agencies • Employees act as gatekeepers to business owners and managers • Lying about the owner not being there to avoid outsiders • Mistrust affects ability to relay knowledge to business owners
How relationships and trust are formed by the alliance's project manager	• Changing the "sales pitch" between businesses, depending on culture • Finding a common problem/enemy for businesses to relate to • Using the family as a gateway to the owner—get to know the kids • Acting on problems immediately when informed

possible with the business owners in the community in order to distance herself from misconceptions that she was a "government official," which she was not, that could interfere with many immigrant business owners' willingness to trust her.

LESSONS LEARNED

Overcoming the aforementioned challenges meant that I needed to be flexible enough to change the project's focus midstream in order to work within the parameters of new constraints. In addition, it also meant that I had to be humble enough to admit my and my team members' mistakes regarding our original methodological choices to our community partner. I learned five important lessons while carrying out this project, which I have taken with me to later research projects.

The first lesson was that when doing participatory research, it is important to make sure you *participate* with your partner. In the beginning, we were not listening to the CDC program manager because we thought that, as graduate students in sociology, we knew more about cultural barriers than she did. I ended up learning the hard way that the people who are most familiar with the community on the ground level most likely know more about how to approach people than an outside researcher.

A second lesson I learned was that *qualitative data* can save you when your original design falls apart. By including field notes within my second research design proposal to my Institutional Review board (IRB), I was able to collect rich data on business owners in the community even after the original concept for a survey design completely fell apart. If I had not done this, there was no way that I would have been able to get another proposal completed in time to collect and analyze data for my deadline. It is for this reason that I am a firm believer in mixed methods. Qualitative data can be a great backup when quantitative designs do not pan out, and this technique has proved useful in later projects where I have used qualitative data to substantiate weak quantitative findings. In the end, it just makes you more flexible, which is important when doing participatory research.

The third lesson I learned was that maintaining *good documentation* throughout the research process is important. By taking detailed notes and keeping all correspondence I was able to use my documentation as additional qualitative data to support my findings.

A fourth lesson I have taken away from this project is that a *lack of data* from a failed attempt can sometimes be used to support the end findings. In this specific case, although the original design fell apart, I was able to report the poor response rate on my team's phone surveys as support for the cultural barriers and mistrust of outsiders existing in the community. Including these data in my presentations on the project instead of completely scrapping them was a smart move, and I received a lot of positive feedback for doing so.

In the end, *being open* with my partner to the largest extent possible, the fifth lesson, was the best move I made. By doing this, I ended up gaining the respect of the CDC staff members by keeping them informed and sticking to the project no matter how embarrassing the initial results and team issues were. Consequently, I was asked to help them on a second, larger project in the community, which ended up being another great learning experience and received official recognition by the city government. I also made a lot of great contacts that have proved useful in future research projects.

TO READ FURTHER

Bamberger, M., Rugh, J., & Mabry, L. (2006). *Real world evaluation.* Thousand Oaks, CA: Sage.

Bamberger, Rugh, and Mabry provide a practical approach to evaluation that describes many of the barriers evaluators face in practice and gives suggestions for how to overcome them. The authors also give an explanation of the value of mixed methodologies in evaluation research.

Stoeker, R. (2005). *Research methods for community change.* Thousand Oaks, CA: Sage.

Stoeker gives a straightforward explanation of the differences between academic and applied research and lays out the fundamentals of community-based research methods.

REFERENCES

Bamberger, M., Rugh, J., & Mabry, L. (2006). *Real world evaluation.* Thousand Oaks, CA: Sage.

Logan, J., & Alba, R. (1994). Ethnic economies in metropolitan regions: Miami and beyond. *Social Forces, 72,* 691–724.

Maly, M. T. (2005). *Beyond segregation: Multiracial and multiethnic neighborhoods in the United States.* Philadelphia: Temple University Press.

Maly, M. T., & Leachman, M. (1998). Rogers Park, Edgewater, Uptown, and Chicago Lawn, Chicago. *Cityscape: A Journal of Policy Development and Research, 4,* 131–160.

Patillo, M. (2007). *Black on the block.* Chicago: University of Chicago Press.

Stoecker, R. (2005). *Research methods for community change.* Thousand Oaks, CA: Sage.

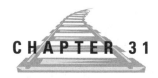

CHAPTER 31

Where Did All the Bodies Go?

HARRY S. SHANNON

BACKGROUND OF THE STUDY

Many blue-collar jobs entail exposures to airborne contaminants such as dusts, fumes, or vapors. Some have been proven to cause diseases; for example, asbestos exposure leads to higher rates of lung cancer, as well as asbestosis and mesothelioma, a rare tumor (Wagner, 1994). If you breathe in fine particles they will deposit in the lung, so it's not surprising that this is a prime target organ for acute and chronic toxic effects of exposures (Christiani & Wegman, 2000). Quite often, the exposures workers get on the job are the same as those the general public has—but the concentrations in the work environment are typically much higher. Workers can be the "canary in the mine," providing an unwitting early warning system for toxic effects; thus, it's thanks to studies of workers that asbestos in buildings is treated with caution.

We were asked to do a study at a workplace where the product—found in many homes—could break into very small particles that could reach the alveoli (air sacs deep in the lungs) when inhaled. There was concern that the exposure could cause lung cancer and maybe other lung diseases. Our job was to see if this was indeed so.

We could have done a prospective cohort study: identified workers in the plant, measured the exposures they were getting at work, asked them for information about smoking habits, and so forth, and followed them over time to see how many developed lung cancer as compared with some control group. The problem in such situations is that everyone wants an answer immediately or sooner. To do a truly prospective study with lung cancer as the outcome would take 30 years or more.

The standard approach to deal with this problem is to do the study *historically* using records (Checkoway, Pearce, & Crawford-Brown, 1989). From the company's records, we find the names of people who had worked there in the past, get information about their exposures, and track down who has died and from what diseases. We then compare their death rates with those of a comparison group—usually the general population, since those data are collated by government agencies and so are easily obtained. This is still a cohort study. In effect, we go back 30 or 40 years in a time machine to identify the cohort, then return to the present day, identifying new cases of death or disease in cohort members along the way. We also find out who started to work at the company in the meantime—if exposures have decreased over time with improved technology and ventilation, more recent hires should be at lower risk.

How We Initially Did the Study

We began by setting up a small steering committee with management and union representation. This is mainly a political precaution, rather than scientific; it ensures that when we're finished people won't say, "Well, of course you got the answer you did; you were doing the study for the company [or the union]." It takes extra time, but we're convinced this safeguard is worthwhile in the end. We also have to explain what we're doing in lay terms. In my experience, this can be much harder than passing peer review—and the people who are affected by the research are going to ask some very tough questions. But, as a character in *Cat's Cradle*, by Kurt Vonnegut, said "Dr Hoenniker used to say that any scientist who couldn't explain to an eight-year-old what he was doing is a charlatan" (Vonnegut, 1963). The committee members are, of course, much more sophisticated than 8-year-olds, especially on these issues, and if we can't explain to them what we're doing, we have a problem! Moreover, their suggestions and ideas improve the study, and they can open doors for us when we need it.

With the committee, we decided that we would include anyone who had worked in the plant for at least 30 days between 1948, when the plant opened, and 1977. We could get the information we needed from the company's medical department. It had records of people who had worked there, including age, address, and details of the specific jobs they had done. We extracted and computerized this information. We hired two summer students to trace the people who had left the company, which was most of the cohort. They used phone books, street directories, current workers, and so on, to find what had happened to the leavers—in particular, whether they had died or were still alive.

(Occasionally this approach tells you more than you want to know. One of our tracers thought she had found one person; I'll call him John Doe. She phoned the home number. Mrs. Doe answered: "Yes, that's my husband, you can call him at work." She provided the number and our tracer called his employer and asked for Mr. Doe: "Oh, he called in sick today." We concluded that John Doe was alive and very well.)

We also contacted Statistics Canada, which has complete records of deaths in Canada since 1950, and it provided the official causes of death. (Nowadays, we would identify deaths and their causes via computerized record linkage with the agency's files.)

The analysis computed standardized mortality ratios (SMRs). Based on the person-years "at risk" of each person, and taking account of the age- and calendar-specific death rates in the provincial population, we compared the observed and expected numbers of deaths from all causes and from specific causes (Breslow & Day, 1987). The SMR shows the ratio of observed to expected deaths, so we get an SMR of 1 if mortality is spot-on normal for the population. There are pros and cons of using this approach, which I won't go into here. It's enough to say that if there's a sizable increase in mortality risk, this method will show it, with an SMR well above 1.

THE CHALLENGES

We eagerly looked at the computer printout, but discovered a big problem. The SMR for total mortality was only about 0.5, suggesting that the number of deaths was only 50% of that expected, and so was the SMR for just about every individual cause of death. We joked that the company's reaction would be to consider advertising its factory as a health spa; it might even be able to get people to pay them to work there. But we knew the results could not be correct. By chance, one or two causes might have many fewer than expected deaths, but this couldn't be right for virtually all of them. We double-checked everything we could, but the impossible numbers stood up.

We finally had to own up to members of the steering committee, and we spent an uncomfortable time with them looking for an explanation. Eventually, we discovered what had gone wrong. The medical department records were incomplete. The department kept the records of people who had left in its office, in part so that if the leavers returned and sought reemployment, the staff could readily check their history with the company. People who had died obviously wouldn't want to be rehired, so some years before the former nurse had archived a lot of the records and they were no longer readily available in the medical department.

OVERCOMING THE DIFFICULTIES

We put on old clothing and dug around in the company's vaults. Finally, we managed to find boxes that seemed to be what we were after. They contained more records. But once bitten, twice shy. We had to be sure that this time we had it right. We realized that we needed to find lists of employees that were contemporary at various dates in the past, so we could be sure we had the full cohort. We kept rummaging through the dusty nooks and crannies and came up with different sources, including seniority lists. Seniority lists are made up for the union and record how long a person has worked for the company. This information is important in the union–company contract—for example, if people are to be laid off, the decisions about who has to leave are determined by seniority. This means that these records have to be very accurate. We found seniority lists at various points in time—we could be sure that workers with even moderately long employment would have been on at least one of the lists. Even then, we couldn't be sufficiently certain about records before 1955. Moreover, new workers didn't qualify for union membership and addition to the seniority list until they had worked for 90 days. So we could include only people with at least 90 days' employment from 1955 onward. But at least we were convinced that, with these new eligibility criteria, we had a complete cohort.

However, another limitation arose. We didn't have full job histories on some people—all we knew was that they had worked in the plant. Nor was there much information on past dust concentrations, and the records were sparser the farther back we looked. In the end, all we could say was when people had worked at the plant and for how long. Our analysis was thus the archetypal "exposed" versus "not exposed."

LESSONS LEARNED

Double- (and triple-) check that your population is complete. There are all sorts of reasons why records are not complete, and many are not obvious. One worrying aspect of this case history is that if the deficit in deaths had not been so large, we might never have realized we had a problem. In that sense we were lucky. We were also fortunate that we had developed a good rapport with the steering committee. I have worked with some committees in a much more difficult atmosphere, with a great deal of tension between union and management. If this had happened in one of those situations, I think we'd have been accused of all sorts of malfeasance.

Another good source of information can be payroll data (which we couldn't use in this study). As my former mentor Molly Newhouse used to say: "Whenever money changes hands, there are good records." And even if you have good records, find an independent source or two for comparison.

TO READ FURTHER

The topic of completeness of historical occupational cohorts has received surprisingly little attention. This is presumably because the construction of a cohort is dependent on where the study is conducted. The location can affect what records are available, confidentiality provisions and privacy legislation, unionization, and other issues. Typically, authors state the source of data for developing the cohort, without providing details of how they can be certain the records are complete.

Marsh, G. M., & Enterline, P. E. (1979). A method for verifying the completeness of cohorts used in occupational mortality studies. *Journal of Occupational Medicine, 21,* 665–670.

Describes how reports filed with the U.S. Internal Revenue Service for tax purposes can be used to establish the cohort's completeness.

Enterline, P. E., & Marsh, G. M. (1982). Missing records in occupational epidemiology. *Journal of Occupational Medicine, 24,* 677–680.

The authors discovered missing records after they had established a cohort; they describe how they verified the completeness and remedied errors. (The original cohort included 16 plants. At one, the "inactive records" had been buried in a landfill and the owners offered to dig them up. The authors decided against this and omitted the plant from the study.)

REFERENCES

Breslow, N. E., & Day, N. E. (1987). *Statistical methods in cancer research: Volume 2. The design and analysis of cohort studies.* Lyon, France: International Agency for Research on Cancer.

Checkoway, H., Pearce, N., & Crawford-Brown, D. J. (1989). *Research methods in occupational epidemiology.* New York: Oxford University Press.

Christiani, D. C., & Wegman, D. H. (2000). Respiratory diseases. In B. S. Levy & D. H. Wegman (Eds.), *Occupational health: Recognizing and preventing work-related disease and injury* (4th ed., pp. 477–501). Philadelphia: Lippincott Williams & Wilkins.

Vonnegut, K., Jr. (1963). *Cat's cradle.* New York: Delacorte Press.

Wagner, G. R. (1994). Mineral dusts. In L. Rosenstock & M. R. Cullen (Eds.), *Textbook of clinical occupational and environmental medicine* (pp. 825–837). Philadelphia: Saunders.

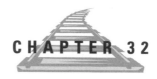

CHAPTER 32

Measures for Improving Measures

KATHERINE MCKNIGHT
PATRICK E. MCKNIGHT

BACKGROUND OF THE STUDIES

In the social and behavioral sciences, measurement does not receive the attention it deserves. Methodologically oriented reviewers frequently focus on experimental control, sample selection, or data analysis. Rarely do reviewers focus on the quality of the measures beyond the required blurb about "the" reliability and "the" validity of the chosen measures, as if these were intrinsic properties of a given measure, devoid of the context and purpose of their use. A brief statement reporting a statistical index of reliability and validity seems to suffice, without much explanation as to the context in which those indices were obtained and whether that context is applicable to the proposed use of the measures in the given study. Yet research depends on reliable and valid measurement; failure to capture all relevant variables in a reliable and valid manner leads to weak inferences. If we want to understand the relationship between parental IQ and a child's math achievement, for example, we must measure both variables reliably and validly. Furthermore, we ought to measure intervening variables that might influence the relationship (e.g., variables that indicate educational, social, and nutritional development). Weak inferences often lead researchers to stop pursuing viable research questions, to pursue errant relationships, or to attend to variables that produce only spurious relationships. None of these outcomes move science forward. We end up wasting precious resources and gain nothing in the process. Measurement, therefore, holds an influential position in the process of scientific progress. The purpose of this chapter is to highlight three common problems researchers encounter when measurement has not received adequate attention: inadvertently adding "noise" or error to our measures, inadvertently adding bias to our measures, and changing the nature of what we are measuring by the act of measuring it. We use examples from real studies in which we have participated or which we have reviewed for funding. These examples are meant to be illustrative—not exhaustive—so that readers can appreciate the potential consequences of poor measurement planning. The three examples illustrate problems associated with poor scale development, problematic item wording and response options, and use of repeated assessments to assess change. The details of these studies are purposefully vague to avoid the identification of a given study as well as its investigators. These examples are not intended to belittle or blame, but rather to illustrate common problems when measurement is not appropriately attended to during the study design phase.

THE CHALLENGES

Creating Noise through Poor Item Development

Sometimes researchers need to create measures of key variables because appropriate measures are not available. Unfortunately, many of us have not been well trained in measurement development or psychometrics, and therefore we resort to mimicking common practices without regard to their appropriateness. When doing so, we fail to anticipate problems associated with measurement design, such as the introduction of "noise" or measurement error to the variables on which we are focused. The first example illustrates the common problem of interpreting responses to scale options that are, at best, ambiguous. In this study, people who had participated in mediational processes were given a survey to capture their perceptions. The problem occurred in the interpretation of responses to a series of items that measured agreement with a given statement on a scale ranging from 1 to 10, where 1 = "Strongly Disagree" and 10 = "Strongly Agree." For example, to measure the extent to which a respondent trusted another party, a survey item asks the respondent to indicate the degree to which she agreed with a statement such as "I fully trusted the other party." Respondents were asked to rate all items on the aforementioned 10-point scale. When investigators reviewed the survey responses, they were unsure how to interpret the scores, particularly from the middle of the scale. Did the middle of the scale represent the point at which respondents shifted from mildly disagreeing to mildly agreeing with a statement? (And what would be the difference between mildly disagreeing and mildly agreeing anyway?) Did it represent the no-man's land of "neither agree nor disagree" so commonly found in the middle of such scales? Did it mean vastly different things to different people? How were they to characterize a mean of 5.8 on the scale if no one knew how respondents interpreted the scale? Moreover, was the level of agreement with the statement indicative of the feature (trusting the other party) in the first place? To interpret results, we need to understand if the respondent used the scale to indicate the extent to which she trusted the other party or the extent to which she agreed with "fully" trusting the other party. In the latter case, strongly disagreeing (a score of 1) would indicate strong disagreement with the characterization of "fully" trusting the other party versus, in the former case, not trusting the other party at all.

A critical task for the investigators was to report performance data to stakeholders, including those who funded the study. Items assessing satisfaction with the process, belief in its utility, perceived success of the process, and so on, were included in the survey to assess performance. However, these items made use of the same 10-point Disagree/Agree scale and they were worded to assess agreement with a particular statement. As the previous example illustrates, conclusions about performance were difficult to draw. Investigators wanted to characterize the proportion of participants with low, moderate and high satisfaction with the process. However, interpreting what low, moderate, and high scores meant, using the given response options, was difficult. The scores reflected level of agreement with a given statement; yet again, it was unclear how respondents interpreted the scale. The investigators were not comfortable in claiming that a given proportion moderately agreed with a given statement, because scores ranged from 4 to 7, for example. Perhaps some respondents were not sure whether they agreed or not. Perhaps others thought the scale moved immediately from disagreement to agreement when it moved from 1 to 2; perhaps they thought it shifted to agreement when it moved from 5 to 6. Because it was unclear how respondents used the scale, it was not clear how to report performance results and multiple interpretations were plausible. Clearly, this is not a comfortable position for investigators when reporting results to the funding agency.

Another problem with the 10-point scale involved interpreting exactly what it was that the respondent was agreeing or disagreeing with. Some items were written in such a way that the response could have indicated agreement/disagreement with several factors. Consider an example: "The process was efficient and fair." A respondent may rate this item lower on the scale because the process was efficient or fair, but not both. A respondent could use the same rationale for using the higher end of the scale. In addition, a lower rating might reflect that the process was neither efficient nor fair. As this example illustrates, it can be virtually impossible to interpret ratings for such items, not only because of the problems discussed previously with the scale itself, but because of the wording of compound items, in which several dimensions (e.g., efficiency and fairness) are being rated at the same time. If program personnel want to understand respondents' views regarding efficiency and fairness, it is best that these two dimensions are rated separately.

The use of an ambiguous response scale and confusing wording of items both introduce "noise" or error into measurement. Adding error means reducing reliability. When respondents are unsure of how to use the given response options or how to interpret a set of items, it is less likely that they will respond to those items in a consistent manner. Reliability is a measure of consistency in how a measure is used, whether it be over time (test–retest reliability), across judges (intraclass correlation), within scales (internal consistency), or in other ways. To enhance the consistent use of a given measure, a clear set of response options and unambiguous item wording are critical.

Overcoming the Difficulties

Fortunately, the investigators were given a second chance to collect data and to revise the survey. Several important changes were made to the 10-point scale and to the wording of the items. First, stakeholders identified the important dimensions of the mediational processes that needed to be evaluated for the purposes of the study. Next, separate items were written for each dimension, rather than for combinations of dimensions, to clarify for respondents what they were rating. Finally, the scale itself was changed from a confusing continuum of disagreement/agreement with a statement to a continuum reflecting low through high magnitudes of the dimension itself. Instead of wording an item to indicate level of agreement with the statement "The process was efficient and fair," two separate items were written, asking the respondent to indicate "the extent to which the process was efficient" (0 = "not at all" to 10 = "completely") and "the extent to which the process was fair" (same scale). Because of the change, it was clear to the respondent that the low end of the scale meant less of that dimension (e.g., less efficiency or fairness) and the high end meant more of that dimension. In addition to the anchors "not at all" at the low end and "completely" at the high end, project personnel requested a label in the middle of the scale at "5" to indicate "moderately" to help respondents use the scale as intended. Those changes eased the concerns about how respondents might interpret the middle scale and, as a consequence, investigators felt comfortable in reporting that scores in the midrange of the scale reflected moderate amounts of the dimension being rated.

Lessons Learned

The moral of this story is to think very carefully about the items we choose to use prior to collecting data for a study. If we need to measure the magnitude of a given variable—for example, efficiency, fairness, trust—we need to word items and design response scales so it is clear to respondents how to interpret the scale and what dimension they are rating. Asking for level of agreement with a statement about a particular variable is not advisable as a means for measuring its magnitude. It is several steps removed from simply rating the variable itself along the more intuitive continuum of *none* to *a lot*. Moreover, combining variables or dimensions in a single item for a single rating is confusing for the respondent and the researchers. Important variables should be identified and rated separately. Analyses may indicate that the variables can be combined statistically (e.g., as part of a common factor), but that should be determined only if they are measured independently and in an interpretable manner.

Creating Bias through Poor Item Development

The previous example illustrated how poor item development can add error or decrease reliability of measurement. In this example, we illustrate how poor item development can add *bias* to measures, thus weakening validity and threatening statistical inference. This example comes from a study of the needs of a group of Native Americans to inform the design of appropriate services for that population. In this study, the investigator designed a survey that assessed a variety of needs, including job training, health and wellness, education, and so on. The first part of the survey consisted of demographic information, including age, gender, and education history, among other items. After a few weeks of data collection, the investigator held a focus group to get feedback about the clarity of the items and instructions, item wording, and response options. Several focus group participants were visibly upset by the response option that indicated *not* graduating from high school. As these participants explained, they had had a long and unfriendly relationship with the Bureau of Indian Affairs (BIA) with respect to BIA school policies. Because of the negative history, education background, particularly regarding school dropout, was a reactive item for them; that is, the item drew an emotional reaction that affected their response to it and, unfortunately, to the rest of the survey. These participants explained that the item probably affected a large portion of a given sector of the population similarly. Perhaps that explained the rather noticeable amount of missing data in the demographic section of the surveys that had been collected.

Reacting negatively to response options such as "did not graduate" is not as uncommon as it might seem. Our experience, as both survey respondents and data analysts, impressed upon us that reporting personal data can be unpleasant and sometimes aggravating for some people. As investigators, we found more than just a few comments in the margins of our surveys indicating "none of your business!" or asking why we needed the information. Personal data such as age, weight, and income tend to be sensitive issues for a subset of the population and are therefore more likely to generate negative reactions and, in some cases, missing data. Wording items and response options carefully can decrease the likelihood of a negative reaction. Survey researchers, for example, often use age brackets (e.g., 20–29, 40–49, 65+) rather than actual age to reduce sensitivity to reporting. The range of the brackets ought to be determined by the type of information that is necessary. If income is an important variable and specific income bands have been shown to be related to the outcomes of interest, the use of those bands would be advisable instead of making up your own brackets. One should consider the width of the bands or brackets that would not only decrease reactivity on the part of respondents, but would be useful for the research questions at hand. Wide brackets (e.g., $0–$50,000 annual income) can be so imprecise as to be uninformative.

Overcoming the Difficulties

Fortunately, the focus group was held early in the data collection phase, so changes could be made to the survey. The investigator asked the focus group members to help reword the item and response options to get the needed information in a nonreactive way. The item was changed so that respondents were allowed to select the highest grade they had completed, which eliminated options such as "did not graduate." In this way, it was still clear whether a respondent completed high school, and the concerns of the focus group members were appeased.

Lessons Learned

As the present example illustrates, whether developing items or using existing ones, investigators ought to pay attention to the wording and the response options to decrease the likelihood of missing data. Systematically missing data of the kind discussed in this example is a source of response bias that can have a severe effect on measurement validity and statistical inferences based on such measurement (McKnight, McKnight, Sidani, & Figueredo, 2007). Anticipating problems is always recommended. One way to do so is to conduct a focus group with individuals from the targeted population to get their feedback. Asking them about how items are worded, how the questionnaire/survey is perceived, how response options are presented, can help researchers avoid some of the problems described here in these examples. Exit interviewing is another useful strategy when data are collected in person. As respondents return the completed questionnaire, data collectors can randomly select individuals to provide feedback about the questionnaire. This method has the added benefit of preventing missing data by ensuring that questionnaires are completed when returned and that any confusion is cleared up for the respondent so that he or she can complete the items.

Field-testing items online is also possible—respondents can test the questionnaire items and provide their feedback online. This approach makes most sense if the questionnaire will be delivered online because issues may arise that are unique to an online, versus paper-and-pencil, format. Web survey software has specific formats for item responses that may not be an issue in the paper-and-pencil version, and vice versa. For example, as of this writing, some Web survey software does not have the option to create a horizontal continuum with anchors at the low and high ends (e.g., "poor" to "excellent"), along which a respondent can select a point to indicate the magnitude of the dimension he or she is rating. Instead, the investigator has to create response options vertically, using whole numbers that the respondent can select. Visually, the horizontal format seems to provide better cues to the respondent about rating along a continuum than does the vertical format. With a paper-and-pencil version, presenting the continuum horizontally is not an issue. As another example, built-in skip patterns (e.g., "If not applicable, skip to item 10") can be confusing for those responding to a paper-and-pencil survey, but not when responding online, where the computer will automatically move to the next appropriate item based on previous responses. Thus, field-testing a survey online and then collecting data using a paper-and-pencil format, or vice versa, would likely be less helpful for anticipating problems with the survey and decreasing the likelihood of missing data.

There are many more reasons why responding to a questionnaire can be problematic for subsets of respondents. This example is meant only to illustrate some of the more common problems. McKnight et al. (2007) provide a more in-depth discussion of ways in which measurement can either induce or reduce missing data.

Repeated Measures

Measurement in longitudinal studies can be particularly difficult for several reasons. It is well known among longitudinal researchers that use of the same measure repeatedly with the same participants can be problematic for assessing change in a targeted variable. Problems occur when responses to a given measure change because of familiarity with the measure rather than because of actual change in the variable that is being assessed. "Familiarity" with the instrument can reflect a variety of processes, such as habituation to a measure (e.g., anxiety is reduced, or perhaps increased, the second or third time a respondent takes the same math test), learning (e.g., scores improve between math assessments because of learning how to take the test), and boredom (e.g., the respondent becomes careless after responding to the same 50 items the second or third time). Problems occur when changes are attributed incorrectly, perhaps to an intervention rather than to habituation, learning, or boredom with the assessment, for example. In their discussion of threats to internal validity, Campbell and Stanley (1966) refer to this threat as "testing."

To illustrate problems associated with familiarity with repeated measures, we present an example from a study using repeated assessments of mental health symptoms with patients at a local hospital. In this study, patients were asked to complete a checklist that measured the severity of relevant symptoms of psychiatric distress several times over the course of a year. Researchers expected that these symptoms would abate over time owing to a variety of services the patients received, but instead, the scores looked worse as the study progressed. Initially, the researchers interpreted these changes as reflecting real changes in psychiatric distress. However, the researchers began to suspect that something was awry when one of the investigators was privy to a conversation among several study participants about the assessment itself. Patients were noting that the same assessment was used throughout the hospital and in other research studies and that therefore they had become well acquainted with the checklist and, in essence, learned the symptoms of several diagnostic categories. They speculated that perhaps some of their peers were "faking" high scores because more severe symptoms entitled them to more benefits.

Overcoming the Difficulties

Changes in outcome variables due to familiarity, habituation, learning, boredom, or other reactions to repeated measures is a serious confound in longitudinal studies. In this particular study, it was not clear whether patients truly were exhibiting worsening psychiatric symptoms or whether they were learning the symptoms that enabled them to increase their scores. If the worsening scores were due to learning, it was not immediately clear what to do about it. There were no other similar assessments conducted via the study with which to compare, and investigators did not have access to medical records, where other symptom assessment results may have been recorded. Alternate assessments could have been used to corroborate the scores on the study's measure of psychiatric symptoms.

Lessons Learned

Methodologists have discussed approaches to decreasing the likelihood of confounds associated with familiarity with repeated measures. Common solutions include using alternate forms of a particular measure, such as versions A and B of a math test, to decrease the likelihood of learning the credited responses or becoming bored with the same items. Another common solution is to lengthen the time between assessments to decrease the chances of remembering or memorizing responses to items. It is not likely that either solution would have helped in this situation. Apparently the patients were learning the symptoms of diagnostic categories with the multiple clinical assessments they underwent that had nothing to do with the study. Moreover, policies regarding those diagnoses and patient benefits were outside the control of investigators but served as powerful incentives for some, which could have led to higher scores. Lengthening time between assessments would not have been terribly helpful either because it would likely have been counteracted by the multiple psychiatric assessments these patients underwent elsewhere as part of the treatment regime at the hospital.

Several other approaches may have been helpful in conducting this study to prevent the problem of change due to a learning effect resulting from repeated exposure to a specific measure. Dispersing the items that measured psychiatric symptoms across a larger questionnaire that included other study variables may have served to detract respondents from the assessment purpose of the specific mental health items. For example, a demographics item measuring ethnicity might be followed by an item from the psychiatric assessment, followed by an item addressing health status, and so on. If the patients were familiar with the psychiatric assessment from other settings, dispersing the items might help to make it less recognizable and/or make it less obvious that one objective of the questionnaire was to obtain a mental health score, which it seems some of the patients wanted to increase in order to obtain more benefits.

Another approach that might have been successful in reducing a learning effect is to design the study to obtain information from a source other than the participant—using either unobtrusive (Webb, Campbell, Schwartz, & Sechrest, 1966) or indirect measures. In this example, it would have been helpful if investigators had access to medical records in which a trained clinician unassociated with the study had carried out a thorough assessment of psychiatric symptoms. Verifying the outcome with another unobtrusive source also could have been helpful. Provided that all the required permissions were in place, investigators might have interviewed the patients' clinicians or loved ones or another appropriate source about the symptoms. Indirect measures such as observations by other hospital staff members who interacted with the patients might help corroborate self-reported claims of psychiatric distress.

A secondary problem illustrated by this study, but no less important than the learning effect, is the apparent assumption on the part of the study participants that the data gathered will be used outside the study—in this case, for decision making about their patient benefits. An approach that might have been successful for avoiding such assumptions is a more targeted informed consent process. The investigators might have averted the problem of the worsening scores by making it very clear to the study participants that the data collected would not be shared with the hospital or anyone outside the study, and therefore could not be used to inform decisions about their benefits. Of course, investigators cannot anticipate all the ways in which participants might perceive their study data to be used. However, it is always a good idea to spend time during the study consent process to make it absolutely clear to participants, both verbally and in written format, how the study data will and will not be used, and to verify that the participants understand the information. Potential participants often have ideas about the "real" reason behind a study and how their data could be used against them. Strong efforts to prevent or at least minimize such fears from the outset are likely not wasted.

CONCLUSIONS

There are many ways in which measurement problems can take a given study "off the rails" from its intended purpose. In this chapter, only three general examples are given: problems with item wording and response options that lead to increased error, problems with item wording and response options that lead to increased bias, and problems with repeated assessments that lead to threats to statistical inference. It should be clear from these examples that the problems go beyond aggravating a few respondents or having a few who "game the system." Measurement problems can lead to unreliable and/or invalid representations of the variables that we wish to understand. Uninterpretable scales, unclear items, reactive items, and unclear change processes hinder our understanding of the variables we study and the relationships between them. If we fail to regard measurement development and/or selection as a critical feature of research design, it is unlikely we will anticipate some of the more serious effects poor measurement can have on study results and the inferential process itself. Careful attention to measurement frequently requires psychometric training and knowledge; however, anticipating problems often requires carrying out commonsense strategies, such as field-testing items before launching the study or hiring someone with expertise in measurement development. From our perspective, investigators without much, if any, formal training in measurement development often convince themselves that they can generate their own measures for a given study—that all it takes is an understanding of the phenomenon to be measured. If only it were so! Measure development would not have its own place in fields such as psychology, education, engineering, economics, and so on, if measurement were so easy. The first example in this chapter reflects only a minute instance of what can go wrong when those lacking measurement expertise develop their own measures. Because measurement is at the heart of science, we cannot afford to ignore its importance nor the consequences of failing to prioritize measurement selection and development when generating our study designs.

TO READ FURTHER

Sechrest, L., McKnight, P. E., & McKnight, K. M. (1996). Calibration of measures for psychotherapy outcome studies. *American Psychologist, 51,* 1065–1071.

Most measurement researchers focus on psychometric properties (e.g., reliability and validity), but in this article these researchers redirect the focus to the implications of the measurements. Understanding how numbers can be interpreted leads to the concept of calibration. A well-calibrated instrument ought not just reflect the underlying property but must also communicate to the user some directly useful information.

Embretson, S. E., & Hershberger, S. L. (1999). *The new rules of measurement: What every psychologist and educator should know.* New York: Erlbaum.

Embretson and Hershberger edited a fine book that details modern psychometric theory, explaining why classical test theory ought to be supplanted by item response theory and Rasch models. Chapters include both theoretical and applied work, which should be interesting to readers with any social science background.

Thompson, B. (2000). Psychometrics and datametrics: The test is not reliable. *Educational and Psychological Measurement, 60,* 174–195.

Thompson reminds us of the limited role psychometrics can play in social science. His thesis is that all tests involve interactions between the test questions and the sample. Researchers who forget that interaction often make the mistake of attributing the psychometric properties solely to the test itself, rather than to the test and the sample.

Cortina, J. (1993). What is coefficient alpha? An examination of theory and applications. *Journal of Applied Psychology, 78,* 98–104.

Cortina does an outstanding job explaining the role and limitations of the most popular estimate of reliability, Cronbach's alpha. Even seasoned psychometricians may benefit from his article, as he offers the layman and expert alike some common sense to an common metric.

REFERENCES

Campbell, D. T., & Stanley, J. (1966). *Experimental and quasi-experimental designs for research.* Chicago: Rand McNally.

McKnight, P., McKnight, K., Sidani, S., & Figueredo, A. J. (2007). *Missing data: A gentle introduction.* New York: Guilford Press.

Webb, E. J., Campbell, D. T., Schwartz, R. D., & Sechrest, L. (1966). *Unobtrusive measures.* Chicago: Rand McNally.

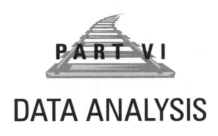

PART VI

DATA ANALYSIS

Much of graduate training is spent learning how to analyze data, whether in courses on multivariate statistics or on interpreting qualitative transcripts. We are taught about the assumptions of the methods and the problems caused by everything from heteroscedasticity to unusually verbose group participants. We are also warned about the bane of all researchers—not enough data—and how this may lead to insufficient power in quantitative research, or a failure to achieve concept saturation in qualitative research. But who ever warns us about *too much* data? How can we ever have too much data? Well, MacLean and her colleagues did. In Chapter 33, they describe a novel illness caused by too much data—analysis-induced narcolepsy. In their case, the data were transcripts of interviews that had to be coded, a difficult task when your eyes are closing. Kairouz and Nadeau (Chapter 34) present an interesting dilemma—the need to merge a number of large administrative databases, with the result that the number of people in each of the cells then becomes too small to preserve anonymity.

Different types of problems are discussed in the next two chapters. Martí-Carvajal (Chapter 35) was trying to do a meta-analysis of a medical intervention, in which it appeared that the drug company kept changing the eligibility criteria for participants in randomized controlled trials in an apparent attempt to compensate for negative results. In the case of Ferraro and Trottier-Wolter (Chapter 36), *they* had enough data, but their test battery didn't; in particular, there were no norms for the groups they were studying, a major problem in a multicultural society, where there are many minority groups with too few members to justify a company's expense in deriving normative data.

The last three chapters in this section take a somewhat different tack and try to keep the research from going off the rails to begin with. In Chapter 37, MacLean and her group explain what software designed for analyzing qualitative data can and, more important, cannot do. However, their points are universal—the silicon "brain" in your computer is not a substitute for the real one between your ears, and careful thought must accompany every step in the analysis process. This point is also made for quantitative data analysis by Davis (Chapter 38) and Glaser (Chapter 39). It is imperative, from the very beginning of a project, to think through what analyses you want; data that aren't collected can't be analyzed, and if you are vague about how the data will be recorded, they may be unanalyzable.

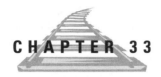

CHAPTER 33

Drowsing Over Data
When Less Is More

LYNNE MACLEAN
ALMA ESTABLE
MECHTHILD MEYER
ANITA KOTHARI
NANCY EDWARDS
BARB RILEY

BACKGROUND OF THE STUDY

What are the conclusions you might draw if you found yourself falling asleep every time you sat down to code and analyze the last half of a large qualitative dataset for one particular study? What would you conclude when you discover the same thing is happening to the rest of the team, or when the same thing occurs when you review the same data for secondary analysis 3 years later? Do you have narcolepsy? No, you have a too large dataset.

In qualitative research there are sound theoretical reasons for small sample sizes, as well as practical ones: Not only are qualitative data resource-intensive to transcribe, code, and analyze, but the purpose of qualitative work is not sample or statistical generalizability (i.e., external validity; Hillebrand, Kok, & Biemens, 2001). When qualitative researchers consider external validity, they are more often concerned with the transferability of findings from the study sample cases to other cases, or theoretical generalizability, (i.e., identification of internal causal mechanisms, and structural similarity to other cases). Neither transferability nor theoretical generalizability requires statistical representativeness (Hillebrand et al., 2001). For qualitative studies, a larger sample does not contribute to the quality of the data and findings and may not be worth the costs. Sometimes "more data mean more participants, more interviews, perhaps even more data sources, and much more work without developing a better study" (Morse, 2000, p. 3).

The study we're presenting was a segment of an applied research project with specific deadlines and deliverables, including local site evaluation reports. It was part of the multicomponent evaluation of a province-wide program supporting community coalition partnerships for a specific public health issue. This chapter addresses the qualitative evaluation activities included in a comprehensive mixed-methods design.

We conducted 68 qualitative, semistructured audiotaped interviews (a mix of telephone and in-person, but mostly in-person, interviews were conducted). The interviews focused on the coalitions in eight communities, and participants were program staff and community members. For most communities, a minimum of seven interviews were done. A purposive sample of voluntary participants was used, representing a range of sectors and successes. Overall, we were able to obtain a balanced number of interviews from organizations of differing mandates, sizes, sectors, and target groups at all sites. To look at success in coalition formation, questions focused on themes and indicators found in previous research to be related to community partnership and coalition-building success, and also probed for new ones. We also wished to determine, from the perspective of the participants, whether the program was actually meeting its goals in terms of changes in health outcomes within each of these communities. Data were analyzed using a content analysis approach and matrix methods (Miles & Huberman, 1994), supported by QSR N5 software (QSR International, 2000).

THE CHALLENGES

Sixty-eight interviews were considerably more than we needed in order to saturate our concepts and themes. The sample size was selected on the basis of a desire to provide some representativeness to the combined findings for the evaluation over all, as well as a need to report site-specific findings. Therefore, we determined that each site required sufficient interviews to provide a snapshot of its process and progress. The team felt an iterative approach to data collection and analysis would not work because the project had short time frames. As a result, all data were collected before we began to do the analysis.

Our data collection and analysis team was composed of three very experienced qualitative researchers. We are used to working through interviews carefully, thoroughly, systematically, confirming and disconfirming findings, reflecting back on the interviews we conducted, building audit trails, always documenting the expected, and looking for the unexpected. We enjoy this. We like talking with people and hearing their stories. We enjoy the intricacies of the analysis. We are even used to the sensation of drowning in a sea of data that engulfs the unwary at midpoint. We rise above it, smiling, with sanity intact (for the most part), and thick reports in hand.

Once again, we proceeded in our usual fashion through a content analysis—each reading a few transcripts, some of those transcripts common to all and some unique to each analyst. We then developed a coding tree using codes identified from the transcripts, the literature and program information. We divided up the interviews by site, so that we would work with interviews we had ourselves conducted in order to be more open to the nuances of the words. Each of us, independently, found we were reaching the limits of absorbing any new information about half-way through our stacks of transcripts. Moreover, the interviews were dry, work-related discussions. With new insights coming few and far between, and no juicy bits to keep us focused, we each found ourselves nodding off as we worked through the long interviews. At our next meeting we admitted this to each other, shamefaced. We felt obligated to use all the transcripts, inasmuch as busy people had made time to come to the interviews and each interview itself had a story to tell.

OVERCOMING THE DIFFICULTIES

In order to fight off the boredom, we redivided the stacks so that we were reading interviews conducted by someone else, hoping this would help. We assumed each interview now would be a fresh experience, full of sparkling new thoughts and vibrant connections. This new approach did not help. We then moved to group coding, so that we were all sitting in the same room and could poke each other across the table. Finally, we made it through all of the interviews, and completed the remaining steps of the analysis with frequent breaks, discussion, and much caffeine.

A few years later, we discovered the need for a secondary analysis of the data for a different purpose. This meant we needed to revisit the original transcripts in detail. As 2 years had passed, and several other projects had intervened, we forgot about the soporific effect of this particular study. We took the transcripts away to work on, and all became sleepy again. Either we had discovered a powerful One-Study Narcoleptic Conditioning Effect, or there were just too many transcripts.

LESSONS LEARNED

It is an old but true cliché: Hindsight is 20/20. The increased generalizability of the findings was not worth the cost, in terms of financial and human resources, of an oversized sample. Qualitative research is not the method of choice when statistical generalizability is sought. If that is what you need, consider quantitative methods. The strengths of qualitative research—the ability to look at a phenomenon in depth, to understand context, and to uncover new ideas—do not require large samples. Indeed, data saturation occurred with half the sample. Essentially, half the interviews we conducted were not necessary to answer the research questions. When you consider the amount of time and mental alertness required for qualitative transcription and analysis, having a sample too large is really a disservice to the study funders and to the research team, assuming all would like to use their time and other resources to best advantage. In fact, for the next phases of follow-up evaluations that were conducted 3 and 5 years later, a smaller sample of qualitative data was used, and instead of interviews, sector-specific focus groups were conducted, reducing the number of transcripts to 10 (9 focus groups and 1 interview transcript; 36 participants) in a second phase and 9 (51 participants) in a third phase. It was thought that the interview process had provided sufficient detail and that now focus groups would provide sufficient viewpoints.

We were not the first, nor, regrettably, the last, to use a sample size that was too large. Although tables for qualitative sample size selection exist, their use is not an exact science. Indeed, Morse (2000), the developer of one set of such tables, cautions researchers who attempt to use qualitative sample size tables that "the number of participants required in a study is one area in which it is clear that too many factors are involved and conditions of each study vary too greatly to produce tight recommendations" (Morse, 2000, p. 5). What else could we (or indeed, should we) have done?

Given that we had collected all these data, did we really need to use them all? Another option, that of selecting only a few interview transcripts from each site to analyze for the cross-site portion of the analysis (perhaps basing transcript selection on a maximum variation sampling approach), also might have worked. However, all interviewees had commented on program-wide issues, and we felt an obligation to review and use what all informants had said, given that they had taken time to speak with us.

We could have done a less intensive analysis of this large sample, just a quick overview of the issues that came up, and skimmed over the data quickly and lightly, without too much detail. But we didn't. After having tried to do so in the past—without success—we now resist this approach. Quick skimming of large data samples can give qualitative research a bad reputation as being impressionistic and unsystematic. It does a disservice to the method, which is designed to do the opposite: to read participants' responses and comments with great attention to detail to ensure that nuances are not missed and are pointed out in the analysis. No, the key to this solution was in the precollection design phase.

Perhaps we could have sampled fewer sites, while keeping the same number of interviews within each site. We could have used maximum variation sampling (i.e., sampling to capture range or diversity; Lincoln & Guba, 1985; Patton, 1990) to select sites, rather than just to sample within sites. Thus, we could have focused our sampling more tightly on wider variations of the sites (e.g., sampled the two most remote, sparsely settled sites and the two largest urban sites, rather than a selection of remote and urban sites).

But this was not an option for us. Using maximum variation sampling over all sites and all participants to make recruitment decisions would have served the evaluation as a whole. However, it would not have met the needs of the individual communities that volunteered for the study and the participants who were waiting for results to feed back into their own specific programs.

What we should have done was to follow the classic qualitative pattern of iterative data collection and analysis—that is, doing a few interviews in a community, pausing to analyze the information, seeing if more data were needed to saturate findings, and beginning the cycle again until no new themes were reported (Dreher, 1994; Strauss & Corbin, 1990). In that way, we could have assessed the quality of the data and adjusted the sample size as we went along (Morse, 2000). But at the time we were designing the study, we thought such a cycle would have required more time than was allotted in the project deadlines. In reality, although it looked as though we were being more efficient by getting all the interviews done and then moving on to analysis, in fact it would probably have been more cost-effective to follow the iterative procedure.

The most useful approach, under the tight constraints of the research contract and with possible difficulty in meeting deadlines with an iterative approach, would have been to work with a maximum of four sites, using maximum variation sampling to select them. With this approach, communicating the sampling intent for the qualitative research component of the study would have been important to do before recruiting sites, as participants at some sites would have wondered why they were not selected for qualitative interviews.

CONCLUDING ADVICE

Our strategic tools at the time of our study were caffeine, group coding, and a sense of humor. Our advice now is to discern when less really is more:

1. Consider qualitative design expertise and literature in developing a qualitative study. There is aid available for identifying factors to take into account in estimated sample size requirements (e.g., Morse, 2000). Qualitative sample size estimation procedures are based on well-established theory and consistent with the goals of qualitative research.

2. Qualitative researchers should communicate to other team investigators the "rules" or guidelines they will use to determine when they have an adequate number of interviews—for example, a saturation of themes from the data.

3. Consider that combinations of factors such as scope, data quality, and so forth, will affect the ideal sample size, and that it is okay to reduce your sample size if you are getting quality data leading to more rapid saturation than expected. Some authors suggest providing an overestimation of sample size in qualitative proposals, inasmuch as you cannot guarantee the sample size needed but will require sufficient funding to collect it if necessary (Morse, 2000). This does not mean you have to collect a sample of this size, unless specified under contract.

4. Use an iterative approach to data collection and analysis, so you don't collect extra data that you then feel compelled to analyze because of feelings of responsibility for the participants' time and effort.

5. If using the iterative approach in item 4, be sure to explain to participants/sites in advance why they may not be included in qualitative interviews, especially if this is part of a mixed-methods study.

6. Calculate the resources required to conduct *one* interview, including administration (booking interview time, travel or telephone expenses), interviewer time, interviewee time (times 2: time spent on the interview + time lost away from her or his regular work), interview transcription hours (usually 4 times the length of the interview), and research analyst hours (including verification of transcript accuracy, reading transcript and coding, and analyzing content). This calculation multiplied by the sample size you are considering will help you to keep in perspective what you are getting into with a large sample size, as well as help you determine your needed resources.

7. Stop data collection when saturation is achieved.

TO READ FURTHER

Morse, J. M. (1994). Designing qualitative research. In N. K. Denzin & Y. S. Lincoln (Eds.), *Handbook of qualitative inquiry* (pp. 220–235). Thousand Oaks, CA: Sage.

Morse, J. M. (2000). Determining sample size [Editorial]. *Qualitative Health Research, 10,* 3–5.

These two should be read in tandem. Morse (1994) gives a good overview and comparison of many qualitative approaches, including sample size. Morse (2000) gives her cautions about using her sample sizes without due consideration of some important elements.

Strauss, A., & Corbin, J. (1990). *Basics of qualitative research: Grounded theory, procedures, and techniques.* London: Sage.

Coauthored by one of the originators of grounded theory (Ansel Strauss), this book discusses how to do theoretical sampling (among many other things).

Miles, M. B., & Huberman, A. M. (1994). *Qualitative data analysis: A sourcebook of new methods.* Beverly Hills, CA: Sage.

This book is a standard first text for quantitative researchers wanting to try qualitative research. It is clear, straightforward, and has a good section on sampling approaches.

REFERENCES

Dreher, M. (1994). Qualitative research from the reviewer's perspective. In J M. Morse (Ed.), *Critical issues in qualitative research methods* (pp. 281–298). London: Sage.

Hillebrand, B., Kok, R. A. W., & Biemens, W. G. (2001). Theory-testing using case studies: A comment on Johnston, Leach, and Liu. *Industrial Marketing Management, 30,* 651–657.

Lincoln, Y. S., & Guba, E.G. (1985). *Naturalistic inquiry.* Beverly Hills, CA: Sage.

Miles, M. B., & Huberman, A. M. (1994). *Qualitative data analysis: A sourcebook of new methods.* Beverly Hills, CA: Sage.

Morse, J. M. (2000). Determining sample size [Editorial]. *Qualitative Health Research, 10,* 3–5.

Patton, M. Q. (1990). *Qualitative evaluation methods.* Beverly Hills, CA: Sage.

QSR International. (2000). *QSR N5.* Available at *www.qsrinternational.com.*

Strauss, A., & Corbin, J. (1990). *Basics of qualitative research: Grounded theory, procedures, and techniques.* London: Sage.

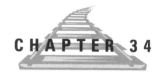

CHAPTER 34

Bigger Is Not Always Better
Adventures in the World of Survey Data Analysis

SYLVIA KAIROUZ
LOUISE NADEAU

BACKGROUND OF THE STUDY

It is not always obvious to us that a good part of our health depends on where and with whom we live. Such is, however, the case. "Places do matter" has become a leitmotiv in health research, expressing the role environments play in shaping health and health differences in the population above and beyond individual influences (Macintyre, Ellaway, & Cummins, 2002). Significant inequalities have been observed between areas for various health outcomes (Yen & Kaplan, 1999), perceived health (Pampalon, Duncan, Subramanian, & Jones, 1999), and a variety of potentially addictive behaviors in adolescents (Ennet, Flewelling, Lindrooth, & Norton, 1997) and adult populations, such as tobacco (Duncan, Jones, & Moon, 1999) and alcohol consumption (Balarajan & Yuen, 1986; Duncan, Jones, & Moon, 1993; Rice, Carr-Hill, Dixon, & Sutton, 1998). Numerous studies have shown that area of residence is associated with health, so that some neighborhoods could possibly be healthier than others (Cox, Boyle, Davey, Feng, & Morris, 2007; Diez-Roux et al., 2001; Kawachi & Berkman, 2003; Macintyre & Ellaway, 2003).

In view of these facts, we decided to investigate the role environments play in shaping the habits of gambling and problem gambling. Gambling was and still is an emergent priority in public health, given the increased prevalence of gambling with thriving venues. Yet the research had been scarce in examining gambling habits, from occasional and inconsequential gambling to pathological gambling, in relation to social and physical environments. Studies had been predominantly anchored in an individual-oriented perspective. Because of the work conducted in our city by our colleagues Galliland and Ross (2005), we knew that gambling venues were more heavily concentrated in poor areas as compared with rich ones on the island of Montreal. Several hypotheses have attempted to explain these differences. Disparities in exposure to gambling between neighborhoods may create differential levels of risk for individuals' developing gambling problems. Ecological factors such as the availability of resources and access to those resources may play a significant role in creating geographical differences. Alternatively, compositional factors such as the concentration of residents with shared health lifestyles might explain the geographical clustering of health outcomes. Furthermore, new conceptual and empirical orientations recognize the overlapping boundaries between individuals and places and the two-way relationship between environments as constraining/enabling structures and individuals as agents continuously shaping the lived environments (Bernard et al., 2007; Giddens, 1984). In accordance with the theory, we were eager to find out if there were more problem gamblers in the poor neighborhoods of Montreal in comparison to the more affluent ones.

In 2002, the prospect of a first-ever national survey including data on gambling and geography was a trigger for our project. In fact, Statistics Canada conducted the Canadian Community Health Survey, Mental Health and Well-Being (CCHS, cycle 1.2; Gravel & Béland, 2005) to provide provincial cross-sectional estimates of mental health determinants, mental health status, including addictions and gambling, and mental health system utilization. With the CCHS, conditions were met to examine neighborhood variations in the prevalence of gambling and to assess individual and environmental determinants of these variations. The CCHS provided (1) a large and representative sample ($N = 5,000$ for the Province of Québec) and (2) postal code information to create neighborhoods units. The number of interviewed households in neighborhoods units ranged from fewer than 5 to more than 20. Moreover, ecological information on neighborhoods could be derived from administrative sources and census data could be merged with the CCHS file. Given the availability of information, we had deemed possible the modeling of individual and neighborhood determinants of gambling and problem gambling simultaneously.

In this context, our main research question was then to explore the role of neighborhoods, as proximal and significant environments, in shaping gambling behaviors and problems among people residing in the census metropolitan area of Montreal. Given its demographic and ethnic diversity, we elected this census metropolitan area as a natural geographical setting to explore our research question. The objectives of our project were (1) to explore neighborhood variations in the prevalence of gambling behaviors and problems and (2) to assess individual and environmental determinants of these variations. The use of multilevel analysis allowed us to quantitatively assess the synergy between individuals and environments in the absence of longitudinal data, and the modeling of nested structures of individuals in neighborhoods. The linking of several other public data banks was necessary, and they were available to accredited scientists, which we were. The reviewers agreed with what they read and we were funded. Little did we know about the challenges that stood before us.

THE CHALLENGES AND SOLUTIONS

We discuss here the general area of data analysis and, more specifically, the challenges of secondary analysis of protected or government-controlled epidemiological data; in our case, the analysis of Statistics Canada data in a Research Data Centre (RDC). There is no doubt that working with such large datasets is stimulating and challenging. However, various problems arose throughout our inquiry. The focus of this chapter is on three major obstacles: (1) the problem of data accessibility and the related issue of hiring staff, mostly logistic in nature, (2) the difficulty of merging various sources of information with the CCHS data file, and (3) the limitations of surveillance surveys to explore comprehensive explanatory models.

The Chicken-and-Egg Problem

The first obstacle in our project was the exceedingly long waiting period to access the CCHS dataset in the RDC and its deleterious effect on hiring (see Chapter 9 for another description of this problem). Generally, to access large survey master files (even those with nonconfidential information), users must go through a three-step procedure: (1) complete a request for access, (2) undergo a security check and a personal record investigation, and (3) sign an under-oath working contract with Statistics Canada. Contracts are meant to ensure respect of confidentiality, data use, and rules for disseminating the results by users. This legal action is extremely important, given the access users will get to confidential information.

It took our team members approximately 5 months to get through the access procedure and start working on the analyses. This period of time constituted almost 25% of the overall funded period of this project and was far beyond the time anticipated in our initial planning schedule. This especially long period translated into repeated rescheduling of project deadlines and, ultimately, a request for extension from the granting agency. Yet, most important, the tedious and time-consuming access procedure was particularly detrimental to hiring and retaining qualified research associates on the project. On top of delays, we had to go through several recruitments of statistical experts, which was also time-consuming, given the rarity of those with the necessary qualifications.

It also became clear that secondary data analysis of large survey data bases is synonymous with cutting-edge statistical expertise. With the greater sophistication of social and health surveys, successfully conducting secondary data analyses of these complex treasures is contingent on a solid knowledge of statistical methods and techniques as well as expertise in the use of statistical software. Even with that expertise, more time is involved in understanding the specific problems that need attention. Yet, given the social aspect of our project, we had to find a research associate who would combine advanced statistical knowledge with a social reasoning flair. In other words, we were looking for a hybrid combination that is rarely available nowadays. The search was long and choices were extremely limited. Recruitment was difficult, involving multiple postings. Finally, by word of mouth, we hit the jackpot with a qualified and motivated social science statistician. We agreed on an approximate starting date, contingent on obtaining access permission, and then submitted an application for our employee at Statistics Canada.

Several months passed while we waited for a response. This situation forced us to repeatedly put on hold the contract with our hard-to-find research associate. We ended up losing this valuable resource and had to restart the recruitment procedure, along with a new request for data access. We felt ourselves trapped in a vicious circle, a chicken-and-egg situation. On one hand, hiring a research associate was mandatory to apply for data access and, on the other hand, the long waiting time for accessing the data was forcing us to postpone the contracts and consequently losing our resource. We contemplated several options and one was deemed acceptable: to hire a part-time research associate to minimize costs while waiting for access approval. Yet the part-time option seemed barely realistic in a booming job market for statisticians.

The time access issue called for two actions. The first action was to require an extension of the project deadline, and the second, more crucial, was to develop an association with a pool of other researchers and other research projects to ensure our ongoing access to a highly qualified statistical expert while waiting for approval for data access. For the first time, as a new investigator, one of us (S. K.) discovered how administrative and human management skills are essential in conducting social research. Being in a well-established research center was extremely helpful to get around this awkward situation. Various research teams in the center combined their efforts to hire a social statistician, who was intended to work as a full-time research associate on specific projects when needed. The joint contributions of the various researchers made it possible to hire a full-time person without penalizing any one specific project. We definitely felt less pressure with delays in accessing the data and were ready to face up front the analyses when access was finally granted.

Missing Links

Initially, our project was designed to reproduce information on individuals and neighborhoods in a hierarchical structure. The CCHS provided a wealth of information on individual gambling habits and a diagnostic measure of pathological gambling. Yet we expected to derive two types of ecological information on neighborhoods from various sources: (1) contextual information, namely, the availability of gambling venues and health and social services from the administrative files (the governmental agency controlling venues and the health authority), and (2) compositional information available through census data on various geographical areas in Montreal. The merging of administrative data, which would have given additional meaning to the results, was found to be impossible. There had been a moratorium on data-merging procedures involving other institutions. In our case, we needed to link the CCHS data with that of two other provincial agencies: one holding information on the locations of gambling venues (Régie des Alcohols, des Courses et des Jeux) and the other holding health data (Agence de la Santé et des Services Sociaux de Montréal). We thus had to give up on one key objective, that is, to examine the impact of gambling availability, density, or any other contextual characteristic of neighborhoods, on individual gambling behaviors. We had to settle for broad demographic compositional characteristics of neighborhoods, which were available through census data.

We decided to use census data as an alternative option but encountered another series of difficulties in accessing the right census data. Again, access to the 2001 census data and the conversion to link it to the CCHS involved an extensive procedure. Our timeline was once again exceeded in merging the CCHS with the census data.

Bigger Is Not Always Better

Once individuals were distributed over small geographical units as proxies for neighborhoods, the inspection of distributions revealed that the CCHS sample was not large enough within geographical units identifying neighborhoods. An analysis of the variability in gambling prevalence and related problems was the most we could hope to do. To preserve confidentiality, units with fewer than five observations could not be modeled in an explanatory model, and such was the case in several instances.

At this stage, we were fishing for alternative geographical units that would be "not too broad and not too small"—that is, units large enough to encompass a sufficient sample and still remain meaningful in terms of their impact on individual gambling behaviors. To top it off, when it became clear that pathological gambling was rarer than expected in the population, the use of small geographical units was definitely abandoned, given the survey sample size. Consequently, we had to find creative statistical techniques to address this additional limitation.

The availability of support from Statistics Canada analysts was tremendously appreciated. Staff in charge of the survey and experts on health and geography provided helpful insights to redefine the geographical units of analysis in a meaningful way. Finally, on the geographical level, we were able to set our analysis at the Census Subdivision (CSD) level, defined as an area that is a municipality or an area deemed to be equivalent to a municipality. On the statistical level, the use of multilevel modeling enabled us to deal optimally with unbalanced sample size within geographical units and to minimize sensitivity to missing cases.

The analysis was deemed optimal, given the administrative, technical, and statistical limitations. However, our ambition to get a more complete understanding of the multilevel determinants of gambling behaviors and problems was undermined. Once again, the complexity of relationships between individuals and their lived environments was not appropriately captured with a broad delimitation of geography and the availability of very limited explanatory factors. The large sample size was definitely a valuable asset in this project. Still, our experience revealed that bigger is not always better. Indeed, survey data are fundamental for monitoring the health of the population and the use of health services. Nevertheless, for comprehensive endeavors, the data may not be as versatile as desired and could limit the options for researchers to explore specific health problems. With a prevalence rate nearing 1%, exploring the relationship between gambling and geography could be a utopian wish even with a fairly large sample size.

LESSONS LEARNED

Have a realistic timeline! Plan enough time to access databases in data centers. For a researcher or a student, time should be factored out in the scheduling equation. For a research team, this issue may affect the hiring procedure.

Be a statistical whiz! Our own experience revealed that secondary data analysis of large survey databases intrinsically requires cutting-edge statistical expertise. Thus, the success of any project using complex population data depends on the mastery of advanced statistical techniques and statistical software. In this respect, the expertise of our team in advanced social statistics helped significantly in finding attractive alternatives when we were faced with major obstacles to achieving the originally planned analyses.

Where does the cycle of research start? One of the key learning experiences in this project was to realize that the cycle of research should sometimes start at the data level. In the case of secondary data analysis, it is often the data that dictate the conceptual content rather than the theoretical model determining the data. We had the sense, at the end of this project, that in order to get the bigger picture at the population level, we lost important details about subgroups, blurring the picture itself. With a population perspective on gambling, the sense of the meaningful determinants of gambling problems was lost. To give meaning to low prevalence rates, large representative samples are needed, as is easy access to the information contained in complementary data banks.

Use monitoring surveys! Large surveys provide a wealth of information on social and health issues. It is our contention that those high-quality databases are not sufficiently used. Despite various obstacles encountered throughout our project on gambling, we were eager to develop new studies with the CCHS. Working with the database was indeed a challenging endeavor, yet an inspiring experience for a thirsty mind.

EPILOGUE

One of us (S. K.) was invited to present the results of this research at a meeting of psychiatric epidemiologists. The results were well received. They were published in a special issue of the *Canadian Journal of Psychiatry* in 2005 (Kairouz, Nadeau, & Lo Siou, 2005). The authors have recently obtained another grant to study gambling from a population perspective. The experience related here should help them solve the inevitable problems that come with generating new knowledge.

TO READ FURTHER

Psychiatric epidemiology in Canada: The Canadian Community Health Survey: Mental Health and Well-being. (2005, September). *Canadian Journal of Psychiatry, 50,* 10.

This special issue of the *Canadian Journal of Psychiatry* provides a collection of articles that describe one of the major health surveys in Canada and a collection of studies generated from the survey data.

Gonthier, D., Hotton, T., Cook, C., & Wilkins, R. (2006). Merging area-level census data with survey and administrative data. *Proceedings of Statistics Canada Symposium 2006: Methodological issues in measuring population health.* Ottawa: Statistics Canada. Catalogue No. 11-522-XIE.

The authors describe the procedure for merging administrative survey data and geographical area-level data.

REFERENCES

Balarajan, R., & Yuen, P. (1986). British smoking and drinking habits: Regional variations. *Community Medicine, 8,* 131–137.

Bernard, P., Charafeddine, R., Frolich, K. L., Daniel, M., Kestens, Y., & Potvin, L. (2007). Health inequalities and place: A theoretical concept of neighbourhood. *Social Science and Medicine, 65,* 1839–1852.

Cox, M., Boyle, P. J., Davey, P. G., Feng, Z., & Morris, A. D. (2007). Locality deprivation and Type 2 diabetes incidence: A local test of relative inequalities. *Social Science and Medicine, 65,* 1953–1964.

Diez-Roux, A. V., Stein Merkin, S., Arnett, D., Chambless, L., Massing, M., Neito, J., et al. (2001). Neighborhood of residence and incidence in coronary heart disease. *New England Journal of Medicine, 345,* 99–106.

Duncan, C., Jones, K., & Moon, G. (1993). Do places matter? A multi-level analysis of regional variations in health-related behaviour in Britain. *Social Science and Medicine, 37,* 725–733.

Duncan, C., Jones, K., & Moon, G. (1999). Smoking and deprivation: Are there neighbourhood effects? *Social Science and Medicine, 48,* 497–505.

Ennet, S. T., Flewelling, R. L., Lindrooth, R. C., & Norton, E. C. (1997). School and neighbourhood characteristics with school rates of alcohol, cigarette, and marijuana use. *Journal of Health and Social Behavior, 38,* 55–71.

Galliland, J. A., & Ross, N. A. (2005). Opportunities for video lottery terminal gambling in Montréal. *Canadian Journal of Public Health, 96,* 55–59.

Giddens, A. (1984). *The constitution of society.* Berkeley: University of California Press.

Gravel, R., & Béland, Y. (2005). The Canadian Community Health Survey: Mental Health and Well-Being. *Canadian Journal of Psychiatry, 50,* 573–579.

Kairouz, S., Nadeau, L., & Lo Siou, G. (2005). Area variations in the prevalence of substance use and gambling behaviours and problems in Quebec : A multilevel analysis. *Canadian Journal of Psychiatry, 50,* 591–598.

Kawachi, I., & Berkman, L. F. (2003). *Neighborhoods and health.* Oxford, UK: Oxford University Press.

Macintyre, S., & Ellaway, A. (2003). Neighbourhoods and health: An overview. In I. Kawachi & L. F. Berkman (Eds.), *Neighbourhoods and health* (pp. 20–42). New York: Oxford University Press.

Macintyre, S., Ellaway, A., & Cummins, S. (2002). Place effects on health: How can we conceptualise, operationalise and measure them? *Social Science and Medicine, 55,* 125–139.

Pampalon, R., Duncan, C., Subramanian, S. V., & Jones K. (1999). Geographies of health perception in Quebec: A multilevel perspective. *Social Science and Medicine, 48*, 1483–1490.

Rice, N., Carr-Hill, R., Dixon, P., & Sutton, M. (1998). The influence of households on drinking behaviour: A multilevel analysis. *Social Science and Medicine, 46*, 971–979.

Yen, I., & Kaplan, G. A. (1999). Neighbourhood social environment and risk of death: Multilevel evidence from the Alameda County Study. *American Journal of Epidemiology, 149*, 898–907.

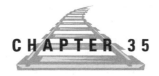

CHAPTER 35

Taking Aim at a Moving Target
When a Study Changes in the Middle

ARTURO MARTÍ-CARVAJAL

BACKGROUND OF THE STUDY

In 2007, the *British Medical Journal* published a narrative review about the treatment of sepsis (Mackenzie & Lever, 2007), a serious medical condition in which an infection causes inflammation throughout the body. It focused on the Recombinant Human Activated Protein C Worldwide Evaluation in Severe Sepsis (PROWESS) study (Bernard et al., 2001). This study was the basis for the Food and Drug Administration's (FDA) authorizing the marketing of activated protein C (APC) as a treatment. The narrative review supported the use of this treatment, even given that the drug has a cost between $ 6,000 and $ 7,000 and that the PROWESS study has come under criticism (Eichacker & Natanson, 2003).

In 2007, my colleagues and I published a Cochrane systematic review to answer the question "What is the effectiveness and safety of recombinant human activated protein C in patients with severe sepsis?" (Martí-Carvajal, Salanti, & Cardona, 2007). We included the original FDA approval document for APC in the Cochrane review. The FDA document showed that the PROWESS study had two phases, perfectly discernible and absolutely different. The sample size of PROWESS (*N* = 2,280) was calculated to determine the efficacy of APC in a global way, not for specific subgroups. However, in the middle of the study, a modification was made to the inclusion criteria; the most important change was the exclusion of patients with septic shock. This amendment was not published by Bernard et al. (2001).

The first interim analysis of the PROWESS study, using the original data, showed that APC was not effective for treating patients with severe sepsis. In the first phase (original data), there was a 28-day mortality rate of 28.3% (102/360) in the experimental group versus 30.2% (109/360) in the control group, and the relative risk (RR) was 0.94 (95% confidence internal [CI] 0.75 to 1.1; p = .57). In the second half of the PROWESS study, using the amended protocol, the 28-day mortality rate was 22% (108/490) in the experimental group versus 31.2% (150/480) in the control group. The RR now was 0. 71 (95% CI 0.57 to 0.87; p = .0001), meaning that there were about 30% fewer deaths in the APC group.

Using sensitivity analysis, we determined the influence of the methodological quality of the various studies of APC and its effect on the relative risk. When the second phase (amendment protocol) of the PROWESS study was excluded from that analysis, the heterogeneity of the results of the different studies fell from 68.5% to 0% and the global RR was 1.01 (95% CI = 0.89 to 1.15; p = .84). This indicated two things: first, that the results from the second phase were completely different from the results of other studies of the drug; and second, that APC had absolutely no effect. Our review concluded that there seems to be no evidence suggesting any benefit associated with APC for treating patients with severe sepsis.

THE CHALLENGES

The objective of the PROWESS study was to demonstrate that APC reduces 28-day all-cause mortality in patients with severe sepsis. To reach this objective, the researchers established inclusion and exclusion criteria regarding which patients would be enrolled in the study. When the researchers saw the results of the first interim analysis (based on 720 patients), they modified those criteria, but the reasons were not described (Food and Drug Administration, 2001).

The randomized controlled trial (RCT) is the cornerstone for studies of treatment effectiveness. This capacity is based on "how closely a trial's participants reflect the general population of patients with the disorder that has been investigated" (Seale, Gebski, & Keech, 2004, p. 558). The findings of an RCT must be applied only to patients with similar characteristics as those who were included in the trial. If the inclusion criteria were broad, the extent of trial's findings will be broad; conversely, if the inclusion criteria were narrow, the implications of trial's findings will be narrow. This is known as the generalizability, or external validity, of the study. External validity must not be confused with internal validity, which means the "results are true," whereas external validity means the "results are widely applicable" (Sackett, 1980, p. 1059). The internal validity is the quantitative component of the randomized controlled trial; the external validity is its qualitative component.

The comparison between the two phases of the PROWESS study (original versus amended) showed that "81 patients or 11% eligible for the original protocol would not have been eligible for the amended version of the protocol. This highlights the fact that the amended protocol did enroll a different patient population compared to the original protocol" (Food and Drug Administration, 2001). The participants were changed, and then a different research study was carried out with the same objective. The PROWESS study has two types of participants sharing the same objective, the same research question, and the same drug.

Why are the eligibility criteria important? First, "Enrolling participants with similar characteristics helps to ensure that the results of the trial will be due to what is under study and not other factors. In this way, eligibility criteria help researchers achieve accurate and meaningful results. These criteria also minimize the risk of a person's condition becoming worse by participating in the study" (National Cancer Institute, 2006). The second reason is that patients enrolled in a study may be different from the potential users of the treatment, and this may affect the outcome (Weiss, Koepsell, & Psaty, 2008), so it is important to know exactly who was or was not enrolled.

Many questions could be asked: Which one of the two phases of the PROWESS study has greater internal validity? How can you understand its external validity? What is the true external validity of the PROWESS study? A small change, a big impact!

OVERCOMING THE DIFFICULTIES

During the course of any RCT, serious or nonserious adverse events can occur, which can be expected or not. In order to reduce the risk for participants or guarantee their safety, all RCTs must be monitored by two committees: an Institutional Review Board (IRB) and a Data and Safety Monitoring Board (DSMB), independent of the sponsor (Piantadosi, 1997). Their mandate is to guarantee that the study is conducted fairly and that participants are not likely to be harmed (Grant, 2004).

The IRB decides when the trial will be reviewed once it has begun, and together with the DSMB, has these functions: first, to decide whether the RCT will continue as initially planned or what changes should be made; second, to stop the trial if the researchers are not following the protocol, the study appears to be causing unexpected harm to the participants, or there is clear evidence that the new intervention is effective, in order to make it widely available (National Cancer Institute, 2006).

Remember that the problem was that APC was not more effective than the control, which was demonstrated during the first interim analysis; therefore, the DSMB has an important role to play. The PROWESS study should either have been continued as it was planned, or stopped early. The researchers could have either tried to determine why APC was not effective, or started a completely different study; they should not have changed the criteria in the middle.

LESSONS LEARNED

I learned with this Cochrane review that decision making in daily clinical practice should be based on the critical appraisal of the literature; that the physicians, academics, and policy makers should interpret the results of an RCT using established guidelines; and that the most important aspect of any study will be, first and foremost, the methodology, and never the discussion.

The research team must remember, first, that any RCT has a Data and Safety Monitoring Board that is an independent committee; second, that the concept of external validity should be carefully examined; third, that any violation of the original protocol creates bias and reduces the internal and external validities; and, fourth *primum non nocere* ("first, do no harm").

TO READ FURTHER

Porta, M. (Ed.). (2008). *A dictionary of epidemiology* (5th ed.). New York: Oxford University Press.

This book is where to begin on the epidemiological research road. It is a key reference for epidemiologists.

Berger, V. (2007). *Selection bias and covariate imbalances in randomized clinical trials*. New York: Wiley.

This book explains how and why participant selection is key in any research.

Egger, M., Smith, G. D., & Altman, D. G. (2001). *Systematic reviews in health care: Meta-analysis in context* (2nd ed.). London: British Medical Journal.

A great source for understanding, almost without any mathematics, what systematic reviews and meta-analyses are.

REFERENCES

Bernard, G. R., Vincent, J.-L., Laterre, P.-F., LaRosa, S. P., Dhainaut, J-F., López-Rodríguez, A., et al. (2001). Efficacy and safety of recombinant human activated protein C for severe sepsis. *New England Journal of Medicine, 344,* 699–709.

Eichacker, P. Q., & Natanson, C. (2003). Recombinant human activated protein C in sepsis: Inconsistent trial results, an unclear mechanism of action, and safety concerns resulted in labeling restrictions and the need for phase IV trials. *Critical Care Medicine, 31*(Suppl.), 94–96.

Food and Drug Administration briefing document: Anti-infective Advisory Committee. (2001, September). *Drotrecogin alfa (activated). [Recombinant human activated protein (rhAPC)]. XIGRIS™ BLA # 125029/0.* Available at *www. fda.gov/ohrms/dockets/ac/01/briefing/3797b1_02_FDAbriefing.pdf.*

Grant, A. (2004). Stopping clinical trials early. *British Medical Journal, 329,* 525–526.

Mackenzie, I., & Lever, A. (2007). Management of sepsis. *British Medical Journal, 335,* 929–932.

Martí-Carvajal, A., Salanti, G., & Cardona, A. F. (2007). Human recombinant activated protein C for severe sepsis. *Cochrane Database Systematic Review, 3,* CD004388.

National Cancer Institute. (2006). *Clinical trials: Questions and answers.* January 18, 2008, from *www.cancer.gov/cancertopics/factsheet/Information/clinical-trials.*

Piantadosi, S. (1997). *Clinical trials: A methodologic perspective.* New York: Wiley-Interscience.

Sackett, D. L. (1980). The competing objective of the randomized trials. *New England Journal of Medicine, 303,* 1059–1060.

Seale, J. P., Gebski, V. J., & Keech, A. C. (2004). Generalising the results of trials to clinical practice. *Medical Journal of Australia, 181,* 558–560.

Weiss, N. S., Koepsell, T. D., & Psaty, B. M. (2008). Generalizability of the results of randomized trials. *Archives of Internal Medicine, 168,* 133–135.

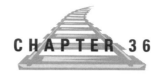

CHAPTER 36

Lack of Normative Data as an Obstacle to Neuropsychological Assessment

F. Richard Ferraro
Kaylee Trottier-Wolter

BACKGROUND OF THE STUDY

Both of us are appreciative of the issues facing researchers studying Native Americans, specifically Native elders. With life expectancy increasing worldwide come the potential ravages of dementia. Age is the leading risk factor (among many others) for dementia onset. Thus, as we age our risk of developing any of a wide array of age-related diseases and disorders increases dramatically. This issue is even more pressing for Native elders, as they are unaccustomed to issues related to dementia and how its effects are far-reaching (individual family, community, tribe, reservation). Although the same issues face other minority groups, Native elders are an often overlooked group despite great advances in longevity and life expectancy.

For the past 10 years or so, I (F. R. F., with the assistance of graduate and undergraduate students) have been attempting to determine appropriate neuropsychological assessment batteries for Native American elders (Ferraro & Bercier, 1996; Ferraro, Bercier, Holm, & McDonald, 2002; Ferraro et al., 2007) in addition to the effectiveness of such batteries. One reason for this is that there are currently no such normative datasets in existence, although there are pockets of data available from the few studies that have collected such normative data. Thus, it becomes difficult to adequately assess or even identify individuals with, for example, dementia within the Native elder community. This issue is further compounded when one attempts to interpret the effectiveness of interventions. This is a significant concern, as life expectancy is gradually increasing in Native elders and they, as a group, are now becoming more at risk for dementia. In many instances, though, no differences have actually been found between Native elders and non-Native elders across a variety of neuropsychological tests (Ferraro et al., 2002; Whyte et al., 2005), raising the issue of the need to have specific norms in the first place.

As an update to the Ferraro et al. (2007) study, my co-authors and I (F. R. F.) have shown that in various samples of Native elders there are few differences, as compared with nonnative elders, on neuropsychological tests, including the Boston Naming Test, the Digit Symbol test, and the Logical Memory test. However, we have observed some tribal differences. That is, across these most recent papers, we tested three different Native American tribes. This is somewhat different from what we did previously (Ferraro et al., 2002), in which we tested only one tribe. In each instance, the Native elders performed within the bounds of nonnative community-dwelling individuals. But the significant tribal differences across some tests underscore the relevance of not assuming that all tribes are the same or that all tribes require similar intervention. Although this is interesting, it leads to more questions about the utility of constructing specific normative data and raises the issue of constructing specific normative data for specific tribes, as well as determining the most effective intervention for a specific tribe. This does not seem like a practical solution, as there are more than 500 identified and registered Native American tribes. It also becomes somewhat of an ethical issue as well. One cannot simply not assess an individual if no normative data exist.

THE CHALLENGES

One of the greatest challenges in cross-cultural neuropsychological assessment is the ability to make accurate assessments and diagnoses on the basis of accurate and reliable normative datasets and then include these assessments in a larger neuropsychological intervention. Without adequate or accurate normative data on the specific population under investigation, one could overestimate or underestimate a diagnosis or include an intervention that may not be as effective as it could be. This can cause problems; for example, a person could be diagnosed with, say, dementia, when no dementia exists. Alternatively, a person may not be so diagnosed when, in fact, such a diagnosis is required. Each of these scenarios leads to additional problems related to adjustment on the part of the patient and his or her family and additional doctor visits. It also, according to Manly and Echemendia (2007), raises issues related to the minimization of the roles of cultural and educational factors in assessment and diagnosis, as well as potentially setting more lenient or less stringent cutoff scores.

OVERCOMING THE DIFFICULTIES

One way to work around the problems is simply to acknowledge the discrepancies and inform those who need to be informed. Alternatively, one could use existing normative data or could collect new normative data using tests initially normed on a sample other than the one under investigation. Finally, one could revise the current tests and adapt them to the sample under investigation. All of these options have some merit. However, some are easier to perform than others. For instance, what is commonly done is that existing normative data are used. This offers the quickest method, and even though there are actually no normative data on the sample in question, examiners can acknowledge this when they report their findings. Interventions can then proceed. Likewise, such a practice is common within many neuropsychological circles, although there are those who advocate for race-specific normative data (Manly & Echemendia, 2007) but at the same time indicate the many problems associated with such a practice. In our own (F. R. F.) research the solution of using existing non-Native normative data was sufficient but at the same time raised additional questions, especially as they relate to the tribal differences some of my previous work had revealed.

LESSONS LEARNED

A currently debatable issue in the area of cross-cultural neuropsychological assessment (Brandt, 2007) is coming up with normative data specific to the cultural/racial group under investigation and then being able to use that information in an effective neuropsychological intervention. At the same time, this is a very controversial issue on several fronts, including the notion that race-specific normative data ignore underlying cultural and educational factors (i.e., literacy) and that setting more lenient, or lower, cutoff scores potentially results in the denial of additional special services for these groups. Would we now advocate constructing specific tribal norms for each neuropsychological test given? No. Rather, we would accept the fact that norms do not exist but attempt to design an intervention that would favor tribal differences.

The problems we have encountered in our cross-cultural research into neuropsychological function in Native elders have not resulted in our wanting to stop this research. Rather, these problems have made us even more aware that solutions to these problems are greatly needed and time is of the essence. Native elders are a fast-growing segment of our population, and with advanced age comes numerous age-related diseases and disorders heretofore unheard of in Native circles. Life expectancy is greatly increasing, and although this increase is encouraging, it poses additional challenges. Blindly applying existing norms is not an adequate solution, and constructing race-specific (or tribe-specific, in our case) is also not adequate. These serve short-term, but not long-term, needs and requirements. The ultimate goal is to provide accurate and informative information to various tribes and tribal members in an effort to create an intervention that can lead to lowered rates of dementia or interventions that result in more people understanding what can be done to offset the problems associated with dementia.

TO READ FURTHER

Gopaul-McNicol, S.-A., & Armour-Thomas, E. (2002). *Assessment and culture: Psychological tests with minority populations.* New York: Academic Press.

This book nicely goes over various testing issues with various minority populations. Included are chapters related to ethical and legal issues, the biocultural perspective, work with populations across the life span (children, adults).

Nell, V. (1999). *Cross-cultural neuropsychological assessment theory and practice.* Florence, KY: Routledge.

This book is one of the classics in this area and relevant for those interested in and called upon to assess neuropsychological function across various cultural groups. This how-to book exposes the reader to issues related to racism and politics associated with neuropsychological assessment, the IQ controversy, and core testing batteries that can be useful with various minority groups.

Yeo, G., & Gallagher-Thomson, D. (2006). *Ethnicity and the dementias.* Boca Raton, FL: CRC Press.

This book examines ethnicity as it relates to various dementias (including Alzheimer's disease), cognitive status, and prevalence rates across various minority groups. Key features include assessment issues, testing protocols, and international psychogeriatrics. The book is ideal for students as well as practitioners.

REFERENCES

Brandt, J. (2007). 2005 INS Presidential address: Neuropsychological crimes and misdemeanors. *The Clinical Neuropsychologist, 21,* 553–568.

Ferraro, F. R., & Bercier, B. (1996). Boston Naming Test performance in a sample of Native American elderly adults. *Clinical Gerontlogist, 17,* 58–60.

Ferraro. F. R., Bercier, B., Holm, J., & McDonald, J. (2002). Preliminary normative data from a brief neuropsychological test battery in a sample of Native American elderly. In F. R. Ferraro (Ed.), *Minority and cross cultural aspects of neuropsychological assessment* (pp. 227–240). Lisse, The Netherlands: Swets & Zeitlimnger.

Ferraro, F. R., McDonald, L. R., Allery, A., Irwin, A., Lambert, P., Sutherland, J., et al. (2007). Mini Mental Status Examination performance in Native

American elderly: Preliminary data. *Journal of Native Aging and Health, 2,* 15–17.

Manly, J., J., & Echemendia, R. J. (2007). Race-specific norms: Using the model of hypertension to understand issues of race, culture, and education in neuropsychology. *Archives of Clinical Neuropsychology, 22,* 319–325.

Whyte, S., Cullum, M. C., Hynan, L. S., Lacritz, L. H., Rosenberg, R. N., & Weiner, M. F. (2005). Performance of elderly Native Americans and caucasians on the CERAD neuropsychological battery. *Alzheimer's Disease and Associated Disorders, 19,* 74–78.

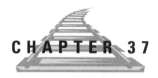

CHAPTER 37

These Data Do Not Compute

LYNNE MACLEAN
MECHTHILD MEYER
ALMA ESTABLE
ANITA KOTHARI
NANCY EDWARDS

BACKGROUND OF THE STUDY

What happens when investigators new to qualitative software plunge in without a clear idea of what the software does and does not do, and what role it plays in analysis? Many investigators assume it will work like quantitative software.

When we have run sessions introducing such programs, *qualitative* researchers holding this incorrect assumption tell us they are appalled at the idea of using qualitative software because they think this approach equates with tabulating data. They may refuse to use the software, as they do not see how it fits with the deep and nonreductionist approach that is the hallmark of qualitative analysis. Some categorically refuse to use software. With *quantitative* investigators new to qualitative methods, the situation is different. Problems occur when the availability of qualitative software leads quantitative researchers to erroneously assume that the data can be analyzed using a quantitative frame of reference.

We illustrate these issues through a variety of incidents experienced over several studies with diverse qualitative software programs, highlighting project management and data analysis issues. As a group, we have considerable experience, together and apart, in being involved in many different kinds of qualitative studies, applied and theoretical, and we use qualitative software regularly. Researchers often come to us with questions or problems. Although the problems tend to be based on incorrect assumptions about the software, they all are likely to end the same way: with frustration and disappointment and a need to spend more resources on training, transcription, coding, and analysis, as either the work needs to be redone, or done by more people, or even just done at all. We wish we had a few really juicy stories to tell, but instead, they mostly play out to the same scenario: Why won't the software work? What do you mean, it won't do that? Now what do we do, we're in the beginning/ middle of analysis? We have to do it with human beings? Maybe all of our human beings? What do you mean we have to redo that first step? We have to step back and train people? We didn't budget for that! The report's due in 2 weeks!

As you can see, the scenarios don't make for much elaboration, but the faulty assumptions do. So, in order to save you some time and money, we present a few common problems that have come our way (or that we have caused ourselves from time to time).

What Qualitative Software Does Do

There are several software programs on the market today that support qualitative analysis. These programs help the researcher to perform some key activities in qualitative analysis, such as organizing, reducing, and displaying the data (Lewins & Silver, 2006; Miles & Huberman, 1994). Software also provides some useful functions such as searching text and indexing information, with greater speed and precision than standard word processing programs, spreadsheets, and, in some cases, graphics programs (Lewins & Silver, 2006). Some software packages have more advanced functions that can link words, images, and/or sounds to each other, to ideas developed by the analyst (both written and schematic), and to external data sources, including Internet sites, documents, and images. Qualitative software facilitates working in teams, allowing people to work on different computers and merge their findings; or to work together on the same computer, but organize their findings efficiently; and/or to provide convenient ways for team members to share their memos of emerging ideas and concerns. It can import and export findings in tabular form by interfacing with word processing packages and spreadsheets. Finally, it assists with tracking the activities in a project, producing reports, and creating audit trails, making the research and analytic process more transparent (Lewins & Silver, 2006). By making some tasks infinitely easier and quicker, software makes it feasible to attempt more systematic, complex questioning of larger volumes of data.

What Qualitative Software Does Not Do

What qualitative software will not do is the final step in all stages of data analysis: drawing or verifying conclusions (Miles & Huberman, 1994). In other words, it won't identify the codes for your data, it won't identify the emergent themes and connect them or disconfirm them, and it won't create a theoretical model or framework for you. The following examples show where people have fallen off-track because of a lack of understanding about what the software doesn't do. We have divided them (rather arbitrarily, given the interconnected nature of this process) into project management and data analysis illustrations.

PROJECT MANAGEMENT

In this section we focus on experiences that have an impact on team roles, staff training, budgeting and resources. Some of these issues are also related to the data analysis itself (isn't everything?), but are mentioned here in terms of their implications for running the project itself and working with team members.

Example 1

In the distant past, our team members have had transcriptionists type in every "umhmm," "uh," or pause, for a study that would *not* be analyzing for emotion, speech patterns, or interpersonal interactions, and so on, but instead was focusing at an informational, content-only level. In one case, the instruction to transcribe everything was deliberate. Other times, this complete transcription was due to lack of clarity in instructions to transcriptionists. In both these circumstances, we found that the "uhs" became very, hmm, distracting, and/or [pause] confusing if they, umm, overlapped with words by another speaker. They, uh, also could make speakers appear less articulate than they actually were [pause, scratching head] (MacLean, Meyer, & Estable, 2004). You would be amazed, like, uh, at how frequently people insert these [pause] interruptions into their speech, and how they can seem to, uh, dominate a transcript. On the bright side, some of the software packages can assist you in removing these items ([pause], you know?).

Example 2

In another study, transcripts of focus groups did not indicate who was a facilitator and who was a participant. Although it was possible retrospectively to identify a facilitator when a question from the interview schedule was asked directly, it was not possible to tell who was asking a spontaneously arising question, or whether the facilitator or a participant was making a comment. The feature of qualitative software that permits comparison of text generated by different sources or "cases" therefore could not be used. Disentangling required going back to the original recordings and retranscribing, adding a couple of weeks to the analysis.

Learning from Examples 1 and 2

Software will not automatically modify or interpret your transcripts. It will read exactly what is in your transcripts, nothing more and nothing less, so training your transcriptionist and providing instructions on how to set up your transcripts are especially important. The software cannot fix basic problems with transcription. Becoming clear on the analysis approach in advance of getting data transcribed and entered in the software program can help ensure that the data that are put into the software are going to work for you.

Example 3

In some projects, investigators have made the assumption that research team roles could be segmented as they can be in more quantitative projects (e.g., a research assistant will enter and clean the data; a statistician will guide the selection of a set of statistical tools that fit the data, and a research associate will conduct the analysis, providing quantitative results for interpretation by the investigators). When applied to a qualitative project, this assumption ended with different people doing the coding, the analysis, and the writing. The result: insufficiently trained coders were drowning in data that they didn't know what to do with whenever the ideas they were reading diverged, even slightly, from the coding definitions they had been given by the project investigators. They did not understand the logic behind the coding, where it came from, or where it was leading in terms of analysis, and so had difficulty making informed decisions about coding variations. Although the coders were skilled in the mechanics of using the software, they did not see the big picture of the analysis, and so coding was flat, not rich. Further, investigators who did no coding themselves sometimes lost their connection to nuances in the data, nuances that generally become apparent during coding and inform distillation and comparative phases of the analysis. As a result, the analysis generally does not go beyond a first level and opportunities for exploring emerging issues more deeply and applying new codes at a second level are missed.

Learning from Example 3

Software will not turn a qualitative study into one that you can manage like a quantitative study. The software may seem to make it possible to segment your study into tasks to be managed solely by different team members, but this is an illusion. Qualitative analysis requires human abstract thought *throughout* data collection, transcription, coding and analysis, and report writing. This requires team members to be involved across all phases of design and analysis. Indeed, many qualitative researchers see all these phases as iterative, adjusting continually on the basis of input from previous phases, and all being integral parts of the same task.

Example 4

In a large sample study ($N \sim 100$), the investigators' expectations were that the software would code, and then analyze, the data for them. The investigators sent a research assistant (RA) to one of us to learn how to do automated coding. Logically enough, the investigators thought that meant that all the coding they had in mind could be automated, including pulling ideas from the transcripts, and not just doing demographic categorizations. They were expecting that coding would then be completed in an hour by the RA using the software. The reality: Because the software could not do this automatically, the assistant had to spend many, many hours coding the data—hours that were not in the budget.

Learning from Example 4

Software will not code the data for you beyond a very superficial auto-coding function. You will still need to budget for significant time and money to get most of your coding done. Depending on the software, auto-coding can be used to import demographic variable tables from spreadsheets and then sort documents along demographic lines; or, for highly structured interviews, to plunk the content that follows specified question headings into predetermined code folders. You still need to code analytically "by hand" into the electronic software files for any but the most structured content analyses.

Example 5

In another study, the RA misinterpreted the instruction to code cases by their demographics. She thought it meant to create demographic categories in which small excerpts of statements by participants about their characteristics were coded (e.g., "My first language is English"), rather than to create node or family categories in which all interviews would be coded in their entirety, based on their first language (e.g., put all the Anglophone interviews in one basket, all the Francophone interviews in another). Not only did this take her longer than the correct task would have, inasmuch as there were software coding functions to automate it, but it also made it impossible to use the powerful matrix analysis functions of this particular software. Again, time-consuming recoding was required.

Learning from Example 5

Software will not compensate for lack of training. Software cannot perform its best with team members or investigators who are not trained in the entire set of software functions, or who are unaware of how qualitative analysis works. Welsh (2002) describes the interplay of software and human involvement as working together to produce the rich tapestry of the research: "The software is the loom that facilitates the knitting together of the tapestry, but the loom cannot determine the final picture on the tapestry. It can ... speed up the process and may also limit the weaver's errors, but for the weaver to succeed ... she or he needs to have an overview of what she or he is trying to produce" (Welsh, 2002, p. 5).

Example 6

However, researchers who fully understand qualitative analysis but who are not technologically minded may be delightfully surprised when their initial misgivings are disproved. Many experienced qualitative researchers chose to struggle on, unaided, for years, coping with tape, scissors, word processing programs, and huge, stuffed, filing cabinets (even huger than those used by qualitative researchers who use software). Several of us began that way ourselves. The patina of quantitative process that software lends to analysis can be off-putting. Fortunately, once these researchers became aware that they would still hold the key role in the analysis, and that they could choose software packages that fit the way they work, they quickly became converts. In fact, such people were often the fastest to pick up the advanced functions of the packages, because they knew where they were directing their activity and quickly saw how the support applied to their work. Sometimes they became concerned that the software would end up driving the analysis (Welsh, 2002). Although this could be true if there were only one kind of software, the variety in packages means that there are functions and structures to support different analysis approaches.

Learning from Example 6

Give software a shot. At least, check it out. Come on. You know you want to.

ANALYSIS

Here we focus on experiences that have had an impact on data analysis specifically. These experiences raised issues for us and the investigators involved in terms of both process and content of analysis.

Example 7

Researchers have thought that the software will analyze the transcripts, codes, or larger theme chunks for them, reading and distilling the ideas within the data, saving them much time and trouble. Unfortunately, they were disappointed. You must construct the codes, the chunks of meaning, and chunks of chunks of meaning.

Learning from Example 7

Qualitative software does not have the capacity to interpret meaning from text: This function requires human abstract thought; in other words, it requires the qualitative researcher!

Example 8

Researchers have hoped that the software will pull out frequent themes, perhaps through word counts, and use some form of hierarchical reasoning based on frequency, or perhaps, proximity data, to connect the ideas. They envisaged that their role would be to review this and correct as necessary. The software cannot do this, and even if it could, it would miss many key and unifying ideas that may be expressed in unusual and idiosyncratic words by only a few people (key informants), widely diverging concepts that could be used in disconfirmation and triangulation, and ideas whose connections flow in unexpected ways. This issue becomes even more apparent when working with qualitative data in different, even multiple, languages. The software, however, can help you compare and map out the ideas. Although of some comfort, this latter ability didn't compensate for the amount of time the researchers thought they were going to be saving.

Learning from Example 8

The software will not tell you how ideas relate to other ideas. It will not develop models or trees or conceptual frameworks for you.

Example 9

Often in mixed-design studies, researchers have wished to triangulate qualitative findings with quantitative findings, not realizing that this triangulation takes place at a conceptual level. They heard that some qualitative software makes use of statistical, spreadsheet or word processing programs, but didn't realize that this was limited to importing tables of cases for auto-coding functions. Although some software can make reports of the number of quotes within and over given themes and groups of themes, export some tables of descriptive statistics about the sample demographics, or even provide exportable tables of quote frequency from matrix operations, it will not match up your qualitative and quantitative data, let alone draw out conceptual links and disconfirmations. We must caution readers that even though the software has some limited capacity for summary quantification, at times even this level of quantification is inappropriate. Its use must be carefully considered, because as soon as findings are reported as frequencies or percentages, readers tend to assume that these are externally generalizable results.

Learning from Example 9

The software will not do statistics for you, beyond descriptive tallying of number of cases, number of quotes in a particular category per interview, mean number of quotes, and the like.

Example 10

The fact that the software is available has tempted people to use large datasets with hopes of quick turnaround times. After all, adding cases (once data are cleaned) to a quantitative study has little impact on analysis time. Some researchers have been surprised (nay, dismayed) that this is not the case with a qualitative study, where each transcript must be read, reread, and coded, perhaps resulting in coding changes for the entire project.

Learning from Example 10

The software will not make adding cases to your analysis an insignificant addition to coding and conceptual analysis time. Be sure to factor in additional analysis time with additional cases (for more detail on sample size in qualitative research, see MacLean et al., Chapter 33, this volume).

There's no escaping it: A rigorous, systematic qualitative analysis will take a long time; it just may take less time when you are assisted by software. The following are suggestions for conducting qualitative research using qualitative analysis software support.

SUGGESTIONS FOR PROJECT MANAGEMENT

- Train transcriptionists to set up the transcript to maximize the features of your particular software. Choose the degree of "verbatim" and participant identification you wish to see, depending on the type of analysis you plan to use (MacLean et al., 2004). Indicate this information in advance to the transcriptionist, and verify first transcripts early on in the process.

- Budget time and resources for coding, recoding, and again recoding, by hand, by human beings.
- Plan on having research staff involved in as many aspects of the project as possible, with at least one person (preferably a principal investigator) involved in all stages from data collection through report writing. If the software is being used by a team of analysts for one study, someone needs to be able to coordinate the team analyses and serve as the main "project" computer site.

SUGGESTIONS FOR ANALYSIS

- Budget sufficient time for the analysis. Check with experienced qualitative researchers if you are new to the approach, so you do not underestimate. If you are an experienced qualitative researcher, but new to software, keep your eyes on your timelines, so you do not get carried away trying advanced functions just for the fun of it. In any case, such activity may not add much to the analysis if not done in a thoughtful fashion (Welsh, 2002).
- Understand the analysis approach you are using before you have data. This will allow you to use the software to its full advantage (and, really, we all should be doing this anyway).
- Plan how the team will work together to draw in everyone's expertise and experience with the data as part of the analysis process. Each human being brings a different set of concepts and constructs to the analysis of qualitative data. See how the software supports teamwork, whether it has merge functions that you will use, or special team memo-ing approaches that might prove useful over distances and sites.

OVERVIEW OF STRATEGIES USED TO ADDRESS THE PROBLEMS: CONSULTING, LEARNING, AND EXPERIMENTING

We were able to fix some of the problems described earlier fairly quickly just through knowledge of the software functions. Sometimes the solutions meant delivering the sad news that humans, in fact, were going to be doing, or redoing, the coding with support of the software, and investigators were going to be spending some hours analyzing the results themselves.

To prevent timelines from flying out the window, choose your software carefully. Determine what various software packages can or cannot do for you in terms of both project management and analysis. Consider which aspects of your work you may choose to continue doing manually (Welsh, 2002). There are many excellent, user-friendly resources to assist you, including articles (e.g., Lewins & Silver, 2006), websites (e.g., the CAQDAS Networking Project website, *caqdas.sc.surrey.ac.uk*), and the software developers themselves.

If you are using software already purchased, then take time to thoroughly understand your software, even if you are not going to be the team member using it most. At the very least, consult with someone experienced with it when you are designing your study. Take time to learn the advanced functions and, ideally, experiment with some existing data before embarking on a new study.

In summary, if you are new to qualitative software, talk to those who have worked with it before; use available resources to understand its functions in the context of your research plans; and make time to "play around" with your software, and see how it feels for you, before you begin to use it for an important project. Then, enjoy yourself!

TO READ FURTHER

Lewins, A., & Silver, C. (2006, July). *Choosing a CAQDAS package: A working paper by Ann Lewins and Christina Silver* (5th ed.). CAQDAS Networking Project. (Retrieved December 16, 2008, from *caqdas.soc.surrey.ac.uk/ ChoosingLewins&SilverV5July06.pdf*).

This is a highly useful article about software considerations for qualitative research.

Miles, M. B., & Huberman, A. M. (1994). *Qualitative data analysis: A sourcebook of new methods.* Beverly Hills, CA: Sage.

This book is a standard first text for quantitative researchers wanting to try qualitative research. It is clear, straightforward, and has a good section on software considerations, although the discussion of specific software is outdated.

Given that analysis software continues to evolve rapidly, readers may find websites more useful. The following two have useful software discussions:

CAQDAS Networking Project (Retrieved December 16, 2008, from *caqdas. soc.surrey.ac.uk*).

FQS—Forum: Qualitative Sozialforschung/Forum: Qualitative Social Research (ISSN 1438-5627), Vol. 3(2). FQS is a peer-reviewed multilingual online journal for qualitative research (Retrieved December 16, 2008, from *www.qualitative-research.net/fqs*).

REFERENCES

Lewins, A., & Silver, C. (2006, July). *Choosing a CAQDAS package: A working paper by Ann Lewins and Christina Silver* (5th ed.). CAQDAS Networking Project. (Retrieved January 9, 2008, from *caqdas.soc.surrey.ac.uk/ChoosingLewins&SilverV5July06.pdf*)

MacLean, L., Meyer, M., & Estable, A. (2004). Improving accuracy of transcripts in qualitative research. *Qualitative Health Research, 14,* 113–124.

Miles, M. B., & Huberman, A. M. (1994). *Qualitative data analysis: A sourcebook of new methods.* Beverly Hills, CA: Sage.

Welsh, E. (2002). Dealing with data: Using NVIVO in the qualitative data analysis process. *FQS—Forum: Qualitative Sozialforschung/Forum: Qualitative Social Research (ISSN 1438–5627), Vol. 3(2).* (Retrieved February 21, 2008, from *www.qualitative-research.net/fqs*)

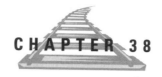

CHAPTER 38

Avoiding Data Disasters
and Other Pitfalls

MELINDA F. DAVIS

Happy families are all alike; every unhappy family
is unhappy in its own way.
—LEO TOLSTOY, *Anna Karenina*

BACKGROUND OF THE STUDY

There are a thousand ways a database can go wrong, and like Tolstoy's
unhappy families, each data disaster is different in its own way. This chapter
describes a variety of database catastrophes that actually happened in medical and behavioral studies. Some of the studies were large, some spanned
many years; others were small intervention studies that were completed in
a few years. Bright, committed people designed and conducted every study.
All of these studies were very costly in time and money, and yet each had at
least one data disaster. The purpose of this chapter is to acquaint you, the
researcher, with some of the ways a database can go wrong, so that you can
avoid such pitfalls in your future studies.

THE CHALLENGES

When the statistician first gets a data file, he or she may need to spend many
hours preparing the data before they can be analyzed. It is the end of the
project, the funding is gone, time is running short, and everyone (the entire

research team, not to mention the funding agency and the clients) wants to know if the intervention worked. At this point in the project, there are a few things no one wants to hear:

- The database manager says, "There's no unique identifier that is on all of the different forms for this study. But that's okay, because there's almost no data in the system."
- You request an exported file from the database, and when you open the file, all of the data fields are text, not numeric.
- The most important variable was never collected.

Most data disasters can be solved. However, it is far cheaper to avoid them than to solve them later. The few nonrecoverable ones are usually due to design and implementation problems. If the treatment was never given, or if the research subjects cannot be recontacted to collect key missing variables, the investigators are out of luck.

A Little Historical Perspective

We pause here to consider a question: Is it just our imagination or are there more data disasters today than in years past? In the dark ages of computers, only the initiated could create databases. Systems analysts sat in back rooms with flowcharts and FORTRAN coding sheets. Keypunch operators using noisy keypunch machines entered and verified data. The limit of 80 characters per card forced researchers to be precise about their variables. Researchers had to make decisions ahead of time. It was not possible to squeeze a variable into the middle of a punch card after the fact.

The advent of desktop computers changed everything. By the mid-1990s, computers came with preloaded database software. Keypunch machines became relics and data could now be entered on personal computers. The new software was flexible and increasingly user-friendly; anyone could create a database. Directors delegated database management to regular staff. Eventually, only large ongoing projects retained expensive staff and procedures (e.g., the Centers for Disease Control and Prevention, 2005–2006). The change was gradual, the initiated slowly retired, and the rigid, uncompromising procedures from the days of mainframe databases gradually died. This set the stage for modern data disasters. Although there are many variations on the theme, a typical data disaster today includes one of the following:

- A student or existing staff member designs the database.
- Data entry takes place at the end of the project.
- No one checks the forms or the data.

The first person to see the raw data is the data analyst, after all of the subjects or patients have completed the study. There is no codebook, and the person who developed this mess has graduated and is now in Timbuktu.

Up to this point, everything has seemed to be fine. The database screens *look* good. There has been a lot of activity—subjects were treated, data collected, forms were entered and filed. However, unless someone from the "old school" designed and maintained the data procedures, the project may come together only by accident. The data analyst is often the first to know that a data disaster is at hand.

OVERCOMING THE DIFFICULTIES

The first step is to develop awareness. It is not easy to tell if a dataset is in trouble. Unless you've been there, you probably won't know what to look for. Here are examples of two data collection forms—a poorly designed one and an excellent form. Figure 38.1 is a composite from a variety of studies and illustrates typical problems. The Physical Exam form does not have a space for the patient's ID or visit number, and there are no restrictions on the data fields. Figure 38.2 is from a federally funded asthma study at the University of Arizona. The study form has space for an ID number and a visit number, indicates field widths for the variables, and provides check boxes with programming codes.

The differences are very apparent in the data files. The poor form results in missing data, text fields that cannot be examined for out-of-range variables, and the file will require significant data cleaning (Figure 38.3). The data collection form has no spaces for the ID and date. The database reflects this mistake; neither field is required, and if either is entered, any format is acceptable. There is no way to link the forms together in the database. The first task will be to clean both of these fields, placing all of the data in the same format.

Physical Exam

Date:

Height:

Weight:

Pulmonary Auscultation:

Nose, Eye, Sinus Problems:

FIGURE 38.1. Physical evaluation form.

	ASTHMA AND GUIDED IMAGERY STUDY PHYSICAL EXAMINATION	For Study Use Only

THE UNIVERSITY OF **ARIZONA.** HEALTH SCIENCES CENTER

Subject ID: __ __ __ __ __ __ __ - __

☐ Initial Exam ☐ 2nd Follow-Up
☐ 1st Follow-Up ☐ Exit Exam

Date: _____ / _____ / _____
Month　　Day　　Year

Subject Name: _____ _____ _____
Last　　　　　　　　　First　　　　　　　　Middle

Measurements

1. Height: ____ ____ ____ . ____ cm　　2. Weight ____ ____ ____ . ____ kg

Pulmonary Auscultation

3. Is chest auscultation clear?　☐₁ Yes　☐₂ No

  3a. If No:　　　　　　　　☐₁ Wheeze

    　　　　　　　　　☐₂ Rales and/or rhonchi

Nose/Eye/Sinus Problems

4. In the past month, has the child had symptoms affecting his/her eyes?　☐₁ Yes　☐₂ No

5. In the past month, has the child had symptoms affecting his/her nose?　☐₁ Yes　☐₂ No

6. In the past month, has the child had symptoms affecting his/her sinus?　☐₁ Yes　☐₂ No

FIGURE 38.2. Asthma study physical evaluation form.

ID	Date	Height	Weight	Pulmonary	ENT
CD	April 1, 2003	149 cm	40 kg	OK	OK
#3		150.00	39.30	Fine	
3	6/10/03	59.1"	89.3	OK	Sinus
	7/13/2003	151.00		OK	—

FIGURE 38.3. Physical evaluation form.

ID	pe_seq	pe_date	pe_ht	pe_wt	pe_ausc	pe_ausc	pe_eyes	pe_nose	pe_sinus
ZZ121292	1	04012003	149.00	40.00	1	8	2	2	2
ZZ121292	2	05032003	150.00	39.30	1	8	2	2	2
ZZ121292	3	06102003	150.00	40.50	1	8	2	2	1
ZZ121292	4	07132003	151.00	41.20	1	8	2	2	2

FIGURE 38.4. Asthma study physical evaluation data.

The next problem is in the height and weight fields. There is no consistency; the weight data can be entered in pounds or kilograms, and height as centimeters, feet, or inches. There is no standard for the number of digits, and even worse, the database allows for words or numbers. The next data cleaning step will be to convert all of the words into numbers, and place all of the height and weight data into the same metric. Data analysis programs cannot calculate averages on words; all of the data must be numeric.

Recording the presence or absence of abnormalities appears to be optional. This may be sufficient for clinical use, but not for research purposes. When a field is left blank, one does not know if the patient did not have that symptom, or if the data were missing. A small study with 60 cases, four time points, and four different data collection instruments will have nearly 1,000 forms. If the abbreviated form in Figure 38.1 is used, there will be 6,000 fields to clean. Obviously, a real study will collect more than six variables per form. Typical data collection forms have 50 or more variables, which translates into more than 50,000 fields to clean.

In contrast, data from the asthma study (Figure 38.4) were consistent and complete. Many excellent examples can be found in large nationally funded databases, such as the Centers for Disease Control and Prevention (CDC) NHANES Study (2005/2006).

RECOMMENDATIONS

In order to avoid or catch database problems before they turn into disasters, consider the following steps.

- Design the database at the beginning of the study and hire an experienced database manager.
- Enlist someone who is naïve to the study to go through the data entry forms and make sure he or she can match every variable on your forms to the database, and ensure that all variables are well documented.
- Test the database using dummy data. Try to simulate data that rep-

resent all of the problems you can think of—no treatments, study dropouts, study restarts, out of range responses, and atypical situations.

Create data analysis files using such dummy data, and then conduct dry runs on the analyses.

- Start entering data as soon as the first case is enrolled.
- Design reports to help manage the project.
- Funding agencies and human subjects committees require reports
- The project staff need to know about activities and their due dates.
- The principal investigator (PI) needs to track project activity. Often the PI will know about enrollment, but little else.
- Run randomization checks to make sure the subjects are being allocated correctly, and monitor study progress.
- As soon as the database has even a small amount of data, request data analysis files and run simple frequency distributions on the data.
- Examine enrollment and treatment data every month.

As for our examples, the asthma project was ready to analyze within hours of the last patient visit. The other projects required many weeks of file preparation before the data could be analyzed.

LESSONS LEARNED

Good data hygiene is boring and about as much fun as flossing. Enrolling clients and providing treatment are more obvious and salient goals. Well-designed forms and databases take little more time to create than poorly designed ones, and the difference between the two is knowledge. Poorly designed forms and databases can result in costly repairs at the end of the study, and lengthy delays.

Like an engine that runs perfectly, a good database operates invisibly, whereas a bad one can stall the project. The following brief checklist covers database topics discussed in this chapter that can be used to improve data integrity.

Database Checklist

☐ Unique case ID
☐ Variable names (eight characters or fewer)
☐ Variable formats (specify text or numeric, and number of decimal places)

☐ Missing and valid values (specify the range of data)
☐ Logic checks (examine the data for logical impossibilities, such as pregnant males)
☐ Database documentation (include coding in database, e.g., 1 = yes, 2 = no)
☐ Required reports
☐ Creation of files for analysis
☐ Planned analyses

ACKNOWLEDGMENTS

This work was supported by grants from the National Institutes of Health National Center for Complementary and Alternative Medicine (No. P50 AT00008) and the Association of University Centers on Disabilities (AUCD)/Centers for Disease Control and Prevention National Center on Birth Defects and Developmental Disabilities (RTOI No. 2004-03-03). Thanks to the diligent work by the Pediatric CAM Center data group at the University of Arizona for the development of the asthma forms and database.

TO READ FURTHER

Statistical Services Centre and the University of Reading. (2000). *Data management guidelines for experimental projects*. Retrieved January 28, 2008, from *www.jic.ac.uk/SERVICES/statistics/readingadvice/booklets/topDMG.html*.

The National Center for Health Statistics provides excellent examples of survey questions and coding. The Statistical Services Center web page includes additional information on data management.

REFERENCE

Centers for Disease Control and Prevention (CDC). National Center for Health Statistics (NCHS). (2005–2006). *National Health and Nutrition Examination Survey Questionnaire (or Examination Protocol, or Laboratory Protocol)*. Hyattsville, MD: U.S. Department of Health and Human Services, Centers for Disease Control and Prevention. Available at *www.cdc.gov/nchs/about/major/nhanes/nhanes2005-2006/questexam05_06.htm*.

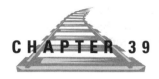

CHAPTER 39

When Interpretation Goes Awry
The Impact of Interim Testing

DALE GLASER

BACKGROUND OF THE STUDY

As an applied statistician and methodologist steeped in training in the social sciences, I have participated in numerous studies from the incipient stage of design construction to interpretation. Even though the ideal scenario is to involve the statistician/methodologist from the beginning of the study, there are many occasions when after-the-fact participation and consultation becomes the case (in fact, there are some quantitative specialists who would claim that this is the rule rather than the exception!). This creates particular havoc when there are problems at the data management stage. I felt somewhat vindicated (and relieved) when Cohen, Cohen, West, and Aiken (2003) asserted that a significant amount of time of a quantitative methodologist's job entails data preparation, cleaning/scrubbing, and other activities unrelated to the actual analysis and testing of models and hypotheses.

It is a well-known axiom that statistical analysis and design are not separate areas, and indeed when I teach research design I often introduce statistical issues, and vice versa when I teach statistics (at both the undergraduate and graduate levels). Thus, it cannot be overstated that the analysis must be congruent with the proposed design, which ranges from the metrics/scaling of the variables up to the specification of the model(s) for more sophisticated multivariate analyses. However, I have been a part of more than a few projects, dissertations, and consultations in which there were formidable gaps between the design and the proposed analysis, and unfortunately, alternative plans had to be investigated to minimize methodological and statistical misinterpretations (Cortina, 2002; Vandenberg, 2006).

DATA MANAGEMENT AND ANALYSIS

There are many examples of how snafus in the methods create havoc for an analysis and/or interpretation (lack of random assignment, omission of relevant variables, etc.). One of the more egregious examples of this that I have seen occurred when a thesis student had as her objective to examine change in a pretest–posttest design. The typical mode of data entry is such that for each measure of time (i.e., pretest, posttest) its own unique array of data is entered column by column. Most important, a unique identifier such as an ID number, a medical record number, and other indication, needs to be given to each individual. At times data are resorted or restructured, or possibly certain individuals become the focus of analysis, thus coding for a unique ID is imperative. In the context of this study, because of logistical constraints, the researcher was not allowed (nor did she plan for) a unique identifier for each participant across time (apparently there were some privacy concerns). Thus, she entered the dependent variable for both occasions in one column with no identifying ID, hence precluding the examination of change. Though this type of data entry, where there are multiple records for each person, may be appropriate for clustered datasets used in techniques such as multilevel modeling, a unique identifier would still need to be entered. Given this unfortunate set of circumstances, we were limited to just comparing the means as an aggregate for Time 1 and Time 2, but we couldn't address the notion of change.

It is clear that this data calamity could have been averted if data management practices had been reviewed before the data were collected. Even with the constraints that were imposed, some type of arbitrary ID could have been fashioned in such a way that patient privacy would still be protected. This is just one example of design and analysis and the intertwining (and sometimes entangled!) nature of such. However, for the purposes of this chapter, I focus on interim/sequential analysis and its impact on a study in which I served as the statistician/methodologist.

INTERIM ANALYSIS: A BRIEF REVIEW

When planning a longitudinal study, there are many challenges with respect to the conceptualization (Widaman, 1991) and analysis of change (Rogosa, 1995), as well as the many contextual facets that need to be considered (Little, Bovaird, & Card, 2007). When in the throes of a longitudinal research project, it is tempting to assess the efficacy of a given intervention as the study progresses. There may be many compelling and competing reasons for "snooping" at the data, some of which may not always stand up to scrutiny by the methodological and statistical community.

In the medically related literature there is much written about interim testing, which may fall under related rubrics such as adaptive interim analyses (Bauer & Köhen, 1994), sequential analysis (Todd, 2007), and/ or group sequential designs (Müller & Schäfer, 2001). With these types of interim analyses, as the study progresses, modification of the design may take place (Bauer & Köhen, 1994), as well as reestimation of sample size (Posch & Bauer, 2000). This plays a key role in clinical trials, for as evidence is amassed in regard to support (or otherwise) for the hypothesis, decisions may be made to terminate the study early (Todd, 2007; Pocock, 1982). As one can imagine, this can be a thorny problem for pharmaceutical studies: If a drug or some other intervention shows early promise, do we hold off on passing on the results to others who may benefit from such an intervention (e.g., control group) until the study reaches the proposed end date? Or do we divulge the promising results before termination? Moreover, with repeated testing, Type I error (the probability of wrongly rejecting a true null hypothesis, that is, saying there is a difference when there isn't) may become markedly inflated if not corrected (Wassmer, 1998). It is obvious that, besides the scientific and ethical (Cannistra, 2004) issues at hand, there may be economic and administrative reasons (Todd, 2007) that drive the use of interim analyses, though it is clear that the consequences (i.e., the advantages and disadvantages) of such a design should be carefully considered (Van Houwelingen, Van de Velde, & Stijnen, 2005; Hommel & Kropf, 2001).

THE CHALLENGES

With this brief background on interim analysis, I discuss a study in which, though my colleagues and I did not employ the statistical rigors associated with adaptive/sequential testing, we definitely executed interim analyses.

In many applied work settings, there may be vested interests across stakeholders in closely monitoring the progress of a research project. The types of projects may range from large-scale multisite randomized comparative experiments, to program evaluations, to more modest quasi-experiments or survey research. Regardless of the scope of the project, the stakeholders may have their own set of objectives, ranging from publicizing the results for mass coverage, maximizing return on investment (or containing costs), and/or publishing in top tier peer-reviewed journals. Sometimes those motivators are complementary and unified in purpose, but often the objectives may be competing or, at worst, antithetical to each other. Whether by financial or political forces (or a hybrid of both), the researchers may find themselves at odds with the funders, administrators, or other interested parties. Prudent politics doesn't always make for sound science.

This was the scenario our research team encountered on a multisite health care project examining the impact of an intervention on certain healthcare behaviors (e.g., awareness of symptoms, mode of self-care behaviors, emotional/physical lability, etc.) for a group of patients suffering from heart failure. This was a 2-year study with data collected every 3 months. Although I would be managing the data (along with the project director) as they were administered and collected, there were no plans to summarize or analyze the findings at each stage of data collection.

(Incidentally, a frequent point of fervent discussion during the course of this study was where to assign data that were not returned in a timely fashion. After the baseline data were uniformly collected, surveys were mailed out every 3 months and we would anticipate [and require] that they be received within 2 weeks' time. However, some respondents sent the Time 2 surveys back closer to the collection date for Time 3 data. Thus, we bandied about whether a specific set of surveys should be assigned to Time 2, or consider Time 2 to be missing and assign it to Time 3, as it was closer to that time point. This is when the flexibility of a multilevel modeling approach [which was discussed but not applied] at that point would have served us well, given that we could have coded for the exact time [Singer & Willet, 2003] and not concern ourselves about treating time as a fixed factor.)

As the first quarter of data collection ended (thus giving us baseline and 3-month data), we were requested by key administrators/executives to furnish a synopsis of the project to date. I assumed it would be descriptive at this juncture (e.g., measures of central tendency, dispersion, etc., and maybe a few bivariate correlations); however, as events were unfolded, I was dismayed to find that an examination of the between-group trajectories (with only two time points) was to be tested for significance. At that time, we were not savvy as to the workings of modifying p values à la sequential testing or adaptive interim testing. Nor were we anticipating that this was to be a quarterly requirement. Hence, the findings were not only presented to the key administrator but also frequently disclosed to other interested parties throughout the institution. Even though interest in our project was appreciated and, to some extent, flattering, we had also discussed among ourselves concerns about the possible pitfalls of early disclosure. If the results were promising, would an overoptimistic disclosure engender false hopes (Type I error)? If the results failed to meet the holy grail of $p < .05$, would the specter of premature termination of the design be looming?

THE RESULTS: TWISTS AND TURNS

With those apprehensions in mind, analyses were conducted on a quarterly basis. When we compared the mean trajectory for the two groups from baseline to the end of the first year for "awareness of symptoms," the group trajectories were in the anticipated direction with the intervention group obtaining a substantively higher level of symptom awareness. Moreover, the interaction for this mixed analysis of variance (ANOVA) design was statistically significant. However, despite the caveats about making any global proclamations about the ensuing results, that being due to the study being only halfway toward completion, much ado was made about the outcomes. Moreover, much to our chagrin, the results were presented to both internal and external audiences.

Following the cautious excitement generated by the first year of interim testing, continued examination of the data was carried over into the second year, although not with as much ballyhoo greeting each of the quarterly results. When the study ended after the second year, the final database was sent to me for data scrubbing and cleaning, examination of univariate and multivariate assumptions, and testing of hypotheses and models. It was at this point that we saw a slight reversal in the trend for the outcome variable "awareness of symptoms" in the second year. Whereas the intervention group showed a modest increase in "awareness," the control group actually had a sharper upward, and unanticipated, acceleration in awareness scores. In fact, when the second year of data was analyzed in isolation, the two-way interaction was not significant, and moreover, the omnibus test of the mixed ANOVA was not significant. Though the simple effects for the group at Year 1 only was still significant, the second year showed a pattern that was neither hypothesized nor anticipated.

POST HOC THEORIZING

After much disgruntled head-scratching and ongoing debate about the unexpected reversal of fortune, amid the broader question of "to what extent (and at what stage of illness) is our intervention effective?" one plausible explanation came to the fore. At the beginning of the second year, a major governmental institution published a healthcare pamphlet that not only was geared to the population that was the focus of our analysis, but also offered suggestions for health promotion that were close (and virtually identical) to our intervention! Thus, it was not unreasonable to assume that the intervention may have bled into the control group, akin to what Shadish, Cook, and Campbell (2002) refer to as "treatment diffusion," and medical researchers call "contamination." If indeed the control group somehow learned about this pamphlet, it would not be unexpected that symptom awareness would manifest some type of accompanying increase. Though this was speculation on our behalf (because of certain constraints we weren't able to conduct follow-up questions about use or knowledge of the pamphlet), it may, in part, explain the reversal of the group trajectories. It is indisputable that the study results would have occurred with or without the interim testing; however, at least the concomitant expectations would not have attained such a high ceiling if the first year of testing had been deferred until study completion.

Lessons Learned

It is after-the-fact speculation to ask: If we had adopted the sequential or adaptive testing mode (i. e., modifying the level of p required for significance because of multiple looks at the data), would such post hoc rumination of the results have transpired? This painfully stark lesson for the research team (and after the fact, the administrators) was the havoc interim testing can wreak when safeguards at each step are not rigidly adhered to. As mentioned earlier in the chapter, it is understandable why those who have a vested (and/or pecuniary) interest in a study would want to be apprised of the progress as the study evolves. But when highlighting of the results becomes part of the unexpected game plan, the research team members may find themselves standing on statistical, methodological, and possibly political tenuous terra firma.

TO READ FURTHER

Todd, S. (2007). A 25-year review of sequential methodology in clinical studies. *Statistics in Medicine, 26*, 237–252.

This is a nice historical review of sequential/adaptive testing that gives the reader a glimpse into the underpinnings and development of interim testing.

Wassmer, G. (1998). A comparison of two methods for adaptive interim analyses in clinical trials. *Biometrics, 54*, 696–705.

Oft-cited article that compares alternative methods in adaptive testing.

REFERENCES

Bauer, P., & Köhen, K. (1994). Evaluation of experiments with adaptive interim analyses. *Biometrics, 50*, 1029–1041.

Cannistra, S. A. (2004). The ethics of early stopping rules: Who is protecting whom? *Journal of Clinical Oncology, 22*, 1542–1545.

Cohen, J., Cohen, P., West, S. G., & Aiken, L. S. (2003). *Applied multiple regression/correlation analysis for the behavioral sciences* (3rd ed.). Mahwah, NJ: Erlbaum.

Cortina, J. M. (2002). Big things have small beginnings: An assortment of "minor" methodological misunderstandings. *Journal of Management, 28,* 339–362.

Hommel, G., & Kropf, S. (2001). Clinical trials with an adaptive choice of hypothesis. *Drug Information Journal.* Retrieved December 7, 2007, from *findarticles.com/p/articles/mi_qa3899/is_200110/ai_n8971643.*

Little, T. D., Bovaird, J. A., & Card, N. A. (Eds.). (2007). *Modeling contextual effects in longitudinal studies.* Mahwah, NJ: Erlbaum.

Müller, H.-H., & Schäfer, H. (2001). Adaptive group sequential designs for clinical trials: Combining the advantages of adaptive and of classical group sequential approaches. *Biometrics, 57,* 886–891.

Pocock, S. J. (1982). Interim analysis for randomized clinical trials: The group sequential approach. *Biometrics, 38,* 153–162.

Posch, M., & Bauer, P. (2000). Interim analysis and sample size reassessment. *Biometrics, 56,* 1170–1176.

Rogosa, D. (1995). Myths and methods: "Myths about longitudinal research" plus supplemental questions. In J. M. Gottman (Ed.), *The analysis of change* (pp. 3–66). Mahwah, NJ: Erlbaum.

Shadish, W. R., Cook, T. D., & Campbell, D. T. (2002). *Experimental and quasi-experimental designs for generalized causal inference.* Boston: Houghton Mifflin.

Singer, J. D., & Willet, J. B. (2003). *Applied longitudinal data analysis.* Oxford, UK: Oxford University Press.

Todd, S. (2007). A 25-year review of sequential methodology in clinical studies. *Statistics in Medicine, 26,* 237–252.

Vandenberg, R. J. (2006). Statistical and methodological myths and urban legends. *Organizational Research Methods, 9,* 194–201.

Van Houwelingen, H. C., Van de Velde, C. J., H., & Stijnen, T. (2005). Interim analysis on survival data: Its potential bias and how to repair it. *Statistics in Medicine, 24,* 2823–2835.

Wassmer, G. (1998). A comparison of two methods for adaptive interim analyses in clinical trials. *Biometrics, 54,* 696–705.

Widaman, K. F. (1991). Qualitative transitions amid quantitative development: A challenge for measuring and representing change. In L. M. Collins & J. L Horn (Eds.), *Best methods for the analysis of change* (pp. 204–217). Washington, DC: American Psychological Association.

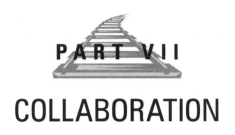

COLLABORATION

Some studies are small and simple enough for one person to carry out the whole process, from the conceptualization, through the design, recruitment, implementation, data collection, analysis, and write-up. Increasingly, though, especially in the health sciences, complexity rules the day. Rarely does one person have the requisite knowledge in the content area, quantitative and qualitative methods, statistics, health economics, and other subjects needed for successful execution of the project. Further, once we leave the lab and enter the real world, it is often necessary to collaborate with other institutions (e.g., schools, the community) because that's where the participants are, or there are not enough patients with rare disorders in any one setting. These can be difficult shoals to navigate, as different organizations have differing cultures, rules, regulations, and timelines. Researchers are often driven by the granting cycle, which dictates when funds become available and by which date they must be spent. Schools run by the academic year, and other institutions, such as businesses and hospitals, by either the calendar or the fiscal year, and none of these coincide with one another. Moreover, outside the university, research is low on the priority list and, in extreme cases, is viewed as an imposition that is intrusive, eats into the staff's time, and may even be a threat if it is seen as possibly revealing problems within the institution.

The first two chapters in Part VII describe projects in a school system, and were actually initiated at the behest of the area school system.

However, for both Roberts (Chapter 40) and Bledsoe (Chapter 41), factors within the system nearly derailed the project. Fortunately, the interventions were merely shunted off onto a siding temporarily, although neither got back on the main track. But let's end on a high note. In Chapter 42, Yantio describes a project carried out in Cameroon, which successfully educated an advisory board about the culture and techniques of evaluation in order to educate youth in the country about sexually transmitted diseases. A good place to end.

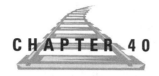

CHAPTER 40

What Happened to Cooperation and Collaboration?

NASREEN ROBERTS

BACKGROUND OF THE STUDY

Studying the prevalence of mental health problems in adolescents is important for prevention and program planning. Epidemiological studies have the potential to elucidate the need and provide the necessary support for program development to meet this need. At present there are no epidemiological studies of adolescents between 16 and 18 years of age in Canada. Although the Ontario Child Health Study (OCHS; Offord et al., 1987) and the Quebec Child Mental Health Survey (QCMHS; Breton et al., 1999) examined the prevalence of psychiatric disorders in community samples, the Ontario study had an age cutoff of 16 years, and the Quebec study of 14 years. Despite the early age cutoff, the overall 6-month prevalence of psychiatric disorders was 18.1% for the OCHS (Waddell, Offord, Shepherd, Hua, & McEwan, 2002) and 12.7% for the QCMHS. Thus, there is a paucity of Canadian data for 16- to 18-year-old adolescents, which has led to extrapolating from studies conducted in the United States despite differences in a number of key factors such as healthcare provision, racial mix, and regulations about firearms. The overall prevalence of diagnoses in children and adolescents based on the text revision of the fourth edition of the *Diagnostic and Statistical Manual of Mental Disorders* (DSM-IV-R), which is the current classification system for mental disorders in North America, is generally about 8–22% for studies conducted in the United States (Gould, Greenberg, Velting, & Shaffer, 2003). In July 2001, the American Academy of Child and Adolescent Psychiatry (AACAP) under its "Official Action," endorsed Direct Case-Finding as "excellent and cost-effective" as well as a highly sensitive way to identify at-risk children and adolescents in the school setting. The use of screening questionnaires was deemed useful in screening normal, high-risk, and clinic populations (American Academy of Child and Adolescent Psychiatry [AACAP], 2001).

Data from Statistics Canada in 1997 showed that among 15- to 18-year-olds there were 529 deaths from unintentional injuries and 261 deaths from suicide. There were 3,674 hospital admissions due to suicidal attempts in this age group, a rate of 18.3 per 100,000 (Health Canada, 1997). This is second only to deaths due to motor vehicle accidents in this age group.

The purpose of our study (conducted by myself and my supervisor for my master's thesis) was to assess the prevalence of mental heath problems in high school students in Kingston in response to a request from the school board for an expedited psychiatric assessment program. We felt that it was essential as a first step, we establish need and the extent of the need to enable us to weigh the costs and benefits of implementing a new program in our area. We knew from extant literature that the prevalence of mental health problems may vary in the population from 6 to 22%, depending on factors such as sociodemographic characteristics, catchment area, and type of school. Our second step was to find an efficient method of identifying those students who would need the expedited service.

We chose a two-stage cross-sectional design for our study of high school students in this midsize city in Ontario. Our primary goal was to estimate the number of the students potentially in need of further psychiatric diagnostic assessment on the basis of the 12-month-period prevalence of child and adolescent psychiatric disorders. A secondary goal was to evaluate the construct validity, accuracy, and yield of the Diagnostic Interview Schedule for Children Predictive Scales-8 (DPS-8; Lucas et al., 2001) screen against the gold standard National Institute of Mental Health–Diagnostic Interview Schedule for Children (NIMH-DISC; Shaffer, Fisher, Lucas, Dulcan, & Schwab-Stone, 2000) for any child and adolescent psychiatric diagnosis.

The study was conducted in the middle of the first semester to allow for settling in after summer holidays and a couple of months before the end-of-semester examinations. The first stage was to administer a short self-report computerized screen, the DPS-8, to all grades 9 to 12 students in three local high schools in different demographic areas. The DPS-8 is composed of 49 questions addressing common psychiatric symptoms. Alas, only one of the three schools participated (woman proposes, God disposes; more about this elsewhere). The DPS-8 screen takes 40 minutes to complete and generates a report that predicts the possibility of being assigned a diagnosis by the structured diagnostic interview, the NIMH-DISC. In the second stage, all students who screened positive for a possible diagnosis were to be administered the gold standard NIMH-DISC diagnostic interview in its computerized voice version. This version provides each item on the computer screen while simultaneously reading it aloud through the earphones. This instrument is self-administered and generates DSM-IV diagnoses based on a preprogrammed algorithm. Both the DPS-8 and the NIMH-DISC have established reliability and validity (Leung et al., 2005; Shaffer et al., 2000). Owing to the lamentable number of schools and participants, we decided to administer both the screen and the diagnostic interview to all students who had parental consent and assented to the study.

THE CHALLENGES

Who would ever have thought that "collaboration"—the 21st century's most overused buzzword—would present a challenge? Of course, had we conducted a literature search we would have discovered what a bumpy ride lay ahead for us. "Collaboration" sounds all warm and fuzzy, but what a hornet's nest it can be; just read some of the myriad of articles on "barriers to collaborative work." You will discover the five problematic "p" factors that make this a daunting gauntlet: people, professional cultures, policies, politics, and practicalities (Taras, 2005).

In our case we were confronted with three categories of barriers to collaboration: personal, systemic, and environmental (Anderson, McIntyre, Rotto, & Robertson, 2002; Armbruster, 2002), all of which worked to pose a substantial challenge to the successful conduct and completion of our study.

On a people/personal level, despite having requested the additional program, the number of meetings held and the discussion with different levels of school bureaucracy made it obvious that some staff members felt there was a threat to their professional integrity and management philosophy and thus were openly resistant to collaboration. We waited 8 weeks after presenting our proposal to the school board senior administration only to be told that the principals of the schools wanted to meet with us for further questioning. So back to everyone's scheduler to synchronize a date; the earliest was 7 weeks later! This meeting had the flavor of a beheading, with many principals obviously opposed to the study in their schools. Then everything went on hold for the summer holidays and we waited to hear which three schools would participate.

By the second week of September we were getting antsy, so we called to find out our fate and were informed that only one school principal had agreed to participate and that he required us to meet with the Parent Teacher Association (PTA) to get agreement for the project in that school. We met and reassured everyone that our motives were honorable and that we were doing this for better service provision and access. Hurrah, we had lift-off!

But—and a big *but* at that—the selection of the school had not been random. The school board had gotten consent from a school that had more than the usual special behavioral and educational programs for high-needs adolescents from a socioeconomically deprived background. This may have been in an effort to get services for these students. The power of the study is undermined by the smaller numbers, 662 rather than 2,500 students whom we could have had access to if we had three schools (which we had requested) from different areas in town. This would given us a representative sample from all types and sizes of schools and may have improved the generalizability of the study results.

On a systemic level there was certainly resistance to the project, which may have been a function of a combination of factors, such as poor internal and external communication due to differences in professional language, turf, or training, or simple lack of skills, experience, desire, or time to collaborate and support the study. On an environmental level, emotional and behavioral problems are not only defined differently by psychiatric services and the educational services, but they also involve the differing opinions and ideas about whether behavior and emotional problems fall within the realm of science and disease or are social phenomena due to rotten parenting. Throw in the stigma associated with mental health problems, and you have a huge hurdle to overcome even with those who are ostensibly well educated and aware; leave aside the underprivileged families with a multitude of biopsychosocial limitations. The school had 662 adolescents, of whom only 222 participated in the initial phase. It is of note that presentation of the study by some of the frontline teachers had an implied negative spin when they sent the kids, who had parental consent and had assented, to complete the questionnaire in the computer rooms: "You don't have to do this questionnaire; it is entirely up to you."

The final straw was when we were precipitously asked to stop the study and had 3 days to finish up. The explanation was that this was taking too long and was exceedingly disruptive to the school's routine. It was our feeling that the principal bowed to the pressure of his classroom teachers, as he himself and his guidance counselors were very collaborative from the outset.

OVERCOMING THE DIFFICULTIES

I am truly from some hardy stock (or perhaps just a masochist) not to have blown a blood vessel, or worse, gone berserk, at one of those meetings after months of facing hurdle after hurdle to any collaboration and experiencing not insubstantial negative, hostile vibes at many meetings.

I had decided that I was "in for a penny, in for a pound" and that one school was better than none. I gratefully accepted the offered school and started the process of regular daily meetings with the school's coordinator and tried hard to troubleshoot by offering to meet individually with parents and teachers who had concerns or were opposed to the study. Each time we ran into resistance, I went to the school and met with the persons involved and tried to resolve the issue without being reduced to a screaming wreck. The school personnel had access to me through my cell phone, and I was able to be at the school in 5 minutes (the advantages of a small town). When I was asked to stop the study, I tried unsuccessfully to persuade them to grant a reprieve for another week. I then contacted the remaining students to see if they were willing to come to the hospital to complete the testing; surprisingly, a few agreed and did complete the study.

LESSONS LEARNED

Don't conduct studies in school (just kidding). This is perhaps better for your own physical and mental health, but not really an option if we want to change the trajectory of the lives of those at risk. We need to have early identification and intervention for those at risk of mental health problems, which impair functioning and pose a monumental burden for the person and the state.

I had presumed that I had a collegial and collaborative relationship with the school board—not an entirely wrong presumption, given my ongoing close contact with the director of educational services. However, in hindsight, I should have met with the principals myself and explained why the study was necessary, why it should be conducted in the schools, and what would be the advantages for their students and schools. This would have avoided the principals' seeing me as being imposed on them by the administration, and I may have had constructive dialogues allowing me to respond their reservations, concerns, and biases. This should have been followed up by a meeting, not only with the PTA but also with the classroom teachers, to inform them and solicit their support and encouragement for the students to participate.

We had been asked to let the classroom teachers inform students about the study and distribute the consent forms to their class. I think it would have been much better if we had given the preamble and handed out the consent forms to the students ourselves; it would have taken 10 minutes, would have been consistent throughout the classrooms and minimized the possibility of subliminal subversion owing to the views of the individual teachers.

Does it sound as though I got nothing from this exercise? Wrong; I got my master's on the first go, with minimal changes, had two major professional journals accept two articles from this study, and most important, I was invited to submit this chapter.

TO READ FURTHER

Taras, H. L. (2005). Promoting multidisciplinary relationships: A pragmatic framework for helping service providers to work collaboratively. *Canadian Journal of Community Mental Health, 24,* 115–127.

This article offers a practical approach to help mental health professionals identify barriers to teamwork and create solutions to those barriers.

Hall, K. L., Feng, A. X., Moser, R. P., Stokols, D., & Taylor, B. K (2008). Moving the science of team science forward: Collaboration and creativity. *American Journal of Preventive Medicine, 35*(Suppl. 2), S243–S249.

This article identifies several promising directions, including operationalizing cross-disciplinary team science and training and fostering transdisciplinary cross-sector partnerships.

REFERENCES

American Academy of Child and Adolescent Psychiatry Official Action Committee. (2001). Practice parameter for the assessment and treatment of children and adolescents with suicidal behavior. *Journal of the American Academy of Child and Adolescent Psychiatry, 40*(Suppl.), 24S–51S.

Anderson, J. A., McIntyre, J. S., Rotto, K. I., & Robertson, D. C. (2002). Developing and maintaining collaboration in systems of care for children and youths with emotional and behavioral disabilities and their families. *American Journal of Orthopsychiatry, 72,* 514–525.

Armbruster, P. (2002) The administration of school-based mental health services. *Child and Adolescent Psychiatric Clinics of North America, 11,* 23–41.

Breton, J. J., Bergeron, L., Valla, J. P., Berthiaume, C., Gaudet, N., Lambert, J., et al. (1999). Child mental health survey: Prevalence of DSM-III-R mental health disorders. *Journal of Child Psychology and Psychiatry. 40,* 375–384.

Gould, M. S., Greenberg, T., Velting, D. M., & Shaffer, D. (2003). Youth suicide risk and preventive interventions: A review of the past 10 years. *Journal of the American Academy of Child and Adolescent Psychiatry, 42,* 386–405.

Health Canada. (1997). *Leading causes of hospitalization and death in Canada.* Available at *www.hcsc.gc.ca/hpb/lcdc/publicat/pcd97/mrt_mf_e.html.*

Leung, P. W., Lucas, C. P., Hung, S. F., Kwong, S. L., Tang, C. P., Lee, C. C., et al. (2005). The test–retest reliability and screening efficiency of DISC Predictive Scales—Version 4.32 (DPS-4.32) with Chinese children/youths. *European Child and Adolescent Psychiatry, 14,* 461–465.

Lucas, C. P., Zhang, H., Fisher, P. W., Shaffer, D., Regier, D. A., Narrow, W. E., et al. (2001). The DISC Predictive Scales (DPS): Efficiently screening for diagnoses. *Journal of the American Academy of Child and Adolescent Psychiatry, 40,* 443–449.

Offord, D. R., Boyle, M. H., Szatmari, P., Rae-Grant, N. I., Links, P. S., Cadman, D. T., et al. (1987). Ontario Child Health Study: II. Six-month prevalence of disorder and rates of service utilization. *Archives of General Psychiatry, 44,* 832–836.

Shaffer, D., Fisher, P., Lucas, C., Dulcan, M., & Schwab-Stone, M. (2000). NIMH Diagnostic Interview Schedule for Children—Version IV (NIMH DISC-IV): Description, differences from previous versions, and reliability of some common diagnoses. *Journal of the American Academy of Child and Adolescent Psychiatry, 39,* 28–38.

Taras, H. L. (2005). Promoting multidisciplinary relationships: A pragmatic framework for helping service providers to work collaboratively. *Canadian Journal of Community Mental Health, 24,* 115–127.

Waddell, C., Offord, D. R., Shepherd, C. A., Hua, J. M., & McEwan, K.(2002). Child psychiatric epidemiology and Canadian public policy-making: The state of the science and the art of the possible. *Canadian Journal of Psychiatry, 47,* 825–832.

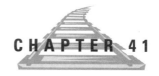

CHAPTER 41

Presto! It's Gone

When a Study Ceases to Exist Right before Your Eyes

KATRINA L. BLEDSOE

BACKGROUND OF THE STUDY

Conducting research is a difficult endeavor, even under the best circumstances. Yet the public is often unaware of the great lengths to which one must go to obtain pithy statements such as "four out of five doctors recommend ... " Such conveniently simple and user-friendly summations are the result of many months or, dare I say, years of work. Between deciding on the topic, the research questions to be answered, the types of methods that should be used to answer those questions, the venue in which those methods will be executed, how the data will be analyzed, and so on, it is a wonder that any research study sees the light of day. But what happens when things go awry? What happens when a study starts out with the best of intentions and almost flawless planning and then falls apart, or worse, ceases to exist at all?

Even under the best of circumstances, such as with an experimental design in a laboratory where variables, environments, and extraneous factors can be controlled (e.g., Cosby, 2008), studies can be challenging beyond what was originally anticipated. If this is the case, then research in unusual or difficult circumstances can be even more daunting. For instance, studies conducted in practical settings such as schools often have other issues to consider, such as resistance to participating on the part of the target population, low response rates among participants, and the political climate of the community in which the study is being conducted (e.g., Mertens, 2007; Bledsoe & Graham, 2005). No matter how well the research is conceptualized, other factors such as sociohistorical context (e.g., the history of the city) and the political climate (e.g., red or blue state) can and often do dictate (1) the kind of research that will be conducted, (2) the manner in which it will be conducted, and (3) whether the research findings will see the light of day or be used (e.g., Quinn Patton, 1997).

Perhaps one of the most pressing concerns for the United States is the relationship of health and weight gain. The issue of obesity has become a national concern for health organizations such as the Centers for Disease Control and Prevention (CDC) because of the sharp increase in obesity among youthful populations. The CDC estimates that over a 20-year period, the American population's body mass index (BMI; normal BMI, 25.5–29.0), has increased an estimated 2%, from 33% in 1980 to 35% in 1999 (Centers for Disease Control and Prevention [CDC], 1999). However, in the same population, *obesity* (defined as BMI greater than or equal to 30.0) has almost doubled, from approximately 15% in 1980 to 27% in 1999 (CDC, 2008). For adults, this is sobering; for youth, it is disconcerting. Approximately 15% of the nation's youth are significantly overweight (CDC, 2008), and these statistics are of special concern for adolescents of color. In urban communities adults of color are at significantly greater risk for negative health consequences and outcomes such as heart disease. For instance, Johnson (2002) found that in comparison to their white counterparts (35%), African Americans are more likely to be obese (44%). For Latino populations the figure is even more sobering: more than 50% are considered to be overweight and/or obese (Levy & Beeman, 2003, as cited in Sanchez-Sheperd, 2005). Poor nutrition, weight gain, and obesity can have long-term outcomes for these communities. For example, African Americans are three times more likely to suffer from heart disease than any other group. Long-term outcomes extend to offspring as well; both African American and Latina women are two times more than whites likely to lose a child to poor nutrition as a result of lack of prenatal care (Department of Youth and Family Services, 1998). Thus, there is an urgency to deal with these challenging issues.

This chapter describes the TOPS project, a school-based research project and program evaluation focused on improving nutrition and preventing obesity among diverse urban-based adolescents at a local high school (which, to preserve anonymity, I simply call "the high school") in a city in central New Jersey, and details the experiences my team and I had in trying to salvage a mixed-methodology field experiment.

TOPS was designed as a response to what the high school recognized as a growing problem among adolescents within the school community. Specifically, the teachers' network (known as TTN) recognized a national trend in its own community: the expanding waistlines of its predominately Black and Latino students. Appalled, TTN conceptualized a program to combat the trend of a growing number of overweight students at the high school. The program, informally known as the "Obesity Project," was part of a larger agenda to provide information and actionable strategies focused on health and well-being for the high school's students and their families. The desire of TTN to have an evidenced-based intervention led it to seek collaboration with the city's local liberal arts college.

TTN wanted to address two objectives. The first was to understand the needs and challenges of an increasingly diverse community by providing scientific evidence of an associative link between cultural identity (how one identifies with his or her culture) and physical health behavior outcomes. The second objective was to make sure that the designed health promotion program not only educated, but also addressed the dynamics (e.g., attitudes and behaviors) that encourage and *discourage* healthy nutrition behavior among adolescents, especially urban adolescents of color.

When the project began it had a host of collaborators from the high school, one from the city health department, and a couple from one of the local hospitals. My college research group, the evaluation team, was asked to join the collaborative group as researchers and evaluation consultants. TTN had designed an intervention (albeit haphazardly) that provided students three opportunities: (a) to engage in physical exercise, (2) to gain a healthy attitude toward healthful living and nutrition, and (3) to develop a generalized understanding of physical and mental health. TTN had received funding from the school district, which in turn had received funding from the state to implement the program.

Students involved in the TOPS program were a subset of the larger campus community and were part of the medical arts academy, a learning community dedicated to training students interested in some aspect of the medical profession. In all, the community boasted a population of approximately 400 students. The program entailed students becoming involved in activities such as "spirit walks" (community walks that promoted the "spirit" of exercise and physical health); watching and discussing the implications of films such as *Supersize Me* (Spurlock, 2004), and keeping food diaries.

Because of TTN's desire to conduct scientifically based research, the study was designed to be a longitudinal field experiment. Specifically, the evaluation team was interested in following the members of one cohort (the freshman class) throughout their high school careers. The study was conceptualized in four phases. Phase 1, the collection of baseline data, was to include but not be limited to, obtaining physical measurements, calculating steps walked in a day, and so forth; obtaining attitudinal data via the use of survey measures (to explore or establish the variables of cultural socialization, health practices, nutrition, and their relationship to obesity); and content analysis of daily food diaries (food eaten, mood while eating). These measures included Phinney's (1992) Multi-group Ethnic Identity Measure,

Oyserman, Gant, and Ager's (1995) Ethnic Identity Scale, and the CDC's (2008) health survey, among others. In addition, the team developed physical measurement scales and daily diary reports

Phase 2 focused on program development. The goal in this phase was to fine-tune program activities and to measure the implementation and process of the program intervention. During this phase participants were to be randomly assigned to experimental conditions (those who were formally in the program versus those who were not) and provided the intervention. In addition to gathering periodic data from participants (to enable comparisons from the 9th to the 12th grades and assess change), the evaluation team wanted to conduct measurements of the actual implementation of the program, including the number of students served, and measurement of the effectiveness of program strategies.

In Phase 3, the program assessment and behavior and attitude change phase, the goal was to address two aspects. First, the evaluation team wanted to assess the overall effectiveness of the program (e.g., are students engaging in healthier nutrition behavior than prior to the intervention?) using an experimental design, and compare baseline data and postintervention data. Second, the team wanted to use the data collected during this phase to establish correlational and predictive relationships between variables such as cultural identity, nutrition health practices, and long-term weight gain.

Finally, Phase 4, the information dissemination stage, was to be devoted to disseminating information in a variety of venues, including local, state, national, and professional.

THE CHALLENGES

"Funding has been put on hold," said TTN's evaluation team contact grimly. TTN and its collaborators sat numb at the meeting. "But the superintendent says it's likely we *may* see funding again in a couple of years. We're going to keep doing what we're doing, though." By the end of the meeting, there was a sense of renewed camaraderie among members of the group. Promises were made to continue the project and to divert funding from other pockets of the high school budget to the program, and to the research. Community collaborators promised to attend the next weekly meeting.

When the evaluation team arrived at the high school the following week, only the chair of TTN (who also served as the team contact) was in attendance. That day was the beginning of the death and disappearance of the TOPS study. Meetings began to occur only sporadically; the evaluation team often arrived at the high school only to find that the meeting had been canceled. Program strategies became nonexistent, student participation decreased dramatically, and former sponsors of activities such as the "spirit walk" pulled their funding and support. In short, the intervention/ program (and by default, the study) was disappearing before the team's eyes. Thus, there was no intervention to assess or, for that matter, any reason to assess students. Both the evaluation team members and the contact became despondent about the program, the research, and the disintegration of both.

Despite defunding and the loss of collaborators, as well as of potential participants, the problem remained: Urban ethnic students were at risk for experiencing the long-term effects of being overweight and obese.

OVERCOMING THE DIFFICULTIES

As mentioned, the study had all but died and disappeared, yet the problem of obesity at the high school remained. Several meetings with the team's evaluation contact yielded a different strategy for (1) regaining funding, (2) reconceptualizing the program and intervention, and (3) continuing the research. First, it was decided that the focus should not be on assessing the intervention per se, but on articulating the problem for students (and, by extension, their families) and on planning a more coherent intervention to address that problem. By taking this approach, it was decided that the research, rather than the intervention, would be the vehicle by which to regain funding.

The first step was to gather baseline data not only from the students but also from their teachers, families, and the general environment. The evaluation team concentrated efforts on the students of the medical arts academy, rather than trying to tackle and extend data collection to the entire student body (which was the ultimate goal). The team developed parent and teacher surveys and conducted a site mapping of the city to identify the environmental and community factors that encouraged or discouraged unhealthful eating patterns. Thus, the data collection was not concerned with conducting a field experiment, but instead focused on setting the stage to conduct one in the future.

The second step was twofold. First, the team began meeting with faculty, staff, and administration to discuss their opinions and actions concerning obesity within the high school population. Second, new community collaborators who reflected the new environmental focus were invited to be a part of the research (e.g., a municipal land use group, a community environmental housing organization), and the evaluation team considered using technology such as geographical information systems to provide a mapping of the city's environment, including elements such as eateries, groceries, and convenience stores.

In the third step the evaluation team began meeting with students regularly, via the use of focus groups, to gather data and information about the kind of intervention to which student participants would respond. Those focus group discussions served two purposes. First, they connected the evaluation team (made up of college-age research assistants) to the high school students and vice versa. Second, they provided needed data to establish a context for any possible intervention design.

Analyses of the baseline data were useful in (1) providing descriptive information concerning the population and its surrounding environment (for example, it was established that more than a third of the high school sample was considered to be obese), (2) articulating possible factors that might prohibit or, conversely, enhance physical health within cultural communities (e.g., students in the sample viewed obesity through a cultural lens), and (3) discerning the kinds of interventions to which student participants would respond (e.g., it was found that students indicated that they would like to attend cooking classes). Such analyses provided the school district concrete evidence as to why the high school should receive funding for the intervention (and, by extension, the research designed to provide evidence of the success of the intervention). Consequently, funding (albeit not full funding) was reestablished and an intervention was developed in collaboration with the environmental community organization (e.g. reviving the spirit walks, adding cooking classes).

LESSONS LEARNED

The TOPS project provided great lessons for the evaluation team, and we pass along our lessons learned as words to the wise in doing field research. First, in doing community-based research, one must be flexible. We advise designing both a plan A and a plan B of research. Plan A should be the best case scenario—what would work if all the stars are aligned in the universe. Plan B should be the realistic design, based on one's knowledge of the community, the participants, and the political climate. We encourage researchers to consider the kinds of questions that can be answered within the context of the community in which the research is being conducted. We also encourage them to be open and willing to adjust the design, perhaps switching from gathering inferential information to gathering descriptive information (or vice versa). In addition, baseline data can be very informative, and can establish a foundation for an experimental study at a later date. Above all, we encourage the community-based and field researcher to keep a cool and level head. One of the guarantees of research is that something is likely to go "off the rails," even under the best of circumstances, so be prepared to get it back on track!

TO READ FURTHER

Bledsoe, K. L., & Graham, J. A. (2005). Using multiple evaluation approaches in program evaluation. *American Journal of Evaluation, 26,* 302–319.

This article describes the use of several evaluation approaches in one study, and how these approaches determine the kinds of methodological designs that can be used.

Cook, T. D., &, Campbell, D. T. (1979). *Quasi-experimentation: Design and analysis issues for field settings.* Boston: Houghton-Mifflin.

This book describes the use of quasi-experimental designs in field settings. It discusses advantages and disadvantages of using quasi-experimental methodology, as well as analyses that can be considered in the use of these designs.

Cosby, P. C. (2008). *Methods in behavioral research* (9th ed.). New York: McGraw Hill.

This book is a quick reference to basic research methodology and analyses.

REFERENCES

Bledsoe, K. L., & Graham, J. A. (2005). Using multiple evaluation approaches in program evaluation. *American Journal of Evaluation, 26,* 302–319.

Centers for Disease Control and Prevention. (1999). *National Health Interview Survey* (NHIS). Retrieved May 24, 2008, from *www.cdc.gov/nchs/about/major/nhis/hisdesc.htm.*

Centers for Disease Control and Prevention. (2008). *Nutrition and physical activity.* Retrieved May 24, 2008, from *www.cdc.gov/nccdphp/dnpa/obesity/defining.htm.*

Cosby, P. C. (2008). *Methods in behavioral research* (9th ed.). New York: McGraw Hill.

Department of Youth and Family Services. (1998). *Blue Ribbon Panel report.* Trenton, NJ: Author.

Johnson, L. P. (2005). Smoking cessation, obesity and weight concerns in black women: A call to action for culturally competent interventions. *Journal of the National Medical Association, 1997,* 1630–1638.

Mertens, D. M. (2007). Transformative considerations: Inclusion and social justice. *American Journal of Evaluation, 28,* 86–90.

Oyserman, D., Gant, L., & Ager, J. (1995). A socially contextualized model of African American identity: Possible selves and school persistence. *Journal of Personality and Social Psychology, 69,* 1216–1232.

Phinney, J. (1992). The Multi-group Ethnic Identity Measure: A new scale for use with adolescents and young adults from diverse groups. *Journal of Adolescent Research, 7,* 156–176.

Quinn Patton, M. (1997). *Utilization-focused evaluation: The new century text* (3rd ed.). Thousand Oaks, CA: Sage.

Sheperd, S. (2003, March 21). Study of obesity among Latinos finds more than 50% overweight. *Memphis Business Journal.* Retrieved May 31, 2008, from *memphis.bizjournals.com/memphis/stories/2003/03/24/story4.htmlhttp:// www.cdc.*

Spurlock, M. (Producer/Writer/Director). (2004). *Supersize me: A film of epic portions* [Film]. Available from Showtime Networks, Inc.

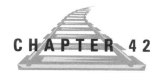

CHAPTER 42

Building Stakeholder Capacity to Enhance Effectiveness in Participatory Program Evaluation

DEBAZOU Y. YANTIO

BACKGROUND OF THE STUDY

Objectives, Implementation Structure, and Achievements of the ADAP

The Adolescent Development and Participation (ADAP) Program was jointly initiated in August 2000 by the government of Cameroon and the United Nations Children's Fund (UNICEF). Between 2003 and 2007, the objective of ADAP was to contribute to the creation of a legal, institutional, and community environment that would favor the development and participation of youths in and out of school settings and trigger a reduction in their vulnerability to sexually transmitted diseases (STDs) and the human immunodeficiency virus (HIV) because of risky sexual behavior. In order to achieve the program objective, we expected four results:

1. At least 25% of adolescents in the target areas would have acquired relevant knowledge and skills and adopted less risky behavior in regard to STDs and HIV/AIDS;
2. At least 50% of youths in the target areas would have access to community-based youth-friendly educational and health services, including counseling and voluntary testing for HIV;

3. A legal, institutional, and community environment that promotes the development and health of teenagers would be set up; and

4. Fifty percent of teenagers would participate in decision-making processes in the target areas and their concerns would be considered in national policy.

The ADAP program is currently implemented in 6 of the 10 provinces of the country. The decision on whether to scale up the program to reach remote areas of the country has to be made on the basis of the evaluation results.

The ADAP program activities are organized around two projects and subprojects. Project 1 centers on counseling and prevention of STDs and HIV/AIDS. Its two subprojects consist of (1) learning relevant knowledge and adoption of risk-reduced behaviors by teenagers and (2) setting up a model to deliver quality youth-friendly educational and health services. Project 2, life skills, also has two subprojects: (1) creating a legal, institutional, and community environment that empowers teenagers and favors their participation in decision making and (2) promoting the participation of teenagers in decision making processes.

Project 1 is built on a model to deliver the services and to enhance and improve the abilities youths need to prevent HIV/AIDS at the communal level: the information, education, and counseling (CIEE) center. This model is based on five sets of activities: (1) setting up the infrastructure base required to deliver educational and health services at the communal level, (2) developing the geographic coverage of the youth population in the target councils, (3) implementing a standard situation analysis and planning procedure encompassing a risk and vulnerability mapping (CRV) of the council and a 10-step behavioral analysis resulting in an action plan for the council, (4) action research to improve program operations, and (5) promoting human resources, especially youth peer educators. Teenagers use the life skills acquired in the framework of Project 2 to map the risk and assess vulnerability, conduct an analysis of youth behavior, and design an integrated communication plan to be implemented as part of the ADAP program.

Origin, Time Frame, Purpose, and Approach of the Evaluation Research Project

As planned in 2004, an external evaluation was carried out from February 2004 to November 2005. Its purpose was to look at the processes implemented under the ADAP program, draw relevant lessons, improve the delivery of services to youths under the CIEE model, and prepare to scale up the delivery of STDs and HIV/AIDS-related education and health services to in- and out-of-school youths, ages 10 to 24, across the country.

Specifically, the evaluation research project aimed at (1) understanding the strategic approaches and methods used to structure and implement the delivery of information, education, and counseling services to youth; (2) analyzing operations to identify (a) elements for possible replication in the scaling-up scenario, (b) elements for a proposal of national response against HIV/AIDS, (c) directions of ADAP program reorientation at a planned midterm review, (d) case materials for publication; and (3) suggesting operations domains with reasonable fundraising potentials.

The evaluation of ADAP program implementation covered (1) structure and administration of program activities, (2) quality and coverage of the services delivered, (3) sustainability of the ADAP program approach, (4) participation of youth and other stakeholders, and (5) monitoring of the program.

The approach to this external process evaluation was participatory, as agreed upon by the stakeholders we consulted during the preparation phase of the evaluation project. This approach was adopted because the purpose and aims of the evaluation clearly gave priority to the participation and learning of the program stakeholders in order to inform further decision making regarding the implementation and development of ADAP program operations. Therefore, consideration of the opinions and concerns of the different stakeholder categories is critical to a successful implementation of the ADAP program in the coming years. However, some quasi-experimental features were included in the evaluation methodology to ensure validity and to enhance credibility of the evaluation results. A multisite proportional stratified sampling and the administration of a questionnaire were integrated into the evaluation design. CIEEs were stratified into in- and out-of-school centers in each of the six provinces of the intervention area. This addition was made necessary because the evaluation also aimed at generalizing the results and eventually justified a scaling-up of the program model and activities to other parts of the country and across African regions where UNICEF carries out similar interventions. Overall, a mixed-method approach was selected for the ADAP program evaluation project.

THE CHALLENGES:
INADEQUATE CAPACITY OF PROGRAM STAKEHOLDERS

As stated earlier, the participation of stakeholders in the planning and conduct of the evaluation was decided upon as a strategy to ensure greater use of the results and strengthen participation in ADAP program implementation for better services to teenagers. The participation of stakeholders, including the youth peer educators who implement ADAP program field activities, was planned in various stages of the evaluation research: orientation, planning and supervision, data collection, validation of the results, and use of evaluation results. Different stakeholder involvement was organized in different instances: the evaluation advisory committee for Stages 1, 3 and 4, and local evaluation task teams for Stages 2 and 4. The evaluation advisory committee was responsible for various tasks: to oversee and endorse the evaluation plan, timeline, and terms of reference; identify and hire the evaluation facilitator; propose the set of evaluation questions; provide feedback and advice to the facilitator; support pilot testing of the evaluation tools; validate and endorse the findings of the evaluation; contribute to the interpretation of the findings; and provide recommendations to stakeholders involved in implementing the program activities. The local evaluation task teams had the responsibility to facilitate contacts with respondents, to provide relevant documentation and information to the evaluation facilitator and enumerators, and to share and discuss the evaluation results in the council they come from and belong to.

The composition of each group was tightly defined during the consultative process of the preparation phase of the evaluation. The evaluation advisory committee gathered 27 representatives of ADAP program stakeholders: youths, line ministries, nongovernmental organizations, United Nations (UN) agencies, and so forth. It was agreed that at least 40% of the membership be youths. These representatives were nominated by the organizations they represented.

To exercise responsibility and fulfill their functions, it was assumed that members of each group had some basic knowledge and skills in evaluation research design and practice, especially the members of the advisory committee. This assumption came to be far too optimistic, and experience revealed that most members of the evaluation advisory committee and local evaluation task teams didn't have such assets. In reality, most members had little or no technical knowledge of program evaluation. This created barriers to effective design and implementation of the evaluation project. The evaluation advisory committee had difficulties in focusing the research by defining a reasonable set of evaluation questions, making knowledgeable assessments of the techniques and tools proposed by the external consultant, and planning and budgeting evaluation activities. The members of the advisory committee were unable to phrase their program-related questions into evaluable ones, to prioritize the initial set of questions, or to retain a few questions to be investigated during the evaluation.

OVERCOMING THE DIFFICULTIES

I decided, after consultation with the client—in this case, the government of Cameroon and UNICEF—to introduce selected capacity-building activities into meetings of the evaluation advisory committee. These included distributing and encouraging the reading of the Organization for Economic Cooperation and Development (OECD) *Glossary of Key Terms in Evaluation and Results-Based Management* (2002) and adding evaluation learning objectives and activities to the agenda of advisory committee meetings. The learning package was designed to equip the advisory committee members with the knowledge and skills required to set evaluation questions, validate the protocol of the evaluation study, validate the findings, and plan the implementation of the changes to the program. The advisory committee was thereafter able to hold several technical meetings to assess the evaluation instruments and proposed plan to the satisfaction of the UNICEF staff and project manager. Following the implementation of the evaluation activities, members of the advisory committee were also able to proofread the report and suggest valuable modifications. Although not all members of the advisory committee are still with the ADAP program, those who remain are strongly involved in carrying out the changes recommended as part of the evaluation results. Overall, one can state that increasing the knowledge base and skills of the members of the advisory committee was instrumental in achieving more effective participation at all stages of the evaluation process.

LESSONS LEARNED AND RECOMMENDATIONS

Evaluation of the ADAP program in Cameroon has shown that lack of evaluation culture and inadequate evaluation knowledge of stakeholders on the evaluation committee is a major constraint to successful participation in evaluations. Thus, the participation of the stakeholders should be planned up front and conditions for successful participation need to be identified and explicitly addressed with appropriate measures.

TO READ FURTHER

Reitbergen-McCracken, J., & Narayan, D. (1998). *Participation and social assessment: Tools and techniques*. Washington, DC: World Bank.

This work provides a useful definition of participation and practical assessment scales. In addition, it discusses a wide range of participatory tools that can be use in designing and conducting participatory program evaluations.

International Fund for Agricultural Development. (2002). *Managing for impact in rural development: A guide for project M&E*. Available at *www.ifad.org/evaluation/guide/m_e_guide.zip*.

This publication sheds light on linking project formulation, annual budgeting, and monitoring and evaluation design.

REFERENCE

Organization for Economic Cooperation and Development (OECD). (2002). *OECD glossary of key terms in evaluation and results-based management.* Paris: Author.

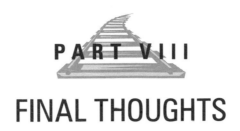

PART VIII

FINAL THOUGHTS

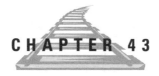

CHAPTER 43

Sometimes It Is the Researcher, Not the Research, That Goes "Off the Rails"

The Value of Clear, Complete, and Precise Information in Scientific Reports

JOSEPH A. DURLAK
CHRISTINE I. CELIO
MOLLY K. PACHAN
KRISTON B. SCHELLINGER

The fault, dear Brutus, is not in our stars, but in ourselves.
—WILLIAM SHAKESPEARE, *Julius Caesar*, Act I, Scene II

BACKGROUND

This book contains numerous accounts of the trials and tribulations they encountered as researchers have tried to conduct their research. We expect that many researchers will blame "outside forces" for such problems. That is, many authors are likely to discuss how administrative and practical snafus, or lack of cooperation, commitment, or support from others, sabotaged part or all of their research plans. Without discounting the validity of these observations, the opening quotation we use from *Julius Caesar* suggests that we are taking a different perspective. The main purpose of this chapter is to discuss a major oversight of many researchers: They fail to report adequately the details of their research projects.

Although there are some exceptions, typically the most respected and influential scientific reports are not only those that follow or improve upon the research methods established in their relevant field of inquiry, but are also those that are objective, precise, clear, and complete. Therefore, thorough reporting of the investigation in question is essential for judging the worth of a particular study and for advancing the discipline. Unfortunately, basic information is often not provided by researchers.

For the past several years, our research team has been conducting reviews of the impact of more than 700 preventive and competence-promotion interventions for youth. We have examined interventions conducted in schools, in community settings, and for families, and although these studies span a wide time period, many have appeared since 2000. Throughout the course of our work, we have been disappointed, irritated, and sometimes amazed to discover how much basic information is missing in reports written by well-trained, sensible, and often highly experienced and well-respected researchers. Moreover, our discoveries are similar to those of reviewers in other areas (e.g., Hoyt & Bhati, 2007; Weisz, Jensen-Doss, & Hawley, 2006). In an attempt to facilitate the collection of crucial information, this chapter has two main aims: (1) to indicate some of the primary data that should be provided in every study and (2) to direct readers to resources that offer specific guidelines on what information to report and how to report it. Because of space limitations, we cannot discuss all the details needed for every type of investigation. Instead, we focus on the Method section of program evaluation or outcome studies (i.e., studies assessing some type of intervention or treatment). Our comments also refer to interventions for school-age youth between the ages of 5 and 18 and their families.

WHAT SHOULD BE REPORTED?

The purpose of the Method section of a program evaluation or outcome study is to describe the intervention or treatment being evaluated in sufficient detail. The reader of any Method section should be able to answer the following questions: Who received the intervention? Who provided it? What were the major elements of the intervention? What measures were used to assess the impact of the intervention assessed? Was the program implemented as planned? In other words, the "w" questions need to be answered: who did what, to whom, what happened, and why does this matter? We focus on participant information and the elements of the intervention here.

Who Are the Participants?

At the very least, research participants should be described with respect to age (expressed in terms of mean, median, and range), school grade (if applicable), gender, socioeconomic status (SES; indicating percentages falling into different strata and criteria used to define SES), race and ethnicity (using percentages and information on criteria used to define cultural groups), and any other unique or relevant characteristics (e.g., recent immigrant, language preference if not English (and/or French, in Canada).

Although the need to report some of this basic information may appear obvious, omissions occur in many studies. For example, of the 723 preventive and competence-promotion interventions in our largest database, 6% of studies did not report the age or grade of the students, 26% omitted information on gender, 38% did not provide *any* information on race or ethnicity, and 55% failed to report *any* information on socioeconomic status. Furthermore, when information for the latter two categories was presented, it was often incomplete and insufficient. For example, some researchers indicated only that the "majority of the sample was white." Sometimes, if authors gave a percentage breakdown according to race/ethnicity, the numbers would not add up to 100% (e.g., 35% were African American and 50% were Caucasian). Similarly, for SES, students might be described as being "mostly from poor families," or the report would say "many" of the students participated in free lunch programs (an inexact proxy for SES). The vast amount of missing data was frustrating and disappointing to our research team because it prevented us from running many potentially useful analyses in an attempt to answer important questions regarding gender, ethnicity, and SES.

Although collecting and providing some of the aforementioned information, such as age, is rather straightforward, reporting on other characteristics such as race/ethnicity or SES is more complicated. For example, although much has been written about the difficulty of collecting data on race and ethnicity, no conclusive and universal definition of these constructs has been established. Moreover, there is no "standard" measure of race or ethnicity, and collecting these data can be done in many different ways, from simply asking participants to report their race, to using measures of acculturation. Unfortunately, the lack of a standard way to collect race and ethnicity information can lead to researchers not collecting these data at all. This is unacceptable. Neglecting to collect information because of the complexity of the construct can have deleterious effects on future replications and mislead readers in their interpretation of the findings. Researchers should always attempt to gather these data, clearly state how groups were defined, and report the data collection methods that were used (Sue, Kuraski, & Srinivasan, 1999).

Although self-report is the most commonly used approach to collect information about race, researchers need to be aware of which categories are most relevant. As of 2003, the very broad U.S. Census categories for *race* include American Indian or Alaska Native, Asian, Black or African American, Native Hawaiian or Other Pacific Islander, and White (U.S. Census

Bureau, 2000). However, there are only two broad categories for *ethnicity*: Hispanic/Latino and Not Hispanic/Latino (U.S. Census Bureau, 2000). Such broad ethnicity categories cannot capture important characteristics of some research samples. For example, important cultural differences can be obscured when participants who speak a similar language (e.g., Spanish) but are from different countries of origin (e.g., Spain, Mexico, or countries in South and Central America) are combined and treated as one group. In addition, new arrivals to the country in which the intervention occurs may differ in levels of acculturation and language preference. In these cases, information beyond that provided by a simple "check which racial or ethnic group you belong to" is important and necessary to collect. Depending on the scope of the research project, simple self-reports of race and ethnicity could be supplemented by measures of acculturation, ethnic pride, or racial identity (see Cokley, 2007; Foster & Martinez, 1995; Phinney, 1996; Roberts et al., 1999; Sellers, Smith, Shelton, Rowley, & Chavous, 1998). This might help clarify the broad constructs of race or ethnicity, particularly in instances where the intervention has been adapted or modified for certain target groups.

Another important, but sensitive, piece of information is SES, which is particularly important for student populations, because SES is frequently associated with educational outcomes (Sirin, 2005). Over the years, SES has been assessed in many ways, through different combinations of parental income, parental education, and parental occupation. This has created an ambiguity in interpreting research findings (Gottfried, 1985; Hauser, 1994; White, 1982). In addition, many empirical studies examining the relations between different measures of SES have found low to moderate correlations between these factors (Bollen, Glanville, & Stecklov, 2001; Hauser & Huang, 1997). That is, not all measures of SES measure the same thing! However, as mentioned earlier in regard to race and ethnicity, researchers should not be fearful of collecting and reporting data simply because there is not a clear standard. Despite the challenge of collecting these data, they should always be reported, along with a rationale for the choice of measures and definitions used.

What Happened in the Intervention?

A detailed description of the characteristics of the intervention is crucial, and research publications should be prepared in enough detail that others could replicate the experiment (American Psychological Association, 2001). Frequently, information on the content of the intervention is reported through manuals or lesson plans that are included in an appendix or made available to interested readers by contacting the author. In addition, basic information on the intervention is needed, such as the general and specific locations in which it was offered (urban, suburban, or rural setting; in schools, clinics, or other community-based facilities), the recruitment and final selection procedures, staff information (training, experience, demographics), mode of delivery (group, individual, phone contacts), attendance patterns (who attended and for how many sessions), duration (the length of each session, how long the program lasted), and implementation (to what extent and in what ways was the program conducted as planned).

In our work we have found that many studies either totally omit critical information or are too vague in their descriptions. For example, among the studies in our database, 15% did not specify the locale of the intervention (e.g., urban, suburban, rural), fewer than half described the relevant training or experience of the staff administering the intervention, 11% did not include details on how many times a week the intervention took place, and 31% did not report enough information to determine the number of sessions included in the program. If these programs were effective, how is the reader to replicate them? If the programs were ineffective, how is the reader to know what went on and what improvements can and should be made? Omitting these data is not only important for other researchers and reviewers, but also becomes an issue of inadequate dissemination.

Information on implementation was also frequently omitted. In a recent review of school-based positive youth development programs, we were disappointed to find that 42% of studies did not even mention implementation (Durlak, Weissberg, Taylor, Dymnicki, & Schellinger, 2008). Once again, when information was provided, it was often insufficient or incomplete. For example, some authors suggested that they monitored implementation and found it to be acceptable, but did not clarify what monitoring methods they used or the specific level or quality of implementation that was achieved. The failure to report on implementation makes interpretation of study findings impossible, because previous research from many different areas indicates (1) that good implementation is not always attained and (2) that there usually is a positive relationship between implementation and outcomes (Durlak & Dupre, 2008). Without data on implementation, it is impossible to judge whether the intervention was actually responsible for any positive outcomes that were obtained, or whether the lack of positive findings was due to poor implementation.

HELPFUL RESOURCES

There are several resources that contain useful guidelines on the information that should be included in publications. The "gold standard" for social scientists is the *Publication Manual of the American Psychological Association* (American Psychological Association, 2001). Two additional guides we recommend are the documents developed by the What Works Clearing-house (*ies.ed.gov/ncee/wwc/*) and the CONSORT group (*www.consort-statement.org/*); there are also various articles addressing specific matters related to ethnicity, SES, and implementation (e.g., Durlak & Dupre, 2008; Foster & Martinez, 1995; Phinney, 1996; Sue et al., 1999).

CONCLUDING THOUGHTS

Full and clear reporting is essential to good research. We implore all researchers to read their reports with fresh eyes before they consider them to be finished. Any reader should be able to discern, at the very least, the basic information about the study in terms of who did what, to whom, and with what results. If someone who has never seen or heard about the program cannot abstract such information, then the manuscript needs a new, more complete draft.

In this chapter, we have attempted to impress upon you the importance of writing clear, complete, and precise scientific documents and have discussed some basic data that should be reported. Thorough reporting is an essential part of the research process, because neglecting to collect and report needed data can result in negative consequences for the researcher, his or her colleagues, and the field at large. The individual researcher should be aware that the absence of essential information can jeopardize the opportunity to publish his or her work. Furthermore, when a researcher or research team (such as ours) attempts to complete a review to ascertain what already has been done in an area of interest, the absence of basic information in a report often means that the study is excluded from the review. As a result, all the hard work the researcher has committed to a project is lost to a larger audience. Most important, a field does not move forward if information is not disseminated fully and accurately, and future experiments cannot benefit from prior work. Thus, neglecting to include just a few lines of critical information on some variables can have serous repercussions.

Finally, it is important to note that researchers are not the only culprits. Journal editors and reviewers are also responsible for upholding reporting standards and should not accept any manuscript for publication that has basic data missing. When submitting a manuscript to the scrutiny of the review process, it is usually far better to impress reviewers and the editor with completeness rather than disappoint or frustrate them with incomplete reporting. Moreover, researchers must be aware of basic reporting standards so that plans to collect necessary data are developed at the beginning of the research process. In sum, Julius Caesar was right: Sometimes it is ourselves, not others or fate, who are to blame.

TO READ FURTHER

Durlak, J. A., Meerson, I., & Ewell-Foster, C. (2003). Meta-analysis. In J. C. Thomas & M. Hersen (Eds.), *Understanding research in clinical and counseling psychology: A textbook* (pp. 243–267). Mahwah, NJ: Erlbaum.

In this chapter, Durlak, Meerson, and Ewell-Foster explain the process of evaluating studies and conducting a meta-analysis. With the increasing reliance by policymakers on meta-analyses, this information is especially useful for researchers who wish their results to be included in the body of literature useful to quantitative reviewers.

Sue, S., Kuraski, K. S., & Srinivasan, S. (1999). Ethnicity, gender, and cross-cultural issues in clinical research. In P. C. Kendall, J. N. Butcher, & G. N. Holmbeck (Eds.), *Handbook of research methods in clinical psychology* (2nd ed., pp. 54–71). New York: Wiley.

This chapter discusses the importance of considering ethnicity, gender, and culture in all sorts of research. Although it is written for clinical psychologists, the ideas pertain to researchers in all fields.

REFERENCES

American Psychological Association. (2001). *Publication manual of the American Psychological Association* (5th ed.). Washington, DC: Author.

Bollen, K., Glanville, J. A., & Stecklov, G. (2001). Socioeconomic status and class in studies of fertility and health in developing countries. *Annual Review of Sociology, 27,* 153–185.

Cokley, K. (2007). Critical issues in the measurement of ethnic and racial identity: A referendum on the state of the field. *Journal of Counseling Psychology, 54,* 224–234.

Durlak, J. A., & Dupre, E. P. (2008). Implementation matters: A review of research on the influence of implementation on program outcomes and the factors affecting implementation. *American Journal of Community Psychology.*

Durlak, J. A., Weissberg, R. P., Taylor, R. D., Dymnicki, A. B., & Schellinger, K. B. (2008). *The impact of enhacing social and emotional learning: A meta-analysis of school based universal intentions.* Manuscript submitted for publication.

Foster, S. L., & Martinez, C. R. (1995). Ethnicity: Conceptual and methodological issues in child clinical research. *Journal of Clinical Child Psychology, 24,* 214–226.

Gottfried, A. (1985). Measures of socioeconomic status in child development research: Data and recommendations. *Merrill-Palmer Quarterly, 31,* 85–92.

Hauser, R. M. (1994). Measuring socioeconomic status in studies of child development. *Child Development, 65,* 1541–1545.

Hauser, R. M., & Huang, M. H. (1997). Verbal ability and socioeconomic success: A trend analysis. *Social Science Research, 26,* 331–376.

Hoyt, W. T., & Bhati, K. S. (2007). Principles and practices: An empirical examination of qualitative research in the *Journal of Counseling Psychology*. *Journal of Counseling Psychology, 54*, 201–210.

Phinney, J. S. (1996). When we talk about American ethnic groups, what do we mean? *American Psychologist, 51*, 918–927.

Roberts, R. E., Phinney, J. S., Masse, L. C., Chen, Y. R., Roberts, C. R., & Romero, A. (1999). The structure of ethnic identity of young adolescents from diverse ethnocultural groups. *Journal of Early Adolescence, 19*, 301–322.

Sellers, R. M., Smith, M. A., Shelton, J. N., Rowley, S. T. A., & Chavous, T. M. (1998). Multidimensional model of ethnic identity: A reconstruction of African American racial identity. *Personality and Social Psychology Review, 2*, 18–39.

Sirin, S. R. (2005). Socioeconomic status and academic achievement: A meta-analytic review of research. *Review of Educational Research, 75*, 417–453.

Sue, S., Kuraski, K. S., & Srinivasan, S. (1999). Ethnicity, gender, and cross-cultural issues in clinical research. In P. C. Kendall, J. N. Butcher, & G. N. Holmbeck (Eds.), *Handbook of research methods in clinical psychology* (2nd ed., pp. 54–71). New York: Wiley.

U.S. Census Bureau. (2000, April 20). *Racial and ethic classifications used in Census 2000 and beyond*. Retrieved January 10, 2008, from *www.census.gov/population/www/socdemo/ race/racefactcb.html*.

Weisz, J. R, Jensen-Doss, A, & Hawley, K. M. (2006). Youth psychotherapy outcome research: A review and critique of the evidence base. *Annual Review of Psychology, 56*, 337–363.

White, K. R. (1982). The relationship between socioeconomic status and academic achievement. *Psychological Bulletin, 91*, 461–481.

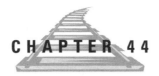

CHAPTER 44

Final Thoughts
A Healthy Dose of Realism

SOURAYA SIDANI
DAVID L. STREINER

That Murphy's law will strike any study and at any stage of the research process is a certainty. The stories told in this book present ample proof of this assertion. What makes the picture even bleaker is that by no means are the stories exhaustive. No matter to whom we mentioned that we were putting this book together, they inevitably said, "Have I got a story for you!" Take a moment to reminisce about the studies in which you were involved in various capacities, beginning with your experience as a student working as a research assistant or coordinator, moving to your participation on a study as a coinvestigator or principal investigator, and ending with your role as a consultant. We are sure you remember encountering a situation in which something went wrong, no matter how benign it was, such as running out of pens or questionnaire copies. Well ... you came face-to-face with Murphy's law. Were you prepared to face such obstacles? Probably, not really "well" prepared. Why? The answer is simple: because of the prevalent perspective on research.

That perspective is characterized by a tendency to forget and not report, at least publicly, about situations where Murphy's law operated. This perspective is well illustrated with the description, in books and published reports, of research as a straightforward, smooth, and uneventful process that strictly adhered to the original study design and was implemented as planned. Further, it is clearly reflected, even embedded, in the belief held by some in the scientific community, and clarified by one contributor to this book, that high-quality empirical work adheres to strict a priori protocols. Any deviation from the protocols is unacceptable and has the potential to devalue a study. Accordingly, investigators hesitate to divulge experiences with Murphy's law. Further, even if a researcher were so rash as to admit that the train had derailed, he or she would never put this into a manuscript for fear that the admission would lead to an automatic rejection by the journal editor; after all, journals publish only "good" studies. (In fairness, though, we should say that one Canadian granting agency believes that if a study were carried out exactly as proposed, it would show that the researcher wasn't paying attention; *all* good studies will run into roadblocks or come up with unexpected findings that should be followed through.)

This state of affairs does a disservice to science and to researchers. Much of what experienced researchers know about these laws and the strategies to address them remains unknown to the vast majority of young researchers, or may be passed on verbally to a select few graduate students by mentors who are willing to disclose their experiences. Orally transmitted knowledge may not be well preserved and may not reach those in need. Researchers, particularly novices, are left uninformed or misinformed about what actually happens in the course of a study. This generates unrealistically optimistic expectations about how long it will take to do the study (our advice to students is to make the most pessimistic estimate—and then multiply this by 4; we've rarely been wrong). In addition, researchers may not have the skills required to prepare for and effectively manage situations that may go wrong; they end up learning through experience, at their own expense. Further, not reporting how studies had to be changed means that the same mistakes will be made by others, resulting in wasted effort, time, and resources. (Although, cynically, we can quote the economist Charles Wolf Jr., who once said that "those who don't study the past will repeat its errors; those who do study it will find other ways to err.")

This book is the product of our concern with this state of affairs and our attempt at documenting the unwritten scientific heritage related to experiences with Murphy's law. The goal was to present a more realistic perspective on research, which can only serve to assist researchers, seasoned and novice, to acquire the knowledge and skills to succeed even when Murphy's law strikes. The realistic perspective is based on the premises that much research in health, behavioral, social, and educational sciences is (or should be) done in the context of the "real world" if it is to be relevant and applicable to practice, and that the reality of research process is different from the prespecified research protocols, which are often formulated in the ivory towers of academia. The realistic perspective involves a clear, explicit, and "courageous" acknowledgement of Murphy's law, a submission that the real world is full of surprises or unexpected and uncontrollable events that do not conform to the strictness of research, a realization that maintaining the rigor of research and the validity of conclusions is not achieved with a blind, unquestioned adherence to a priori protocols but requires judicious flexibility in implementation and sharing of experiences regarding what went wrong, and how it was addressed, for the sake of learning.

So, what have we learned from reading the stories in this book? Although contributors summarized specific lessons learned from their individual experiences, we can draw some more general points from these stories that can be useful to researchers working in various fields and using different research approaches and methods. The points encompass acknowledging, preparing for, and addressing or managing Murphy's law.

ACKNOWLEDGE THAT MURPHY'S LAW EXISTS

Acknowledging a problem is the first step toward resolving it. Similarly, admitting that Murphy's law is a certainty and that it can strike anywhere and at any time during the course of research, is necessary for devising and using strategies to successfully avoid or address it. The experiences described in this book confirm that Murphy's law can—and will—strike at any one stage or at many stages of the research process, even (or especially) at stages when it is not expected: during the formulation of the research problem or question, obtaining funding, and reporting the results. Acknowledging that Murphy's law will strike boils down to the following advice: Anticipate challenges—things will not go smoothly.

BE PREPARED

The motto "Be prepared" has served the Boy Scouts well for nearly a century (as well as providing grist for a humorous song by Tom Lehrer) and should be emblazoned on the wall of every research lab. Expecting that something may (nay, will) go wrong during the course of any study should prompt researchers to prepare to avoid such a difficulty if at all possible and to manage it when it happens. The importance of preparation is well reflected in the statements made by a number of contributors to this book: "Hope for the best, plan for the worst" and "Balance optimism with realism and with perseverance." Preparation demands developing some attributes, adequate planning, and pilot testing the planned study protocol.

DEVELOP SOME USEFUL ATTRIBUTES

Some researchers' attributes appear to form a useful armamentarium in the fight against Murphy's law. The main ones include flexibility, patience, and effective communication; there are probably others, but if you master these, you'll be well on your way.

Flexibility was mentioned in many of the chapters as a critical characteristic underlying researchers' work (other authors most likely felt it was a given, so didn't bother to explicitly mention it). Flexibility is required for engaging in critical thinking when faced with an unexpected situation; it is needed to examine the situation from different perspectives in order to understand what is actually going on that often deviates from what is anticipated; to find alternative, creative solutions; to analyze the strengths and limitations of various alternatives; to select the appropriate solution that is feasible within the constraints of the real world; and to show a willingness to modify the protocol accordingly. Nurturing flexibility demands that researchers be able to let go of their preconceived ideas of how the study *must* be carried out, and the belief that only strict adherence to the study protocol as originally written can achieve high-quality results. Thus, flexibility entails being aware of and sensitive to the features of the real world, the needs of the target population, and the concerns of professionals and the organizations in which the research is done, and being willing to make the necessary changes to accommodate these realities without jeopardizing the validity of the research.

Patience (and plenty of it) is another attribute identified in various chapters as useful to have when things can go wrong. Researchers are advised to "keep their cool." Any strategy or tool to help regain calmness, such as a philosophical attitude, a stress ball, or a bourbon and water, will do. Calmness facilitates the clear thinking needed to select appropriate strategies to manage the situation, to have optimism and energy to carry out the modified plan, and to persevere with implementing the study. If you don't have patience and perseverance, get out of the research game early.

Effective communication is another mandatory skill. As many of the authors pointed out, this means first of all making sure that the information to be conveyed is clear. Speak in your native tongue; not in "psychology," or "nursing," or "evaluation," or any other language. If you find yourself using terms like "vocalities" instead of "views," "discourse" instead of "talking," or "service user" instead of "patient," it's probably worthwhile enrolling in a course of English as a Second Language. Good communication also involves active listening and openness to others, politeness, and respect for others. Effective communication builds rapport and trust between researchers and stakeholders or members of the target population, which makes it easier to discuss issues and to find appropriate solutions.

PLAN AHEAD

Planning spans all stages of the research process, starting with proposal writing and ending with interpretation and dissemination of findings. Having a clear proposal isn't enough if you don't have a realistic timeline in which to complete all phases of the study.

A realistic timeline is one that builds in sufficient time for the research activities. Specifically, ample time is needed in the preparatory phase aimed at setting up the study; obtaining ethics approval can be delayed because of unanticipated and additional requirements imposed by the ethics review board; communicating with stakeholders to build rapport and trust and to gain access to the target population demands effort and time, particularly when the participants are vulnerable or marginalized communities. Murphy's law tells us that the one person whose approval is mandatory for the project to move forward will have just begun a long vacation or be off on extended sick leave, so plan for that. Extensive time and effort are essential for recruitment and screening. This is the case in a variety of situations: For example, if the target population resides in the community at large (i.e., not in institutions), advertising may have to be done through newspapers or agencies. Not everyone who responds will meet the criteria, meaning that a large number of potential participants will have to be screened in order to accrue the necessary sample size. By definition, such extensive recruitment and intensive screening are expensive and should be allotted adequate funding. Many years ago, we formulated our version of a Murphy's law: "Every time you start a study with a clinical population, the disorder disappears." Our first experience of this situation was in a psychiatric emergency room. After tracking who came in and when over a period of 6 months, we began recruiting participants. Two weeks later, another emergency room opened in the city, draining off half of our potential subjects. None of our experiences since then have refuted this immutable law of nature.

A feasible protocol is one that is realistic, has been pilot tested, found acceptable, and can be implemented. Moreover, it should account for real-world constraints. How can this be achieved? Several strategies are proposed to make a protocol feasible, most of which call for the active involvement of gatekeepers, stakeholders, and representatives of the target population in planning the study. As many of the authors point out, knowledge of the target population and of the study context is a prerequisite for using these strategies. This entails understanding the characteristics, beliefs, and values of the group, specifically those that can affect their perception of the research topic (e.g., whether it is a sensitive topic), buy-in of the study (e.g., misunderstanding its intent, or perceiving that the intervention is not consistent with their preferences), and responses to the study methodology (e.g., discomfort with computer use or with group interviews). Learning about the population ahead of time enables researchers to select research topics that are relevant to their concerns and interests, which facilitates buy-in, and to use methods and procedures that are acceptable to members of the target population and consistent with their preferences, which promotes their participation and adherence. In addition to understanding the population, it is important to understand the context of the study, including the structure and culture of the organizations or sites from which participants are recruited, where the intervention is delivered, and data are collected. Knowing an organization's policies and procedures, and the roles and responsibilities of the staff, allows design of the study so that disruption is minimized and the protocol can be followed. Such knowledge of the target population and study context is not only derived from the researchers' expertise, but is also reinforced and expanded through open and clear communication.

Open and clear communication dispels any misunderstanding that gatekeepers, stakeholders, and participants may have about the study. It also shows respect and sensitivity to their needs and concerns, and fosters trust between them and the researchers. This should facilitate developing close collaboration between researchers and the other key players. Collaboration is one major strategy to generate feasible study protocols that account for the characteristics and preferences of the target population and the reality of the research context. You can foster collaboration in a number of ways:

1. Form an advisory committee that includes representatives of the various stakeholders. The role of the committee is to assist in designing a study that is acceptable to the target population and to resolve any problems that may arise while the study is being conducted. Advisory committees are particularly helpful when working with communities with characteristics that are very different from those of the researchers, such as those pertaining to social class, ethnicity, or race.

2. Invite some of the gatekeepers or stakeholders to join the research team and become participants in it. In some of our projects, we have invited the most vocal critics to be part of the team. Few things generate more buy-in than having one's name associated with a project, and all of the research on cognitive dissonance tells us that critics' attitudes will change as they identify with the study. Even if these people don't change, it's better to have them sniping from the inside than taking potshots from the outside.

3. Consult with gatekeepers and stakeholders to discuss the nature of and devise strategies to address any problem arising during study implementation; and

4. Involve gatekeepers as "champions" of the study who are responsible for spreading the word about it to other staff members in the organization, openly expressing support for the study, and encouraging staff members to take part in or facilitate the protocol. Collaboration is promoted if gatekeepers, stakeholders, and participants are regarded as partners in the endeavor, if they can see the relevance or advantages of the study to their

organization and the target population, and if they are rewarded for their involvement in the study in some way, such as through gifts, recognition, or simply being told about the findings.

Whether or not the study was designed with input from gatekeepers and stakeholders, the protocol must be pilot tested to determine if it works in the field. This applies to all aspects of the study—recruitment, screening or eligibility criteria, data collection and measures, the intervention itself, and retention, as well as data entry and management. The pilot testing should be done either as a separate study before the full-scale version starts or as a first phase of the full study. In addition, the pilot testing should include some detective work to identify aspects of the study that are excellent opportunities for Murphy's law to strike. The detective work can take many forms: (1) Close and careful monitoring of all research activities, either overtly or covertly—members of the research team can observe the research activities and take field notes of any difficulties they spot, or can actually pose as participants to see things from their perspective; (2) formally or informally discussing with the staff any problems they encounter during the study, and eliciting possible solutions from them; (3) holding focus group sessions with gatekeepers, stakeholders, and participants to identify what did and did not work, and what can be done to improve the study. Results of the pilot testing and the detective work can allow refinements in the protocol that make it more feasible, acceptable, and applicable; the ultimate goal is to minimize the chances that Murphy's law will strike during the full-scale study. Doing all this, however, does not absolutely guarantee a smooth and uneventful ride. So, what else can be done?

MANAGEMENT

Despite developing the necessary attitudes and careful preparation, Murphy's law can still strike unexpectedly (that's probably another one of his laws). The advice here is: "Do not despair. There is light at the beginning, throughout, and at the end of the tunnel." How so? Two general strategies can be useful: early detection (the beginning of the tunnel) and problem solving (throughout the tunnel) to manage the laws' effects successfully (the end of the tunnel).

Early detection is important, as it is easier to deal with and control a problem in its early stage, when it is still circumscribed, than when the problem is full-blown, extensive, and invasive. Close monitoring of all stages of the research is the hallmark of early detection. Monitoring can take several forms, including but not limited to (1) site visits; frequent and regular meetings with the research staff; periodic checks of specific research activities such as number of people recruited from the various sites, how many were found eligible and enrolled, completeness of the records and data (e.g., responses to questionnaire), availability of all materials and equipment needed for the study, and whether it's working; (2) meetings with gatekeepers, stakeholders, and the advisory committee (if applicable); and (3) interim data analysis. These monitoring activities should point to areas of strengths and, more important, concerns: aspects of the study where Murphy's Law can strike. Once problem areas are identified, the second strategy can begin—problem solving.

Problem solving is a systematic process aimed at finding a solution to an issue. It starts with clearly identifying the problem, which involves determining its nature, the factors or situations that contribute to it, and possible consequences. This detailed understanding of the issue is necessary to recognize its impact on the study and the specific aspects that have to be changed. Problem solving continues with finding alternatives, as mentioned in several chapters of their book. These alternatives consist of different but complementary ways of carrying out an activity, such as sampling (e.g., random digit dialing and network sampling), recruitment (group and individual contact), and data collection (computer and paper administration of questionnaires). The advantages and disadvantages of each alternative should be explored and the most appropriate ones selected. We encourage researchers to find alternative strategies with comparable effectiveness and to use them in combination. This advice is consistent with the principle underlying *critical multiplism*, an approach to research advanced by Cook (1985). In a nutshell, critical multiplism consists of judiciously selecting and using more than one method for conducting research, whereby the methods reflect different perspectives. Similarly, we encourage researchers to choose different but complementary strategies for each research activity. Of course, each strategy may introduce some sort of bias (e.g., random sampling may not reach enough people in a particular subgroup; network sampling may lead to self-selection bias); however, by using a number of strategies in combination, the bias inherent in one approach can be counterbalanced by the bias in another. The multiple strategies were to manage Murphy's law's strikes should be selected on the basis of their ability to reach the intended goal, their acceptability to the target population, and their feasibility within the context of the "real world" of research. We learn about these through an interplay of (1) empirical evidence, and not the uncritical acceptance of research methods, most of which are based on expert opinion and convention; (2) discussions with gatekeepers, stakeholders, and representatives of the target population; and (3) actual trial of the strategies in pilot studies. Incorporating multiple strategies in the protocol is a sound approach to manage Murphy's law—if (or should we say "when") something goes wrong with one approach, the others can compensate for this, saving the situation and the study. Isn't multiplism worth the effort?

FINAL THOUGHTS

Although it is certain that Murphy's law will strike, we never know where and when it will do so. This unpredictability can take many researchers off guard. They may not be well prepared to respond appropriately and promptly, and this may adversely affect a study. We hope this book has helped researchers realize the certainty and universality of Murphy's law and, as with many unjust laws, work to repeal its impact.

REFERENCES

Cook, T. D. (1985). Postpositivist critical multiplism. In L. Shotland & M. M. Mark (Eds.), *Social science and social policy* (pp. 21–62). Beverly Hills, CA: Sage.

Index

About the Editors

David L. Streiner, PhD, began his professional life at McMaster University in Hamilton, Ontario, Canada, where he was in the Departments of Clinical Epidemiology and Biostatistics, and Psychiatry and Behavioural Neurosciences, and Chief Psychologist at the McMaster Medical Centre. After 30 years, he retired for 1 day before beginning at the Baycrest Centre as Assistant Vice President of Research and Director of the Kunin–Lunenfeld Applied Research Unit. Dr. Streiner also holds faculty appointments at the University of Toronto as a Full Professor in the Department of Psychiatry and in Public Health Sciences, the Faculties of Nursing and Social Work, and the School of Rehabilitation. He retired again after 10 years and is now a Senior Scientist at Baycrest and guru-in-residence with the Child Health Research Institute at McMaster. He is the coauthor, with Geoffrey Norman, of four books: *PDQ Statistics; PDQ Epidemiology; Biostatistics: The Bare Essentials;* and *Health Measurement Scales: A Practical Guide to Their Development and Use;* and, with John Cairney, has edited a book, *Psychiatric Epidemiology in Canada.*

Souraya Sidani, PhD, began her research career as a graduate student at the University of Arizona and climbed the ladder of academia (reaching the level of Full Professor) during her 13-year tenure at the Faculty of Nursing, University of Toronto. She did not have an opportunity to retire like her mentor David Streiner, for even half a day, before assuming her current position of Canada Research Chair, Tier One (i.e., senior), in Health Interventions Design and Evaluation at Ryerson University. She is a content-free methodologist, with expertise in quantitative research methods, including measurement and theory-based program evaluation, and an interest in determining the effectiveness and utility of various designs and methods. Dr. Sidani's present research focus is on exploring the influence of preferences for treatment on study enrollment, adherence to treatment, attrition, and outcome achievement, and on comparing alternative designs (random vs. preference trials) and methods for outcome assessment (serial vs. perceived change) on the validity and clinical relevance of findings. She has coauthored two books: *Evaluating Nursing Interventions: A Theory-Driven Approach* and *Missing Data: A Gentle Introduction.*

Contributors

Amy Amidon, PhD, is a Postdoctoral Fellow at the Veterans Medical Research Foundation in San Diego.

Steve Balsis, PhD, is Assistant Professor in the Department of Psychology at Texas A & M University in College Station, Texas.

Philippe A. Barrette, PhD, is a psychotherapist and a workplace consultant to family businesses, government, and the private sector in Ancaster, Ontario, Canada.

Katrina L. Bledsoe, PhD, is Project Director of the national evaluation of the federally funded initiative "Comprehensive Community Mental Health Services for Children and Their Families Program" and a senior research manager at Walter R. McDonald & Associates, Inc., in Rockville, Maryland.

Dianne Bryant, MSc, PhD, is a clinical epidemiologist; Director of Empower, a data management and methods center; Assistant Professor in the School of Physical Therapy, Faculty of Health Sciences, and Department of Surgery, Division of Orthopaedic Surgery, Faculty of Medicine and Dentistry, at the University of Western Ontario in London, Ontario, Canada; and part-time Associate Professor in the Department of Clinical Epidemiology and Biostatistics at McMaster University in Hamilton, Ontario, Canada.

John Cairney, PhD, is McMaster Family Medicine Professor of Child Health Research and Associate Professor in the Department of Psychiatry and Behavioural Neuroscience at McMaster University in Hamilton, Ontario, Canada. He is also Associate Director of Research in the Department of Family Medicine at McMaster University and adjunct Senior Research Scientist in the Health Systems Research and Consulting Unit at the Centre for Addiction and Mental Health. His interests are in population mental health, developmental disorders in children, and survey design methods.

Brian D. Carpenter, PhD, is Associate Professor in the Department of Psychology at Washington University in St. Louis, Missouri.

Christine I. Celio, MA, is a doctoral student at Loyola University in Chicago. She has a BA in psychology from Stanford University, an MA in sociology from Stanford University, and an MA in clinical psychology from Loyola University.

Claudio S. Cinà, MD, MSc, FRCSC, is Professor in the Department of Surgery at the University of Toronto and an associate member of the Department of Clinical Epidemiology and Biostatistics at McMaster University in Hamilton, Ontario, Canada.

Catherine M. Clase, MB, BChir, MSc, FRCPC, is Associate Professor in the Department of Medicine and an associate member of the Department of Clinical Epidemiology and Biostatistics at McMaster University in Hamilton, Ontario, Canada.

Melinda F. Davis, PhD, is a Research Assistant Professor in Psychology at the University of Arizona in Tucson. Her statistical and methodological research interests include method variance and the analysis of change. She is a data analyst and methodologist who collaborates with researchers on the design and analysis of observational and clinical studies.

Mandeep K. Dhami, PhD, is a Senior Lecturer at the Institute of Criminology, University of Cambridge, United Kingdom. Her background is in psychology and criminology. Her research interests include human judgment and decision making (especially legal decision making), risk, psychology of imprisonment, and restorative justice. Dr. Dhami is a Fellow of the Society for the Psychological Study of Social Issues, Division 9 of the American Psychological Association.

Joseph A. Durlak, PhD, is Professor of Psychology at Loyola University in Chicago. His primary research interest area is the use of meta-analytic procedures to evaluate prevention and promotion programs for youth.

Nancy Edwards, RN, PhD, is Professor in the School of Nursing and Department of Epidemiology and Community Medicine, University of Ottawa, Otawa, Ontarioa, Canada. She holds a Nursing Chair funded by the Canadian Health Services Research Foundation, the Canadian Institutes of Health Research, and the Government of Ontario. She is Scientific Director of the Institute of Population and Public Health, Canadian Institutes of Health Research.

Alma Estable, MSW, is a Qualitative Research Consultant with the University of Ottawa Community Health Research Unit and a principal of Gentium Consulting, a community-based social research firm in Ottawa, Ontario, Canada.

Brent E. Faught, PhD, is Associate Professor in the Department of Community Health Sciences at Brock University, St. Catharines, Ontario, Canada.

F. Richard Ferraro, PhD, is Director of the General/Experimental PhD program at the University of North Dakota. In 2007 he was awarded the Chester Fritz Distinguished Professorship, the highest honor bestowed on a faculty member.

Françoise Filion, RN, MScN, is Research Coordinator and Professional Associate for pediatric pain research projects at McGill University and a faculty lecturer in the Faculty of Nursing at the Université de Montréal.

Julie Fleury, PhD, RN, FAAN, is Associate Dean for Research and Director of the PhD Program at Arizona State University, Phoenix.

Dale Glaser, PhD, is a principal of Glaser Consulting and adjunct faculty/lecturer at San Diego State University, Alliant International University, and the University of San Diego, where he instructs undergraduate- and graduate-level statistics, research methods, and psychometric theory.

Elizabeth A. Goncy, MA, is a doctoral student in clinical child psychology at Kent State University. She is also pursuing a minor in quantitative psychology.

John A. Hay, PhD, is Professor in the Department of Community Health Sciences at Brock University, St. Catharines, Ontario, Canada.

Melanie A. Hwalek, PhD, is an applied social psychologist and the Founder and CEO of SPEC Associates in Detroit, Michigan.

C. Céleste Johnston, RN, DEd, FCAHS, is James McGill Professor at McGill University and Codirector of the Groupe de Recherche Interuniversitaire en Interventions en Sciences Infirmières du Québec (GRIISIQ).

Anthony S. Joyce, PhD, is Professor in the Department of Psychiatry at the University of Alberta and Director of the Psychotherapy Research and Evaluation Unit in the outpatient service at the Walter Mackenzie Health Sciences Centre in Edmonton, Alberta, Canada.

Sylvia Kairouz, PhD, is Assistant Professor in the Department of Sociology and Anthropology at Concordia University in Montreal. Her research program focuses on the psychosocial determinants of addictive behaviors, mental health, and comorbidity among youth and adult populations.

Colleen Keller, PhD, RN-C, FNP, is Professor and Director of the Hartford Center for Geriatric Nursing Excellence at Arizona State University, Phoenix.

Christopher Koch, PhD, is Professor of Psychology and Director of Assessment at George Fox University in Newberg, Oregon.

Anita Kothari, PhD, is Assistant Professor in the Faculty of Health Sciences at the University of Western Ontario in London, Ontario, Canada. She also holds a Career Scientist Award from the Ontario Ministry of Health and Long-Term Care.

Chantale Marie LeClerc, RN, MSc, GNC(C), is Senior Director of Planning, Integration, and Community Engagement at Champlain Local Health Integration Network in Ottawa, Ontario, Canada. She was formerly the Chief Nursing Officer at SCO Health Service in Ottawa, Ontario, and served as Coprincipal Investigator on the Abilities Focused Morning Care Approach study. Her research interests include care of older persons, particularly those with dementia, and the organization of health care services.

Lynne MacLean, PhD, is Research Associate at the Community Health Research Unit, University of Ottawa, where she leads the Qualitative Team. She has previously worked as a government researcher and a mental health practitioner.

Arturo Martí-Carvajal, MD, MSc (ClinEpi), was Coordinator of the Venezuelan branch of the Iberoamerican Cochrane Network. He is Professor in the Department of Public Health at the University of Carabobo, Valencia, Venezuela. His research interest is systematic reviews in the area of hematology.

Katherine McKnight, PhD, is Director of Evaluation for Pearson K–12 Solutions, an organization dedicated to working with schools to enhance instruction and student learning. She also teaches graduate statistics as Adjunct Assistant Professor at George Mason University in Fairfax, Virginia.

Patrick E. McKnight, PhD, is Assistant Professor in the Department of Psychology at George Mason University in Fairfax, Virginia. He is a quantitatively oriented psychologist who collaborates with researchers in many disciplines within and outside social science. His research interests are the evaluation of outcome measures and data-analytic techniques in the areas of health services and behavioral health.

Mechthild Meyer, MEd, is Qualitative Research Consultant with the University of Ottawa Community Health Research Unit and a researcher with Gentium Consulting, a community-based research firm in Ottawa, Ontario, Canada.

Julian Montoro-Rodriguez, PhD, is Professor of Sociology and Executive Member of the Institute of Child Development and Family Relations at California State University, San Bernardino. His research program focuses on family caregiving.

Dominique Morisano, PhD, is a Postdoctoral Clinical Research Fellow, Schizophrenia and Addiction Psychiatry Programs, Centre for Addiction and Mental Health (CAMH) and the Department of Psychiatry, Faculty of Medicine, University of Toronto, Toronto, Ontario, Canada.

Louise Nadeau, PhD, is Professor in the Department of Psychology at the Université de Montréal. She is also Scientific Director of the Centre Dollard–Cormier / University Institute on Dependencies and a researcher affiliated with the Douglas Hospital Research Center. Her work in addictions focuses on psychiatric comorbidity, alcohol and gambling addiction, and, in particular, driving under the influence of alcohol.

Geoffrey R. Norman, PhD, is Professor and Assistant Dean in the Department of Clinical Epidemiology and Biostatistics at McMaster University in Hamilton, Ontario, Canada. His research focuses on the cognitive aspects of medical diagnosis.

Molly K. Pachan, MA, is a doctoral student in clinical psychology at Loyola University in Chicago.

Julie Hicks Patrick, PhD, is Woodburn Associate Professor and Director of Undergraduate Training at the West Virginia University Department of Psychology in Morgantown, West Virginia. She is a core member of the Life-Span Developmental Program. Her research focuses on cognitive and social processes in middle and late life.

Adrianna Perez, MS, RN, is a PhD student in nursing and healthcare Innovation at Arizona State University in Phoenix.

Kathleen W. Piercy, MSW, PhD, is Associate Professor in the Department of Family, Consumer, and Human Development at Utah State University in Logan, Utah. She teaches courses in family relations, gerontology, and qualitative methods. Her research program focuses on family caregiving and health services provision to older adults. Dr. Piercy is a Fellow in the Gerontological Society of America and currently edits the Practice Concepts section of the journal *The Gerontologist*.

José Quirino dos Santos, PhD, is Professor of Anthropology at Universidade de São Paulo, Brazil and a Visiting Professor in the Department of Preventive Medicine at the Universidade Federal de São Paulo.

Barb Riley, PhD, is a Scientist at the Centre for Behavioural Research and Program Evaluation at Waterloo University in Waterloo, Ontario, Canada, and Advisor in Knowledge Development and Exchange for the Public Health Agency of Canada. Her career focus is building systemic capacity to generate and use relevant evidence to inform population health programs and policies.

Nasreen Roberts, MD, FRCPC, is Director of the Child and Adolescent Psychiatric Emergency Service and Associate Professor at Queens University in Kingston, Ontario, Canada. Her chapters in this volume are based on her recent experiences as a part-time master's student in the Faculty of Community Health and Epidemiology at Queens University.

Michelle E. Roley, BA, is a recent graduate of Kent State University with a degree in psychology. She is currently employed as Lab Manager for the AAKOMA Project and CBT-RP Study in the Department of Psychiatry and Behavioral Sciences at Duke University Medical Center in Durham, North Carolina.

Brian R. Rush, PhD, is Codirector of the Health Systems Research and Consulting Unit, Centre for Addiction and Mental Health, and Professor in the Department of Psychiatry, Faculty of Psychiatry, University of Toronto, Toronto, Ontario.

Kriston B. Schellinger, BS, is a doctoral student in clinical psychology at Loyola University in Chicago.

Julie M. Dergal Serafini, MSc, is a doctoral candidate in the Faculty of Social Work, University of Toronto, and a graduate student in the Kunin–Lunenfeld Applied Research Unit (KLARU) at the Baycrest Centre, Toronto, Ontario, Canada.

Harry S. Shannon, PhD, is Professor in the Department of Clinical Epidemiology and Biostatistics and the Program in Occupational Health and Environmental Medicine at McMaster University, Hamilton, Ontario, Canada, and Adjunct Scientist at the Institute for Work and Health in Toronto.

Alissa Sherry, PhD, is Associate Professor in the Counseling Psychology Program at the University of Texas at Austin. She specializes in constructivist perspectives in attachment and diversity issues, as well as in the teaching and practice of psychological assessment.

Souraya Sidani, PhD (see "About the Editors").

Gregory C. Smith, EdD, is Professor and Director of the Human Development Center at Kent State University. His research program focuses on informal caregiving arrangements in later-life families. He is a Fellow in the Gerontological Society of America and Associate Editor of the *International Journal of Aging and Human Development*.

Karen A. Souza, MA, is a research assistant at the Institute of Criminology, University of Cambridge. Her research interests include sentencing, community justice interventions, and prisoner assessment.

S. Melinda Spencer, PhD, is a 2006–2008 Kellogg Health Scholar and Assistant Professor in the Department of Health Promotion, Education, and Behavior at the University of South Carolina. She received her doctoral training at West Virginia University in life-span developmental psychology with Julie Hicks Patrick. Her research focuses on racial/ethnic health disparities in older adulthood.

Victoria L. Straub, MA, CSSBB, is Chief Operating Officer of SPEC Associates in Detroit, Michigan, and a specialist in quality information and evaluation systems for nonprofit organizations.

David L. Streiner, PhD, CPsych (see "About the Editors").

Anna Tabor, MA, is a doctoral student in clinical psychology and a graduate research assistant at George Fox University in Newberg, Oregon.

Kaylee Trottier-Wolter, BA, is a second-year graduate student in the Clinical Psychology program at the University of North Dakota.

Manfred H. M. van Dulmen, PhD, is Assistant Professor in the Department of Psychology and Affiliate Faculty Member of the Institute for the Study and Prevention of Violence at Kent State University.

Robert van Reekum, MD, FRCPC, is a neuropsychiatrist and Assistant Professor in the Department of Psychiatry at the University of Toronto. His research interests relate to behavioral changes in people who have suffered an illness or injury to their brains.

Scott Veldhuizen, BA, is a research analyst at the Centre for Addiction and Mental Health in Toronto and a graduate student in the Department of Applied Health Sciences at Brock University in St. Catharines, Ontario, Canada.

Dennis Watson, MA, CSP, is a PhD candidate in sociology at Loyola University in Chicago, and University–Community Research Coordinator at the Center for Urban Research and Learning. His primary areas of interest are applied/clinical sociology, mental health, and health services.

Debazou Y. Yantio, MA, is Ingénieur Agronome with the Ministry of Agriculture and Rural Development in Cameroon. He is currently a task team member of the Network of Networks on Impact Evaluation Initiative, chaired by the Department for International Development, United Kingdom, and is a founding member of the Cameroon Development Evaluation Association. He also serves on various committees of the African Evaluation Association.